HEALTH LEARNING CENTER
Northwestern Memorial Hospital
Galter 3-304
Chicago, IL

HEARING LOSS

Determining Eligibility for Social Security Benefits

Committee on Disability Determination for
Individuals with Hearing Impairments

Robert A. Dobie and Susan B. Van Hemel, *Editors*

Board on Behavioral, Cognitive, and Sensory Sciences
Division of Behavioral and Social Sciences and Education

NATIONAL RESEARCH COUNCIL
OF THE NATIONAL ACADEMIES

THE NATIONAL ACADEMIES PRESS
Washington, D.C.
www.nap.edu

THE NATIONAL ACADEMIES PRESS 500 Fifth Street, N.W. Washington, DC 20001

NOTICE: The project that is the subject of this report was approved by the Governing Board of the National Research Council, whose members are drawn from the councils of the National Academy of Sciences, the National Academy of Engineering, and the Institute of Medicine. The members of the committee responsible for the report were chosen for their special competences and with regard for appropriate balance.

This study was supported by Contract No. 0600-02-60012 between the National Academy of Sciences and the Social Security Administration. Any opinions, findings, conclusions, or recommendations expressed in this publication are those of the author(s) and do not necessarily reflect the views of the organizations or agencies that provided support for the project.

Library of Congress Cataloging-in-Publication Data

Hearing loss : determining eligibility for Social Security benefits / Committee on Disability Determination for Individuals with Hearing Impairments, Board on Behavioral, Cognitive, and Sensory Sciences, Division of Behavioral and Social Sciences and Education ; Robert A. Dobie and Susan Van Hemel, editors.
    p. ; cm.
  Includes bibliographical references.
  ISBN 0-309-09296-5 (pbk.)
  1. Deafness—Diagnosis—United States. 2. Disability evaluation—United States. 3. Insurance, Disability—United States. 4. Social security—United States.
  [DNLM: 1. Hearing Loss—diagnosis—United States. 2. Disability Evaluation—United States. 3. Eligibility Determination—United States. 4. Hearing Tests—United States. 5. Social Security—United States. WV 270 H4348 2004] I. Dobie, Robert A. II. Van Hemel, Susan B. III. National Research Council (U.S.). Committee on Disability Determination for Individuals with Hearing Impairments.
  RF294.H435 2004
  362.4'264'0973--dc22

                                2004019993

Additional copies of this report are available from the National Academies Press, 500 Fifth Street, N.W., Lockbox 285, Washington, DC 20055; (800) 624-6242 or (202) 334-3313 (in the Washington metropolitan area); Internet, http://www.nap.edu

Cover credit: Nautilid Echo (detail), ©Laura Cater-Woods. Mixed media/fibers (acrylic inks and paints on cotton, embroidered and quilted).

Photo credit: Dan Tilton, Photographic Solutions, Billings, MT.

Suggested citation: National Research Council. (2005). *Hearing Loss: Determining Eligibility for Social Security Benefits.* Committee on Disability Determination for Individuals with Hearing Impairments. Robert A. Dobie and Susan B. Van Hemel, editors. Board on Behavioral, Cognitive, and Sensory Sciences, Division of Behavioral and Social Sciences and Education. Washington, DC: The National Academies Press.

THE NATIONAL ACADEMIES
Advisers to the Nation on Science, Engineering, and Medicine

The **National Academy of Sciences** is a private, nonprofit, self-perpetuating society of distinguished scholars engaged in scientific and engineering research, dedicated to the furtherance of science and technology and to their use for the general welfare. Upon the authority of the charter granted to it by the Congress in 1863, the Academy has a mandate that requires it to advise the federal government on scientific and technical matters. Dr. Bruce M. Alberts is president of the National Academy of Sciences.

The **National Academy of Engineering** was established in 1964, under the charter of the National Academy of Sciences, as a parallel organization of outstanding engineers. It is autonomous in its administration and in the selection of its members, sharing with the National Academy of Sciences the responsibility for advising the federal government. The National Academy of Engineering also sponsors engineering programs aimed at meeting national needs, encourages education and research, and recognizes the superior achievements of engineers. Dr. Wm. A. Wulf is president of the National Academy of Engineering.

The **Institute of Medicine** was established in 1970 by the National Academy of Sciences to secure the services of eminent members of appropriate professions in the examination of policy matters pertaining to the health of the public. The Institute acts under the responsibility given to the National Academy of Sciences by its congressional charter to be an adviser to the federal government and, upon its own initiative, to identify issues of medical care, research, and education. Dr. Harvey V. Fineberg is president of the Institute of Medicine.

The **National Research Council** was organized by the National Academy of Sciences in 1916 to associate the broad community of science and technology with the Academy's purposes of furthering knowledge and advising the federal government. Functioning in accordance with general policies determined by the Academy, the Council has become the principal operating agency of both the National Academy of Sciences and the National Academy of Engineering in providing services to the government, the public, and the scientific and engineering communities. The Council is administered jointly by both Academies and the Institute of Medicine. Dr. Bruce M. Alberts and Dr. Wm. A. Wulf are chair and vice chair, respectively, of the National Research Council.

www.national-academies.org

v

Preface

This report is the product of over two years' work by a committee of 12 diverse experts in hearing and other subjects, convened by the National Research Council (NRC) in response to a request from the Social Security Administration (SSA). The committee was tasked to review the tests and criteria used to determine hearing disability for purposes of eligibility for Social Security benefits. The committee evaluated the tests currently used to determine disability for people with hearing loss and examined other possible ways to assess such disability, including new tests of hearing function. Special attention was given to finding ways to improve the reliability and validity of tests of hearing and to reviewing evidence bearing on the ability of such tests to predict job performance capabilities.

On behalf of the committee, I would like to acknowledge the contributions of a number of people who helped us to complete the work reported here. First, we are grateful to Sigfrid Soli and Carren Stika, who prepared reviews and analyses for the committee. We also wish to thank Sandra Salan, the project sponsor at the SSA's Office of Disability. She and her associate, Michelle Hungerman, provided much useful information on SSA disability programs and procedures. Also at SSA, Susan David and her staff prepared data analyses from SSA statistical files in response to our queries.

In the service and advocacy community, we are grateful to the organizations that nominated speakers and otherwise supported the public forum the committee held on May 7, 2003. We are especially grateful to the forum participants, listed in Appendix C, who gave thoughtful and expert responses to the difficult questions we posed, providing the committee with valuable insights on the issues that are most important to people with hearing loss.

At the NRC, Susan B. Van Hemel was the study director for this project. Special thanks are due to Christine Hartel, director of the Center for the Study of Behavior and Development, for her guidance and support; to Christine McShane, for editing our manuscript with skill and insight; to Eugenia Grohman of the DBASSE Reports Office, who managed the review process; and to Jessica Gonzalez Martinez, our skilled and dedicated project assistant, whose contributions to this study were invaluable. The excellent interpreters from Sign Language Associates who supported all of our meetings, including the public forum, were vital to the success of this project as well. I would also like to recognize the committee members for their generous contributions of time and expertise and for their professionalism. Although members often had disparate opinions, they invariably expressed and discussed them with respect and grace.

This report has been reviewed in draft form by individuals chosen for their diverse perspectives and technical expertise, in accordance with procedures approved by the Report Review Committee of the NRC. The purpose of this independent review is to provide candid and critical comments that will assist the institution in making the published report as sound as possible and to ensure that the report meets institutional standards for objectivity, evidence, and responsiveness to the study charge. The review comments and draft manuscript remain confidential to protect the integrity of the deliberative process.

We thank the following individuals for their participation in the review of this report: Monroe Berkowitz, Program for Disability Research, Rutgers University; Judy R. Dubno, Department of Otolaryngology-Head and Neck Surgery, Medical University of South Carolina; George Gates, Hearing Research Center, University of Washington; Walt Jesteadt, Boys Town National Research Hospital, Omaha, NE; Gerald Kidd, Programs in Communication Disorders, Boston University; Doris Kistler, Heuser Hearing Institute, Louisville, KY, and Department of Psychological and Brain Sciences, University of Louisville; Robert Shannon, Auditory Implants and Perception Research, House Ear Institute, Los Angeles, CA; and Alice Suter, independent consultant, Ashland, OR.

Although the reviewers listed above have provided many constructive comments and suggestions, they were not asked to endorse the conclusions or recommendations nor did they see the final draft of the report before its release. The review of this report was overseen by Dennis McFadden of the University of Texas at Austin. Appointed by the NRC, he was responsible for making sure that an independent examination of this report was carried out in accordance with institutional procedures and that all reviewers' comments were considered carefully. Responsibility for the final content of this report, however, rests entirely with the authoring committee and the institution.

> Robert A. Dobie, *Chair*
> Committee on Disability Determination for
> Individuals with Hearing Impairments

Contents

xi

Executive Summary

The Social Security Administration (SSA) asked the National Research Council (NRC) to survey published research on assessment of hearing and the auditory demands of everyday life, and to advise them whether the process of determining eligibility for Social Security disability benefits for persons with hearing loss could be improved. SSA also asked for recommendations for a research agenda in these areas. The key issue is whether or not standardized tests exist or can be developed "that provide adequate prediction of real-world performance capacities to reflect individuals' auditory abilities and disabilities in normal life situations with average background noise." Such tests would need to be valid, reliable, well-standardized, and "simple and inexpensive to administer in a standard physician's or audiologist's office setting."

The NRC formed the Committee on Disability Determination for Individuals with Hearing Impairment to address these issues. Several important questions are laid out in the committee's scope of work, and the committee's responses, in terms of general answers, appear below:

Question 1: Current SSA procedures use "subjective" (behavioral) tests that present tones and words through headphones and rely on individuals' ability and willingness to report what they hear. Could objective (physiological) measures of auditory function perform better?

Committee Response: Physiological measures may assist in the estimation of the severity of hearing loss in claimants who cannot or will not cooperate in behavioral tests, but for most situations the committee recommends the continued use of the current approach to measuring hearing loss.

Question 2: The validity and reliability of the tests currently used by SSA, as well as their criterion values for disability, may not be optimal. Could other tests (including tests that incorporate background noise) or other criterion values perform better?

Committee Response: In general, for adults, the committee recommends the continued use of the current medical listing of impairments to establish disability, with a modified and specific protocol for speech testing. We also recommend that a battery of tests be administered prior to applying the medical listing criteria, in order to improve the reliability and validity of all stages of the SSA disability determination process. For children, the committee is recommending some changes in the speech perception test battery and criteria, as well as the addition of a test of language competence for children over age 3.

Question 3: At present, as stated in the scope of work, "SSA does not give clear guidance about testing with and/or without hearing aids or cochlear implants for those who use such devices." Should aided testing be recommended, and if so, how should such tests be conducted?

Committee Response: The committee provides several recommendations for testing with cochlear implants and hearing aids.

Question 4: Current procedures attempt to assess only the abilities to detect simple tones and to understand speech. Because identification of nonspeech sounds and sound localization are required in some jobs, should these auditory abilities be tested as part of the SSA disability process?

Committee Response: Since there are no standard clinical tests for sound localization or nonspeech identification, the committee is not recommending such tests.

Question 5: Can research using measures of health-related quality of life help to determine which auditory skills and losses have the greatest impact on the lives of persons with hearing loss?

Committee Response: The committee does not recommend such quality-of-life measures for use in SSA disability determination.

Question 6: Can performance deficits resulting from hearing loss be separated from those resulting from nonauditory (e.g., cognitive, linguistic) factors?

Committee Response: The committee describes some of the influences that nonauditory factors can have on measures used in SSA determination of hearing impairment.

FINDINGS

The committee's efforts to assist the SSA in developing disability tests and criteria that could better predict the ability to work were impeded by two major data voids and one fact of life. The first void was the dearth of available data linking hearing loss to job performance in adults. We found some data on employment of people with hearing loss, but they were sparse, based mostly on self-report of hearing loss with no objective measurement of hearing, and could not support analysis of employment outcomes for varying levels of hearing loss. Because there are as few data to support new criteria as there are to support current criteria, we decided in the end not to recommend significant changes to the SSA disability criteria for adults. Some changes were recommended for the determination of disability in children. Research is needed to develop data to inform future decisions about disability criteria.

The second void, closely related to the first, is the lack of information on the auditory requirements of jobs. Knowledge of these requirements is vital to understanding how hearing loss may affect performance in any given job. Again, research is needed. In the absence of good data, the committee developed basic auditory task descriptions and estimates of the probable effects of hearing loss of various degrees of severity on auditory performance on the job, based on our collective expertise.

The fact of life that most complicated our work is that it is clear to those who study disability that many personal, environmental, educational, and social factors contribute in significant ways to the relationship between a person's hearing ability and the ability to work. The current SSA disability determination process considers only the claimant's measured hearing loss through application of the medical listing criteria in Step 3 of the disability determination process. Thus, the very concept of medical listings as a basis for determining disability is called into question. We stopped short of recommending that all claimants be given the vocational factors assessment of Steps 4 and 5, but this was a decision based primarily on practical and economic considerations. Some committee members think that such a step would improve the determination process.

In light of the above issues, the committee's overall approach was to recommend a battery of tests to be used in Step 2 of the SSA process, largely to provide valuable information that should improve the validity of the determination of disability in Steps 4 and 5. Testing with cochlear implants and hearing aids is also included in the recommended test batteries. In general, the committee retained the current Step 3 (medical listing) tests and their criteria, with modifications to the test protocol for adults. For children, we recommend some modifications to the Step 3 tests and their criteria. We also make recommendations for research to support the development of tests or test batteries that could better predict the ability to work. First, however, we discuss the weaknesses in the current measures and criteria that we were able to address.

LIMITATIONS OF CURRENT FORMULA AND TESTING PROTOCOL

Hearing impairment in adults that qualifies for disability benefits under the existing SSA determination in Step 3 is a loss of hearing that is not restorable by a hearing aid. In Social Security programs, eligibility for disability benefits is all or nothing; there is no partial disability. The current formula specifies the following disability criterion: average pure-tone hearing thresholds (500, 1000, and 2000 Hz) of 90 dB HL or worse for air conduction stimuli and at maximal levels for bone conduction stimuli in the better ear, or speech discrimination scores of 40 percent or less in the better ear. These criteria often fail to identify individuals who may have a disability in the workplace because of hearing loss, particularly those in hearing-critical jobs, and they may classify as disabled some claimants who are able to work, especially successful cochlear implant users. There are several reasons for such failures:

• The existing formula for disability determination for adults does not take into account speech recognition performance at average conversational speech levels, which are likely to be encountered in everyday communication situations.

• The current procedure does not evaluate speech recognition in noise; poor speech understanding in noise may severely impair the ability to function effectively in many jobs that are dependent on oral communication.

• The current procedures and formula do not consider performance with a hearing aid or implantable device. Actual performance with these devices cannot be predicted from unaided performance.

• The current protocol includes neither assessment of sound localization nor the ability to differentiate a change in an acoustic stimulus (i.e., sound discrimination). While these are fundamental hearing abilities, especially in certain hearing-critical jobs, there are currently no standard clinical methods of assessing these auditory functions.

• The current formula does not recognize that individuals with severe hearing losses (71-90 dB HL pure-tone average or PTA) cannot receive spoken communication auditorily without a hearing aid. Many people with 71-90 dB hearing loss have not been successful hearing aid or cochlear implant users and function primarily in the deaf world. Such claimants may be at a significant disadvantage in the workplace.

RECOMMENDATIONS FOR SSA ACTION

In the following sections we present our recommendations for the testing of hearing and the determination of disability based on hearing loss. These changes will improve the validity and reliability of tests for disability determination and will provide additional information on residual function for use in Steps 4 and 5 of the determination process. The text of all recommendations and the rationale supporting them is found in the body of the report and the complete range of recommendations is referenced here.

General Recommendations for All Testing During Step 2 of the SSA Process

• The committee recommends that the standard otolaryngological examination follow the audiological examination (but by no more than 6 months), because a physician cannot provide a competent report without recent audiometric data (see Action Recommendation 4-1).
• The otological examination should be performed by an otolaryngologist who has completed at least five years of residency training following receipt of the M.D. or D.O. (doctor of osteopathy) degree and who is certified by the American Board of Otolaryngology (see Action Recommendation 4-1).
• The audiological tests for determining a disability based on hearing impairment should be conducted by a **clinical audiologist** who holds state licensure (if applicable) or, if no state licensure is available, is certified by the American Speech-Language-Hearing Association (Certificate of Clinical Competence in Audiology, or CCC-A) or by the American Board of Audiology (see Action Recommendation 4-3).
• Equipment should meet American National Standards Institute (ANSI) **standards** or other established standards when no ANSI standards are available. The environment for assessment of auditory threshold should conform to current ANSI standards (see Action Recommendation 4-4).
• Audiometric testing should not be performed within 72 hours of significant noise exposure or if there is recent exposure to ototoxic drugs or, in cases of fluctuating hearing loss, on a day when hearing is noticeably poorer (see Action Recommendation 4-5).

Recommendations for Testing Adults

• In order to capture an accurate assessment of an individual's hearing abilities on a given day, a test battery is recommended (see Action Recommendation 4-2). This approach permits a determination of the validity of the claimant's responses by examining intertest agreement. It is recommended that this entire test battery be completed in Step 2 before a determination of disability is formulated:

—pure-tone thresholds in each ear presented via air and bone conduction transducers;

—speech thresholds under earphones in each ear;

—monosyllable word recognition performance for test materials presented in the sound field at average conversational levels in quiet and in noise;

—tympanometry; and

—acoustic reflex thresholds.

• The committee recommends that SSA require a **checklist** to be completed by the clinical audiologist at the time of testing, as an indication of the quality of the data collected for use in the disability determination process and to provide additional useful information for evaluating a claim in Steps 3, 4, and 5 (see Action Recommendation 4-5).

• The standard **pure-tone threshold** audiometric test is required to determine pure-tone average thresholds at 500, 1000, and 2000 Hz (PTA 512) for each ear. The pure-tone test should be conducted without the use of a hearing aid (unaided). Even if an individual wears a cochlear implant, it is necessary to assess hearing sensitivity bilaterally (see Action Recommendation 4-6).

• A **speech threshold** is a required measure in the test battery for the primary purpose of cross-checking the validity of the pure-tone audiogram and indicating the claimant's ability to detect and recognize speech. If a speech recognition threshold cannot be determined, then a speech detection threshold should be assessed (see Action Recommendation 4-6).

• **Speech recognition** testing should be performed under controlled conditions in quiet and in noise, using standardized monosyllable word recognition test materials that meet the criteria recommended in Chapter 3 (see Action Recommendation 4-6).

• **Objective (physiological) tests,** such as frequency-specific evoked potentials, should be used in place of or as corroboration for behavioral tests for persons who cannot or will not cooperate in behavioral testing (see Action Recommendation 4-6).

• Two **test protocols** are recommended: one for claimants who use hearing aids or cochlear implants and one for claimants who do not. The protocol for users of hearing aids or cochlear implants includes aided testing (see Action Recommendation 4-6).

- The committee recommends that **all information gathered during testing be used to evaluate residual functional capacity.** SSA should examine the claimant's test performance in relation to auditory communication task requirements on the job to help determine the claimant's ability to work in his former job or in other appropriate jobs (see Action Recommendation 4-7).

Recommendations for Testing Children

- **Recommended tests and protocols,** as well as criteria for disability, for infants and children **vary with the age of the child** (see Action Recommendations 7-1 through 7-4; Table 7-2). We recommend that the degree of hearing loss in the better ear that is considered disabling in infants and children should be 35 dB HL before age 6, 50 dB from ages 6 to 12, and 70 dB from ages 12 to 18.
- **Standardized language processing measures** should be administered to compare the child's function at the time of testing to normative data for children of comparable age (see Action Recommendation 7-1 and Table 7-2).
- The recommended **criteria** for determination of disability in children during Step 3 appear in Chapter 7, Table 7-2. To qualify for benefits, children age 3 and older must meet the criterion for hearing level *and either* the criterion for deficit in speech perception *or* the criterion for language processing. For children under age 3, only the hearing level criterion must be met (see Action Recommendations 7-1 and 7-4).
- **Speech perception tests** should be administered in quiet using recorded test materials at 70 dB SPL. Presentation of the speech perception test should be via sound field using personal amplification or cochlear implant if such is used by the child. If no device is used by the child, testing is performed unaided (see Action Recommendation 7-2).
- In general, **average hearing levels** should be determined from pure-tone thresholds at 500, 1000, 2000, and 4000 Hz (PTA 5124) (see Action Recommendation 7-3). Under conditions that warrant using auditory brainstem response (ABR), the ABR thresholds require a minimum of two frequencies, one low (500 to 1000 Hz) and one high (2000 to 4000 Hz) to determine average hearing level. When auditory neuropathy is thought to be present, it will not be possible to determine hearing thresholds by ABR. In those cases, disability should be presumed unless or until proven otherwise by behavioral testing (see Action Recommendation 7-3).

• The committee recommends that SSA require a **checklist** to be completed by the clinical audiologist, as an indication of the quality of the data collected for use in the disability determination process and to provide additional useful information for evaluating a claim (see Action Recommendation 7-5).

RESEARCH RECOMMENDATIONS

The committee developed many recommendations for research that the SSA should support in order to provide a sound scientific basis for future decisions about the determination of disability due to hearing loss. The most important are summarized below, first for adults, then for children, followed by some general research goals. For each recommendation we have referenced the complete text in the report.

Research Recommendations Related to Adult Disability Determination

• Develop and standardize new tests of basic hearing functions—including speech recognition for words and sentences in quiet and in noise, localization, and sound discrimination—that correlate with auditory performance in the workplace (see Research Recommendations 4-1 and 4-2).

• Study speech recognition performance in a variety of listeners with and without hearing loss, both users and nonusers of aids and implants, in acoustic environments and conditions that simulate the workplace (see Research Recommendation 4-3).

• Develop an understanding of the auditory requirements of jobs in the current workplace (see Research Recommendation 4-4).

• Study the effectiveness of hearing aids, assistive listening devices, and workplace accommodations in realistic listening environments, for individuals with severe and profound hearing loss (see Research Recommendation 5-1).

• Determine the prevalence of hearing loss in the workplace and its effects on worker performance, earnings, and mobility (see Research Recommendation 6-1).

Research Recommendations Related to Children's Disability Determination

• Develop standardized speech perception measures for infants and children, in English and other languages, that take into account developmental age and degree of hearing loss (see Research Recommendation 7-1).

- Identify the contributions of environmental factors, such as the linguistic environment in the home and educational settings and educational intervention variables, to the varying outcomes in persons who have been deaf or hard-of-hearing since early childhood (see Research Recommendation 7-2).
- Perform more prospective studies of children using amplification to determine outcomes for communication, socialization, and educational achievement (see Research Recommendation 7-3).
- Develop standard clinical measures that incorporate auditory and visual assessments (see Research Recommendation 7-4).
- Perform research to better understand the true nature of auditory dysfunction in children with slight or unilateral hearing loss and the possibilities for interventions to mitigate such dysfunctions (see Research Recommendation 7-5).

Other Research Recommendations

- Acquire data about the real-world use of hearing aids from a large population of users, separating those with adult-onset hearing loss from those who developed their hearing loss as children (see Research Recommendation 5-1).
- Conduct research to validate tests that purport to measure or predict functional hearing ability in daily life against real-world criteria measured in natural settings (see Research Recommendations 4-8 and 5-3).
- Develop and validate methods to detect and manage exaggeration (see Glossary, Appendix A) of speech recognition problems during administration of speech tests (see Research Recommendation 4-7).

1

Introduction

The Social Security Administration (SSA) asked the National Research Council (NRC) to survey published research on assessment of hearing and the auditory demands of everyday life and to advise them whether the process of determining eligibility for Social Security disability benefits for persons with hearing loss could be improved. The SSA also requested recommendations for a research agenda to address unanswered questions in these areas. The Committee on Disability Determination for Individuals with Hearing Impairment[1] (the committee) was charged with answering these questions.

KEY ISSUES

According to the committee's scope of work, the key issue is whether or not standardized tests exist or can be developed "that provide adequate prediction of real-world performance capacities to reflect individuals' auditory abilities and disabilities in normal life situations with average background noise." Such tests would need to be valid, reliable, well-standardized, and "simple and inexpensive to administer in a standard physician's or audiologist's office setting."

---

[1]Throughout this report we use the term "hearing loss" whenever possible in preference to "hearing impairment." When impairment is meant in a generic sense or is used as a term in referenced documents under discussion (as in SSA regulations and guidance), we use the term "impairment."

The scope of work went on to list several important subsidiary issues, each of which is discussed briefly in this section and extensively in the report:

1. Current SSA procedures use "subjective" tests that present tones and words through headphones, relying on individuals' ability and willingness to report what they hear. Could objective (physiological) measures of auditory function perform better?

2. The validity and reliability of the tests currently used by SSA, as well as their criterion values ("cutoff" levels), may not be optimal. Could other tests (including tests that include background noise) or other criterion values perform better?

3. At present, as stated in the committee's scope of work, "SSA does not give clear guidance about testing with and/or without hearing aids or cochlear implants for those who use such devices." Should aided testing be recommended, and, if so, how should such tests be conducted?

4. Current procedures attempt to assess only abilities to detect simple tones and to understand speech. Since identification of nonspeech sounds and sound localization are required in some jobs, should these auditory abilities be tested as part of the SSA disability process?

5. Can research using measures of health-related quality of life help to determine which auditory skills and losses have the greatest impact on the lives of persons with hearing loss?

6. Can performance deficits resulting from hearing loss be separated from those resulting from nonauditory (e.g., cognitive, linguistic) factors?

Most of these questions have to be addressed separately for adults and children, for two reasons. First, small children sometimes require different testing methods than adults, because of their relative inability to participate in some hearing tasks. Second, adults and children must meet very different standards for eligibility for SSA disability programs. For adults, SSA disability is defined as "inability to engage in any substantial gainful activity by reason of any medically determinable physical or mental impairment which can be expected to result in death or has lasted or can be expected to last for a continuous period of not less than 12 months." For children, in contrast, any stable impairment that is "marked or extreme" may result in eligibility, and SSA regulations explicitly define this statistically rather than in terms of inability to successfully perform the learning tasks of childhood. "Marked" limitation is "the equivalent of the functioning we would expect on standardized testing with scores that are at least two, but less than three, standard deviations below the mean," whereas "extreme" limitation begins at three standard deviations below normal. A child is considered to meet the listings if he or she has extreme impairment in one functional domain or marked impairments in two of six functional domains.

For both adults and children, determination of eligibility is a multi-step process. Step 1 deals with financial eligibility, and Step 2 requires proof of a physical or mental impairment that at least "significantly limits" some activities and is expected to last at least 12 months or to result in death. Step 3 applies "medical listing" criteria to the applicant's impairment; if these are met or exceeded, the claimant is found eligible. Adult applicants not found eligible at Step 3 may still receive eligibility if, after consideration of their age, education, and work experience, as well as their residual capacities, they are found to be unable to perform either the work they have done in the past (Step 4) or any other work in the U.S. economy (Step 5). An additional step is also available for children who fail to meet the medical listing criteria in Step 3. This report addresses the hearing testing that is used in Steps 3-5.

Nature of Current Measures

For both adults and children, SSA now relies on two clinical tests, described in detail in Chapter 3, that are widely used in clinical practice. One of them, pure-tone audiometry, is also well standardized: four American National Standards (American National Standards Institute, 1996, 1997, 2002a, 2003) specify the conditions and methods of testing. The other, speech discrimination (presumably using monosyllabic words, although the SSA regulations do not specify this), is not standardized by the American National Standards Institute, by any national professional association, or by SSA. Speech discrimination tests done by different audiologists frequently differ in several ways that affect the difficulty and the reliability of the test: the word lists chosen, the number of words presented, the intensity (loudness) of the words, male versus female speaker, the use of live voice versus recorded word lists, and whether people who use hearing aids or cochlear implants are tested with or without their devices. Other types of speech tests, using sentences instead of words, with or without background noise, are discussed in Chapter 3; none of these is widely used in the United States at present.

Pure-tone audiometry is a test of auditory sensitivity. The softest sound that can be heard (threshold) is recorded for each ear, for tones ranging from low frequencies (250 Hz is approximately middle C) to high frequencies (8000 Hz is one octave above the highest note on the piano keyboard). A graph of threshold versus frequency is called an audiogram. Audiometry measures the ability to detect simple sounds, and thresholds for the frequencies most important for speech communication correlate approximately with the level of difficulty people experience in daily life (e.g., 25 to 40 dB = "mild" hearing loss, 40 to 55 dB = "moderate" hearing loss, etc.; see Table 3-1 for complete classification of hearing loss). Audiometry does not directly measure other auditory abilities, such as sound recognition, sound localization, and speech recognition. Because of this limitation, scientists and clinicians have sought better ways to assess real-world hearing abilities for over 60 years.

At the beginning of World War II, some otologists thought that speech tests should be used instead of audiometry to determine fitness for duty, but the prevailing expert opinion was that "speech tests are very unreliable" (Fowler, 1941, p. 941). In the 1950s, a committee of the American Medical Association (AMA) hoped that valid and reliable tests of everyday speech understanding would soon be available, ending what they believed to be a "temporary" reliance on audiometric methods of estimating the impact of hearing loss (American Medical Association, 1955). For reasons we discuss below, this never happened.

The AMA continues to recommend pure-tone audiometry for the evaluation of hearing impairment (American Medical Association, 2001), and no state or federal agency uses speech tests to determine eligibility for workers' compensation benefits (the Veterans Administration uses both pure tones and speech for eligibility for disability benefits, but has an alternate procedure using only pure-tone audiometry for cases in which speech tests are deemed unreliable). As in the United States, compensation schemes in Canada (Alberti, 1993), Ireland (Hone et al., 2003), and Australia (Rickards et al., 1996) use pure-tone audiometry. Some programs in the United Kingdom also use pure-tone audiometry (King et al., 1992), but others do not (Niven-Jenkins, 2004). Members of the committee do not know the methods used in other countries.

For a hearing disability to be determined, the SSA medical listing criteria for adults require, for the better ear, either:

1. Pure-tone average (PTA) air conduction threshold, for 500, 1000, and 2000 Hz, (PTA 512)[2] of 90 dB hearing level or greater, with corresponding bone conduction thresholds, or

2. Speech discrimination score of 40 percent or less, at a level "sufficient to ascertain maximum discrimination ability."

The committee was unable to discover the history or rationale for these criteria. In addition, while the references to the better ear and to "maximum discrimination ability" suggest tests done using earphones,

---

[2]Throughout this report, PTA refers to a pure-tone average of 500, 1000, and 2000 Hz (often abbreviated as PTA 512) unless otherwise specified.

without the use of cochlear implants or hearing aids, the medical listings are ambiguous. They mandate neither testing with earphones nor aided testing, but they refer to "hearing not restorable by a hearing aid," and a separate SSA manual (Social Security Administration, 2003b) states that aided testing should be done for individuals who use hearing aids or when there is a "probability that the hearing level can be improved by a hearing aid." The committee has been advised by SSA staff that this policy is generally disregarded, and that when the results of aided testing have been the sole basis for denial of benefits, appeals to administrative judges have usually been successful. Thus, in this report, we assume that the current medical listings (for both adults and children) refer to unaided hearing tests, performed using earphones.

The audiometric criterion level (PTA = 90 dB or worse) is equivalent to "profound" hearing loss in ordinary clinical terminology. People with hearing loss of this magnitude almost always consider themselves "deaf." If the goal is to predict "inability to engage in any substantial gainful activity," the 90 dB criterion will produce both false positive errors (granting eligibility to people who can work) and false negative errors (denying eligibility to people who cannot work). In the SSA process false negative errors in Step 3 can be reversed in Steps 4 and 5 (i.e., the applicant may succeed in obtaining eligibility based on factors including age and experience), while false positive errors in Step 3 are generally irreversible.

Many—perhaps most—adults with severe to profound hearing loss do work, and some who use hearing aids and cochlear implants work in jobs that require frequent speech communication (some of those will be false positives, if the 90 dB criterion is used). Conversely, many people are genuinely disabled by lesser degrees of hearing loss (false negatives). For example, even with well-fitted hearing aids, many people with PTA between 80 and 90 dB understand fewer than 60 percent of words in sentences at conversational levels (Flynn et al., 1998). They would probably have difficulty in many tasks requiring hearing without the assistance of vision, such as using the telephone. Such a person whose job had always required telephone work, and whose age and experience realistically precluded other work, might be unable to work but would fail to meet the 90 dB criterion of Step 3. This person could still be found eligible in Steps 4 and 5.

The committee is unaware of any data, from SSA or other sources, that attempt to quantify the problem of false positive and false negative errors using the current medical listing criteria. Such data, if available, could suggest changes in those criteria. For example, if the percentage of people who reenter the workforce after failing to meet medical listing criteria were found to drop sharply for PTA worse than 70 or 80 dB, this might support a lower (more liberal) PTA criterion.

By requiring absent bone conduction thresholds at the limits of the audiometer, SSA limits the medical listings to hearing loss that is purely or predominantly sensorineural (due to inner ear disorder), rather than a "mixed" hearing loss that could include a large conductive (outer or middle ear) component. The rationale for this requirement is unstated. While it is generally accepted that persons with conductive hearing losses usually function better with hearing aids than people with purely sensorineural hearing losses of the same severity, this may not be true for people with profound mixed hearing losses.

The speech discrimination criterion for adults (40 percent or worse for monosyllables) is more difficult to relate to everyday difficulties. It has long been known that the level "at which 50 percent [of monosyllables] is correctly understood is a little above the level at which we can easily understand ordinary connected speech" (Davis, 1960, p. 191). According to American National Standard ANSI S3.5 (2002b), a score of 40 percent for monosyllables predicts that words in familiar sentences will be understood with greater than 90 percent accuracy, while words in novel sentences will be understood with about 75 percent accuracy (without being able to see the speaker's face). Thus, a 40 percent score for isolated monosyllables would imply at least some difficulty in everyday life for most persons (for example, using the telephone), but not necessarily inability to communicate by speech at work, especially in situations in which the listener can see the speaker's face. Speech discrimination is an important part of the current criteria, because many applicants with PTA much better than 90 dB will have maximum speech discrimination scores (under earphones) below 40 percent. Dubno et al. (1995) have suggested that people with 70 dB PTA have mean speech discrimination scores of 50 percent, and 5 percent of them will have scores below 25 percent.

The SSA speech discrimination listing, like the audiometric listing, will produce both false positive and false negative errors. In addition, speech discrimination scores are subject to additional sources of error: increased problems with reliability, validity, exaggeration (discussed in the following paragraphs), and reliance on a subject's knowledge of the language used in the test (see nonauditory factors below).

Because of lack of standardization, a 40 percent score from one audiologist is not equivalent to a 40 percent score in another office, where the word list, the voice, and the presentation level may all be different. Even under identical conditions, test-retest reliability is worse for speech discrimination tests than for pure-tone audiometry. The 95 percent confidence interval for a 40 percent score is quite wide: 26 to 55 percent (Thornton and Raffin, 1978). This means that if a claimant who scored 40 percent on a single test were subjected to a large number of test repetitions and that person's "true score" is defined as the average of all the individual scores, one can be pretty sure that the true score is between 26 and 55 percent. This assumes the use of a 50-word list for each test (the confidence interval would be even wider when using the 25-word lists typically used in clinical testing).

The validity of monosyllable speech discrimination tests given in quiet, often at levels considerably above the levels of conversational speech, has been severely criticized because most real-world speech involves sentences, with variable types and amounts of background noise. Indeed, reviews of studies comparing pure-tone audiometry with speech perception tests as predictors of subjects' self-report of hearing difficulties have usually found pure-tone audiometry to be superior (Dobie and Sakai, 2001; Hardick et al., 1980; King et al., 1992). (Measures of health-related quality of life could in principle be used instead of self-report of hearing difficulty to validate different types of hearing tests; this potential approach is discussed in Chapter 6.)

It is not yet clear whether other types of speech tests, such as those using sentences, perform better than monosyllable tests or pure-tone tests as predictors of real-world difficulties. Simply substituting sentences for words only begins to address the range of real-world speech communication, which involves many other variables, such as:

1. Background noises of different types, levels, and locations;
2. Speech that varies in complexity, familiarity, level, speed, and even frequency composition (e.g., shouted speech contains relatively more high-frequency energy than spoken speech);
3. Distortion introduced by such transmission systems as two-way radios or by reverberation in enclosed environments;
4. Opportunity to request repeats of misheard words or sentences;
5. Different speakers (men, women, children, different accents, etc.);
6. Opportunity to see the speaker's face;
7. Linguistic and cognitive factors for speaker and listener (see nonauditory factors below);
8. Need to respond quickly; and
9. Duration of the task (need for auditory "stamina").

No published speech test has attempted to capture variations in even half of these factors. As long as 55 years ago, Davis and his colleagues (Davis, 1948) developed a battery of speech tests (the Social Adequacy Index), given at three different intensity levels, in an attempt to capture at least some of this range, but this strategy was abandoned because the tests took too long. Other tests, described in Chapter 3, have used sentences of varying difficulty or presented background noise—of a single type—at different levels. But valid and reliable simulation and prediction of real-world performance with speech tests of reasonable length remains a challenge (Gatehouse, 1998).

Speech tests are also more susceptible to exaggeration than pure-tone tests, an important consideration for medical-legal testing (American Speech-Language-Hearing Association, 1981). Audiologists have many methods to detect exaggeration on pure-tone audiometry, and when behavioral tests cannot be trusted, evoked potentials can be used to estimate the pure-tone audiogram. No such tools have been described that can either detect exaggeration on speech discrimination tests or estimate "true" performance for an uncooperative subject.

The SSA medical listings for children use the same tests as for adults, but with different criteria for pure-tone audiometry. The average threshold for 500, 1000, 2000, and 3000 Hz (PTA 5123) is used, instead of the three-frequency average used for adults. For children below the age of 5, the better-ear criterion is 40 dB; from age 5 to 17, the criterion is 70 dB, unless there is a coexistent speech or language disorder (then it is 40 dB, as for younger children). The speech discrimination criterion, which is applied only to children age 5 and older, is 40 percent, as for adults. The committee was unable to discover the history or rationale behind these criteria.

The committee noted the SSA's interest in knowing whether "objective" hearing tests could replace or supplement the behavioral tests that now are used.[3] These tests (otoacoustic emissions and evoked potentials), discussed in Chapter 3, are extremely useful for such purposes as newborn hearing screening and determining the part of the auditory system that is affected in an individual. For example, they are essential when making a diagnosis of auditory neuropathy. They do not help to estimate the impact of hearing loss in everyday life for an adult who is able and willing to cooperate and to provide valid results in behavioral testing. For small children and uncooperative adults, however, evoked potential tests may provide the best or only available information regarding auditory sensitivity; in such cases, evoked potential threshold estimates can be used in place of unobtainable or unreliable behavioral thresholds.

Hearing-Critical Work and Everyday Activities

Each of the auditory abilities described in Chapter 2 is important in some workplaces. Many workers need to be able to detect simple sounds

---

[3]These test are called "objective" because they do not require that the person being tested provide a voluntary response to a sound stimulus. However, clinical judgment is required in their scoring and interpretation.

such as back-up beepers and fire alarms. Knowledge of a person's audiogram, combined with the intensity and frequency content of both a warning signal and any interfering background noise, will usually permit a valid prediction of that person's ability to hear the warning signal (International Organization for Standardization, 2003). Other workers need to discriminate one sound from another (for example, normal versus abnormal functioning of a piece of equipment) or to localize sounds that may come from different directions. No tests of sound localization or discrimination of nonspeech sounds are in common clinical use.

Most workers need to communicate using speech. Speech communication on the job is at least as variable in difficulty as everyday speech. A lawyer listening to a soft-spoken witness or to several angry people talking at once is performing very different tasks from an air traffic controller guiding airplanes to their runways. Entry requirements for many jobs (e.g., as set by the Department of Defense, the Department of Transportation, and many local police and fire departments) require relatively good hearing, based on pure-tone audiometry. In general, these criteria appear to have been based on expert judgment rather than on evidence relating audiometry to job performance, and these entry criteria vary widely across agencies, even for jobs that are substantially identical. In workplaces covered by the Americans with Disabilities Act, if speech communication is not an "essential function" of the job, "reasonable accommodation" for hearing-impaired persons may include substitution by email, text messaging, occasional use of sign translators for meetings, etc.

Despite the obvious importance of hearing in most jobs, hearing loss—even when severe or profound—is far from an absolute impediment to employment. Most adults ages 18 to 44 (and almost half of those ages 45 to 64) with severe to profound hearing loss are employed (Blanchfield et al., 2001). Similarly, 75 percent of working-age men who described themselves as "deaf in both ears" on the National Health Interview Survey were employed (Houtenville, 2002). Some of these people derive significant benefit from hearing aids and cochlear implants, enabling them to do jobs that require some hearing abilities. Others work in jobs that do not require hearing ability at all or that have been modified to accommodate their disabilities. It seems unlikely that there is any measurable degree of hearing loss that can reliably predict the "inability to engage in any substantial gainful activity" without taking into account a person's age, education, and work experience.

Prosthetic Devices

Until the widespread availability of cochlear implants in the 1980s, persons with hearing loss had to function either unaided or with conventional hearing aids, which are essentially amplifiers that make some inaudible sounds audible. The AMA's *Guides to the Evaluation of Permanent Impairment* (American Medical Association, 2001) and almost all state and federal workers' compensation programs (including the Veterans Administration) base estimation of the impact of hearing loss entirely on unaided testing. While this approach ignores the benefit of hearing aids, it preserves at least a reasonable ranking of severity across individuals. For example, three patients with mild, moderate, and severe hearing loss (unaided) would be expected to have the same relative performance ranking with hearing aids: the patient with mild hearing loss would probably have the best aided performance, and the patient with severe hearing loss would have the poorest aided performance. An exception to this general practice is the California workers' compensation system, which combines aided and unaided tone thresholds into an overall estimate of severity of hearing loss.

Some decades ago, there was considerable enthusiasm for aided speech testing (in a sound field rather than under headphones) as a method of selecting the "best" hearing aid for an individual or estimating the impact of (aided) hearing loss on that person. That enthusiasm has waned considerably. Dempsey (1994, p. 731) has stated "The feeling of a significant number of researchers today is that no particular speech test or speech stimulus has been shown to be a reliable or valid predictor of performance with a hearing aid." Of dispensing audiologists who responded to a recent mailed survey, only about half used aided speech discrimination tests at all; of those who used such tests, most used monosyllables in quiet. Only 3 percent of respondents used sentence tests (Mueller, 2001).

Cochlear implants required a return to aided sound field speech testing, because neither aided nor unaided pure-tone thresholds could predict the degree of benefit an individual received from a cochlear implant. A cochlear implant's external sound processor can be adjusted to produce aided pure-tone thresholds at any desired level, but these thresholds are unrelated to the ability to understand speech, which is extremely variable across individuals (Bilger, 1977; Rizer et al., 1988). Only by self-report or aided speech testing can the performance of different cochlear implant patients or devices be distinguished from one another.

Linguistic, Cognitive, and Other Nonauditory Factors

All behavioral tests, including even pure-tone audiometry, test more than just the ear, requiring an alert and cooperative subject who is able to respond when sounds are heard. When speech sounds are presented, the subject must also possess some knowledge of spoken language in general and of the language being spoken. The importance of this knowledge increases as the type of speech sound moves from nonsense syllables to single words to sentences.

Native speakers find sentences much easier than single words or nonsense syllables, because they can use multiple types of cues to "fill in the blanks" when words and sounds have been misheard. One type of cue involves familiarity with individual speech sounds (phonemes); every language has a limited set of phonemes (English has about 40) selected from a much larger set represented in the world's languages (the International Phonetic Alphabet has over 100 symbols, which can be combined to describe hundreds of different speech sounds). A second type of cue is that some phoneme combinations never occur in a particular language, even in nonsense words ("tsetse," a borrowed word from Bantu, is "illegal" in English). At the level of "real" words, a native speaker knows that if what was heard sounded like "traj," the word actually spoken was probably "trash." Finally, in listening to sentences, all of these lower level clues combine with knowledge of grammar and context; if what was heard was "Cake me out to the ball dame," any native speaker of American English will know what was actually said.

A test of sentence understanding would obviously be more similar to real-world speech communication than a test using tones, nonsense syllables, or words. As one approaches real-world performance, linguistic and cognitive factors become more important (and the state of the ears becomes relatively less important). Children, nonnative speakers, and people who are intoxicated, sick, demented, or just tired perform less well on speech tests than alert, cooperative adults who are native speakers—and the differences in performance are greatest for sentences. Even elderly people without frank dementia have more difficulty remembering sentences than individual words they have just heard (Gordon-Salant and Fitzgibbons, 1997). Any speech test that is proposed for use in disability determination will be vulnerable to these nonauditory effects.

If the job requires speech communication in English, the distinction between auditory and nonauditory problems may be unimportant, but many people who speak English poorly have jobs where other languages are spoken exclusively, and for them a test of ability to understand English is irrelevant to their ability to work.

In routine clinical practice, speech understanding is tested without permitting the subject to see the speaker, yet much of everyday speech, including speech in the workplace, occurs in a face-to-face context, permitting the use of visual cues for "speech-reading." Vision is especially important in difficult listening situations. For example, Grant and Seitz (2000) presented unfamiliar sentences (e.g., "the birch canoe slid on the smooth planks") together with background noise as intense as the sentences to 34 patients with mild to severe hearing loss. When listening without vision, the patients could identify only about half of the key words in the sentences (mean = 49 percent correct, range = 9 to 87 percent), but when they were allowed to see the speaker's face, performance improved markedly (mean = 84 percent, range = 56 to 99 percent). In almost all cases, the addition of vision reduced the number of errors made by more than 50 percent. In another study of patients with hearing loss ranging from mild to moderately severe, speech-reading ability (estimated by the improvement in performance when subjects could see the speaker) was a strong predictor of self-reported disability—almost as strong as PTA or speech threshold in quiet, and much stronger than the ability to understand speech in noise without vision (Corthals et al., 1997). These studies probably did not include people with significant visual impairment, but it seems obvious that people with substantial impairments in both vision and hearing would have greater difficulty in face-to-face conversation than people with equivalent hearing loss and good vision.

In the workplace, training and experience must be added to the list of important nonauditory factors. Specialized vocabulary and frequently used phrases, once learned, make communication on the job easier, especially in the presence of background noise or distortion. Workers who know the job well can often predict, based on the task being done at the time, which of these stereotyped messages is most likely to be delivered. Standardized hearing tests cannot measure these skills.

Even after considering some of the factors described above, individuals vary in the degree of difficulty they report for a given degree of hearing loss. Some deny that they have a problem, while others complain of it (Demorest and Walden, 1984). Additional factors that seem to increase the likelihood of elevated complaint behavior include youth, neurosis, and low intelligence quotient (Gatehouse, 1990).

PREVALENCE AND DEMOGRAPHICS
OF HEARING IMPAIRMENT

Prevalence of hearing loss in the United States is estimated from a number of different sources, which collect their data using varying procedures. The National Health Interview Survey (Pleis and Coles, 2002), which publishes the prevalence of chronic health conditions reported by adults, estimates that 17 percent of adults in the United States, or 34 million people, indicate some hearing difficulty. The prevalence of men experiencing hearing difficulty is greater than the prevalence of women experiencing hearing difficulty, with 20.8 percent of adult men having hearing trouble compared to 14.1 percent of adult women having hearing trouble. In addition, the prevalence of reported hearing loss increases with age: 8.4 percent of the population ages 18-44, 20.6 percent of the population ages 45-64, 34.1 percent of the population ages 65-74, and 50.4 percent of the population age 75 and older report some problems with hearing. These estimates include persons with conductive and sensorineural hearing loss and are not verified directly with audiometric examination.

Hearing loss prevalence is also derived from direct audiometric assessment in representative samples of the population. For example, a population-based epidemiological study conducted in Beaver Dam, Wisconsin, examined vision and hearing in the older population of a predominantly white, non-Hispanic Midwestern town. Among older adults ages 48-92 in this study, the prevalence of measured hearing loss (defined as a PTA 5124 of 25 dB or greater) was 45.9 percent. Prevalence in the subgroup ages 48-59 was 21 percent (Cruickshanks et al., 1998). This rate appears to be congruent with the rate of self-reported hearing loss. The prevalence of severe to profound hearing loss among the U.S. population has also been estimated from national data and ranges from 464,000 to 738,000, with 54 percent of this population over age 65 (Blanchfield et al., 2001).

Among children, the estimated prevalence of hearing loss is 1.26 percent based on family report (National Center for Health Statistics, 1996). Other reports suggest that 5 percent of children 18 years and under have hearing loss (U.S. Department of Health and Human Services, 1991). Measured hearing thresholds in a sample of children ages 6-19 are available from the National Health and Nutrition Examination Survey (NHANES-III). Niskar et al. (2001) suggest that 12.5 percent have noise-induced hearing threshold shifts in one or both ears. Projecting this prevalence rate to the national population suggests that approximately 5.2 million children are estimated to have noise-induced threshold shifts in one or both ears. Among every 1,000 children in the United States, 83 have an educationally significant hearing loss (U.S. Public Health Service, 1990). The total number of students receiving special education services for hearing loss in the United States is 43,416 (Gallaudet Research Institute, 2002). The number of children among this sample with known additional disabilities is 14,588, or 33.6 percent.

The rate of hearing aid and cochlear implant use by persons with hearing loss is relatively low, especially among adults. The total number of persons using a hearing aid in the United States is approximately 4.15 million (12.2 percent), with the majority of users age 65 and older (National Center for Health Statistics, 2002). In the Beaver Dam Epidemiology of Hearing Loss Study, the prevalence of hearing aid use among adults ages 48 to 92 with hearing loss was 14.6 percent (Popelka et al., 1998). In the United States, about 13,000 adults have cochlear implants and nearly 10,000 children have them (National Institute for Deafness and other Communication Disorders, 2004). Among children receiving special educational services for hearing loss, 6.2 percent use a cochlear implant and 62.9 percent use a hearing aid for instructional purposes (Gallaudet Research Institute, 2002).

THE SOCIAL SECURITY CONTEXT[4]

SSA administers benefits programs for people with long-lasting disabilities that severely affect their ability to work or, for children, to perform everyday activities like their peers. Under Title II of the Social Security Act, workers covered by Social Security may qualify for benefits called Social Security Disability Insurance (SSDI, often referred to as DI). Under Title XVI, adults and children whose income and assets are low may qualify for Supplemental Security Income (SSI) disability benefits, which are means-tested. It is possible for a beneficiary to qualify for and receive both SSDI and SSI benefits, and nearly 10 percent of Social Security disability beneficiaries do so.

When children and adults apply for disability benefits and claim that a hearing loss has limited their ability to function, SSA is required to determine their eligibility for disability benefits. (See Appendix A for a glossary of terms used in reference to SSA disability programs.) To ensure that these determinations are made fairly and consistently, SSA has developed criteria for eligibility and a process for assessing each claimant against the criteria. The criteria are designed to make the determination process as objective as possible, but to leave some room for considering individual circumstances. The criteria include duration and severity of the disabling condition, employment and income (and assets for SSI), "medical listings" of conditions that are presumptively disabling, and the vocational factors of age, education, and work experience.

In the case of adults with hearing loss, SSA has medical listings criteria that partially correspond to the conventional audiological definition of "profound" hearing loss (see Chapter 3 for categorization of hearing loss). These criteria are identical for SSDI and SSI benefits. For people who do not meet the medical listings criteria, additional tests of hearing may be used to evaluate functional capacity, but there are no clear guidelines at present for evaluating hearing losses that do not meet the medical listings criteria.

---

[4]Parts of this section describing SSA programs and procedures have been adapted from the corresponding section in an earlier NRC report, *Visual Impairments: Determining Eligibility for Social Security Benefits* (National Research Council, 2002).

SSDI is funded by the Social Security Trust Fund, the same trust fund as the well-known SSA retirement program. It is a contributory plan; that is, one must have worked under and contributed to the Social Security tax program (FICA) to be eligible for these benefits. SSDI covers only working-age adults and their dependents. At retirement age, SSDI beneficiaries transition to the retirement benefits program.

SSI is a means-tested program for old-age assistance, aid to the blind, and aid to permanently and totally disabled adults. Disabled children from families with limited income and resources are also covered under this program. The program considers both income and assets in its means-testing. SSI disability determinations are made using the same process and criteria as the SSDI program. SSI children who are 18 and under are evaluated using a process and criteria different from those applied to adults. Funding for this program is not from the Social Security Trust Fund; SSI is primarily funded through congressional appropriations. Adult eligibility for entitlement under both the SSI and SSDI programs is based on demonstrating that a disabling, medically determinable impairment is present in an individual whose labor earnings capacity has fallen below a set limit, termed substantial gainful activity (SGA). Neither SSDI nor SSI has provisions for variable benefits based on severity of impairment; the claimant either meets the disability criteria or does not.

SSI is the only program of the SSA that covers children with disability. The definition of disability for children is somewhat different from that for adults, and it has been changed more than once in recent years in response to litigation and legislation. Currently, if children do not meet the specifically listed medical criteria defining disability, they must be considered under an equivalence standard. The equivalence of their impairment to the specifically listed medical criteria must be evaluated by its medical or functional consequences; that is, it can medically equal a listed criterion or, using the functional domains cited in the SSA regulations, it can be judged functionally equivalent to the intent of the listings. The methodology used to make this decision is discussed in a later section.

Social Security Disability Determinations and Caseload for Hearing Impairment

Early in this study, the SSA provided the committee with statistical tables on claimants and beneficiaries with hearing impairments for the years 1997-2001 for determinations and 1998-2001 for numbers of beneficiaries. The SSA staff noted that the statistics from which these tables were prepared are subject to various types of error but are the best data available. Over the period 1998 through 2001, the total number of current beneficiaries with a primary diagnosis of hearing impairment, including both SSDI (Title II) and SSI (Title XVI) beneficiaries, increased from just under 100,000 to nearly 106,000. In addition, 10,686 (in 1998) to 21,876 (in 2001) beneficiaries annually received benefits with hearing as a secondary impairment.

SSA did not provide figures for dollar costs of hearing impairment benefits. However, SSA was recently able to provide us with the number of beneficiaries in current pay status (as of May 2004) for hearing and related impairments (vertiginous syndromes, other ear disorders, and deafness), shown in Table 1-1, and with average monthly benefits for all disability beneficiaries. The average monthly benefit for DI disabled workers in 2003 was $844 and the average paid to SSI disabled beneficiaries was $433, but payment amounts specifically for hearing-impaired beneficiaries were not available. If it is assumed that these beneficiaries received the average benefit, then at this time the DI worker beneficiaries, primary and secondary, were receiving over $60 million per month and SSI beneficiaries were receiving a bit over $31 million per month in benefits. (Nonworker beneficiaries are not included in these estimates, because their average benefit was not provided.) This comes to a total of nearly $1.1 billion per year.

For the years 1997-2001, the total number of *claims* per year with a primary diagnosis of hearing impairment showed no major change, varying between 15,400 and 16,600. The percentage of these claims allowed (awarded benefits) increased from 39 percent in 1997 to 47 percent in 2001. The overall number of disability claims has been rising since 2001 (Social Security Administration, 2004), but we do not have the most recent figures for hearing impairment claims. Claim allowance rates are consistently highest for children under age 5 and for older working-age adults.

TABLE 1-1 SSA Beneficiaries in Current Pay Status for the Impairment Codes of Vertiginous Syndromes, Other Ear Disorders, and Deafness, May 2004

Beneficiary Type	Disability Insurance: Workers	Disability Insurance: Auxiliary[a]	Supplemental Security Income
Primary impairment	57,847	9,748	56,838
Secondary impairment	13,543	1,879	14,800

[a]DI nonworker beneficiaries, such as spouses and children.

In parallel with this, the proportion of allowed claimants meeting or equaling the listings is lowest for children under age 5 and for older adults, but is above 90 percent for claimants over age 18 and under age 54 across this time period. This indicates that the youngest and oldest groups are more likely to receive favorable determinations based on vocational factors for adults or on functional equivalence to the listings for children.

Procedures for Determining Disability

SSA reviews all claims for disability benefits using its sequential evaluation process. For adults, the process has five steps; for children, a three-step process is used.

Adults

For adults covered by SSDI and for adult SSI claimants, the disability determination process follows the steps shown in Figure 1-1. The first step of the sequential evaluation process requires that the disability examiner working on behalf of SSA determine whether the claimant is engaged in SGA. Each year the SSA formally establishes an average monthly earnings level that serves to define SGA for disability. For 2004, the monthly SGA limit is $810 for disabled claimants. If the claimant is determined not to be performing SGA, the case goes on to Step 2 of the sequential evaluation process. If the claimant is determined to be performing SGA, she or he is found ineligible for benefits at this step.

At Step 2, the claimant must document through a report or medical records provided by an acceptable medical source that a medically determinable impairment is present that significantly limits his or her physical or mental ability to do basic work activities. Furthermore, medical evidence must support a judgment that the limitations imposed by the impairment have lasted or can be expected to last for at least 12 months or are expected to lead to the claimant's death. If these criteria are satisfied, the claim progresses to Step 3. If the criteria are not satisfied, the claimant is found ineligible for benefits at this step.

Step 3 of the sequential evaluation process uses medical criteria as a screening test to identify claimants who are obviously disabled. In this step, SSA must decide whether the claimant's medically determinable impairment(s) meets or equals in severity the specific medical criteria listed in 20 CFR Part 404, Subpart P, Appendix 1. This decision requires concurrence of a medical or psychological consultant. If the claimant has an impairment that is determined to meet or equal the listed criteria and that level of impairment severity has been demonstrated to have lasted or is expected to last for at least 12 months or to end in death, the claimant is

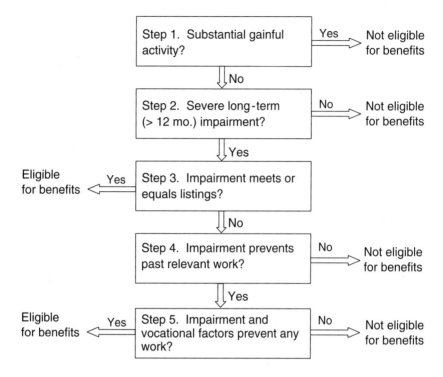

FIGURE 1-1 SSA decision flow for adult disability determination.

found eligible for benefits. If not, the process continues to the consideration of vocational factors in Steps 4 and 5.

At this point in the process, the adjudicative team assesses the residual functional capacity of the claimant. Form SSA-4734-BK, called "Physical Residual Functional Capacity Assessment," is used for physical impairments, and Form SSA 4734 is used when a mental impairment has been identified. These are assessments of what the claimant can do in spite of any physical and mental impairment over a 12-month period of time. The forms require assessment of exertional, postural, manipulative, visual, communicative, and environmental limitations. The auditory functions listed include pure-tone threshold, tested by air and bone conduction, and speech discrimination (test unspecified).

In Step 4, the decision makers must determine whether any of the claimant's physical and mental limitations cited in the evaluations of residual functional capacity precludes the performance of "past relevant work." If the claimant is found able to perform past relevant work in spite of cited physical and mental limitations, he or she is found ineligible for benefits. If the claimant is found unable to perform past relevant work, the claim goes to Step 5.

In Step 5, the SSA uses a defined set of profiles and rules that consider the claimant's age, education, and work experience or skills. A decision is made whether the claimant is capable of performing any work in the U.S. economy. A so-called vocational grid is used as a decision aid, embodying the rules for determining disability. The grid combines the vocational factors and recommends findings for various combinations. Constructed in 1979 based on information from the *Dictionary of Occupational Titles* (Social Security Advisory Board, 2003), the grid reflects SSA's evaluation of the existence of work in the national economy. It was designed to be used in cases of limitations of strength and stamina, for example, to consider whether a claimant is able to perform "sedentary," "light," "medium," or "heavy" work. It is not useful for other functional limitations, for which the assessment must be based on professional judgment. In practice, the claimant's age is quite important in this determination, with older claimants, especially those over 55, not expected to learn new skills to find a job in a new line of work.

If the claimant is found to have a disability under the rules of Step 5, he or she is eligible for benefits. If he or she is found not to have a disability, benefits are denied. If a claimant disagrees with SSA's decision, several levels of appeal are available.

Children

For children (covered only under SSI), a slightly different set of steps is followed, as shown in Figure 1-2.

Steps 1 and 2 are the same as for adults. Step 3 for children is initially the same as for adults. If a child is determined to have an impairment that meets or medically equals the criteria cited in the listings, and that impairment is expected to last for 12 months or to end in death, the child is eligible for SSI disability benefits. Because Steps 4 and 5 for adults are not appropriate for children, an additional decision point has been added to Step 3 of the process for children. Under rules that took effect January 2, 2001, when a child is found to have a medically determinable impairment that does not meet or medically equal a listed criterion, SSA must make a determination of whether the child's impairment(s) *functionally* equals the intent of the listings.

The fundamental decision to be made is whether the functional effects of the impairment(s) are "marked and severe." This is judged mainly on the child's ability to perform in six functional domains compared with normative data based on the ability of an unimpaired child of the same age. The regulations specify the functional domains to be considered and

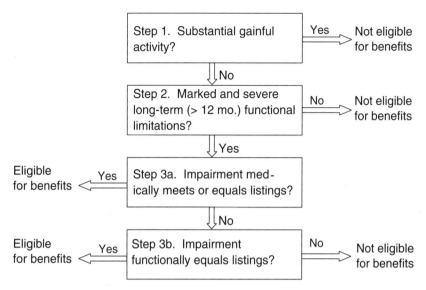

FIGURE 1-2 SSA decision flow for infant and child disability determination.

give examples of age-appropriate levels of functioning for various age groups (20 CFR §416.924-926a). The regulations state that "marked" limitation "is the equivalent of the functioning we would expect to find on standardized testing with scores that are at least two, but less than three, standard deviations below the mean" (20 CFR §416.926a, (e) (ii)). "Extreme" limitation is described in a subsequent section as equivalent to at least three standard deviations below the mean. Box 1-1 shows the six functional domains.

If the child meets the functional equivalence criteria, which may be satisfied by showing marked limitations in two or more domains or extreme limitation in one domain, she or he is judged medically eligible for benefits. If not, she or he is ruled ineligible. All children who receive benefits must have their eligibility reviewed when they reach age 18, based on the adult SSI criteria.

Current Disability Criteria for Hearing

In the discussion of Step 3 of the sequential evaluation process, we mentioned the listing of impairments found in Appendix 1 of Subpart P of 20 CFR Part 404. The hearing listings are based on measures of pure-tone threshold, using air and bone conduction, and on speech discrimination testing.

BOX 1-1
Functional Domains Considered in Determining
Disability for Children

1. Acquiring and using information
2. Attending and completing tasks
3. Interacting and relating with others
4. Moving about and manipulating objects
5. Caring for yourself
6. Health and physical well-being

SOURCE: 20 CFR §416.926a.

Criteria for Adults

The requirements for testing and for documenting hearing loss of adults are as follows (Social Security Administration, 2003a, p. 24):

Loss of hearing can be quantitatively determined by an audiometer which meets the standards of the American National Standards Institute (ANSI) for air and bone conducted stimuli (i.e., ANSI S3.6-1969 and ANSI S3.13-1972, or subsequent comparable revisions) and performing all hearing measurements in an environment which meets the ANSI standard for maximal permissible background sound (ANSI S3.1-1977).

Speech discrimination should be determined using a standardized measure of speech discrimination ability in quiet at a test presentation level sufficient to ascertain maximum discrimination ability. The speech discrimination measure (test) used, and the level at which testing was done must be reported.

Hearing tests should be preceded by an otolaryngologic examination and should be performed by or under the supervision of an otolaryngologist or audiologist qualified to perform such tests.

In order to establish an independent medical judgment as to the level of impairment in a claimant alleging deafness, the following examinations should be reported: Otolaryngologic examination, pure tone air and bone audiometry, speech reception threshold (SRT), and speech discrimination testing. A copy of reports of medical examination and audiologic evaluations must be submitted.

Cases of alleged "deaf mutism" should be documented by a hearing evaluation. Records obtained from a speech and hearing rehabilitation center or a special school for the deaf may be acceptable, but if these reports are not available, or are found to be inadequate, a current hearing evaluation should be submitted as outlined in the preceding paragraph.

The criteria for hearing loss severe enough to be taken as prima facie evidence of disability in adults are (p. 26):

- Average hearing threshold sensitivity for air conduction of 90 decibels or greater, and for bone conduction to corresponding maximal levels, in the better ear, determined by the simple average of hearing threshold levels at 500, 1000, and 2000 Hz.; or

- Speech discrimination scores of 40 percent or less in the better ear.

Criteria for Children

The listings include special provisions for the evaluation of children (Social Security Administration, 2003a, p. 111):

The criteria for hearing impairments in children take into account that a lesser impairment in hearing which occurs at an early age may result in a severe speech and language disorder.

Improvement by a hearing aid, as predicted by the testing procedure, must be demonstrated to be feasible in that child, since younger children may be unable to use a hearing aid effectively.

The type of audiometric testing performed must be described and a copy of the results must be included. The pure tone air conduction hearing levels in 102.08 are based on American National Standard Institute Specifications for Audiometers, S3.6-1969 (ANSI-1969). The report should indicate the specifications used to calibrate the audiometer.

The finding of a severe impairment will be based on the average hearing levels at 500, 1000, 2000, and 3000 Hertz (Hz) in the better ear, and on speech discrimination, as specified in 102.08.

The listing criteria for children are as follows (pp. 111-112):

102. 08 Hearing Impairments

A. For children below 5 years of age at time of adjudication, inability to hear air conduction thresholds at an average of 40 decibels (db) hearing level or greater in the better ear; or

B. For children 5 years of age and above at time of adjudication:

1. Inability to hear air conduction thresholds at an average of 70 decibels (db) or greater in the better ear; or

2. Speech discrimination scores at 40 percent or less in the better ear; or

3. Inability to hear air conduction thresholds at an average of 40 decibels

(db) or greater in the better ear, and a speech and language disorder which significantly affects the clarity and content of the speech and is attributable to the hearing impairment.

As noted above, a child's impairments are considered to be functionally equivalent to the intent of the listings if he or she has "marked" limitations in two broad domains of function (see Box 1-1) or an "extreme" limitation in one domain.

THE COMMITTEE'S APPROACH[5]

Models of Disability

The conceptual model underlying disability determination has been undergoing changes over the past several years, especially since the passage of the Americans with Disabilities Act (ADA) in 1990. One newer conceptualization follows a social model of disability, which postulates that factors both within the individual and in his or her physical and social/cultural environment combine to influence performance and participation in everyday situations. An even newer formulation, the "new paradigm" discussed by Pledger (2003), recognizes a "disability culture" and approaches some issues as matters of civil rights for a minority group. This approach stresses respect for people with disabilities as being capable of self-determination and independent decision making. It also advocates for people with disabilities to be in charge of their own assistance and accommodations, rather than to have others determining what they need.

These newer models replace the earlier stress on disability or handicap and the negative aspects of an individual's situation, emphasizing instead the person's remaining capabilities and how they can best be supported to permit full economic and social participation. They also replace earlier implications that disability was the simple and inevitable result of an impairment. The ADA, based on the social model, represents a commitment in the United States to help individuals with disabilities to participate as fully as possible in the society and the economy.

The social model also underlies the approach now taken by the World Health Organization toward disability and handicap. Whereas *The International Classification of Impairment, Disability, and Handicap* (ICIDH) (World Health Organization, 1980) established definitions for these

---

[5]Some of the descriptive parts of this section have been adapted from the corresponding section in an earlier NRC report, *Visual Impairments: Determining Eligibility for Social Security Benefits* (National Research Council, 2002).

terms, the newer *International Classification of Functioning, Disability and Health* (ICF) (World Health Organization, 2001) is an attempt to fully account for the interactions between the individual and the physical and social environment in determining the participation of an individual with a disability. Further discussion of disability models is presented in Chapter 6, where social and environmental aspects of disability are considered.

Predicting Disability from Clinical Tests

The committee carefully considered the social model as it applies to those with hearing loss, recognizing that the measured severity of hearing loss does *not* inevitably predict a person's disability or handicap. However, this model does pose a dilemma for using the measurement of hearing loss as a surrogate for determining level of disability. In reviewing data on audiological testing and functional status, the working hypothesis was deceptively simple: increasingly severe hearing loss, by some measure, is associated with increasing inability to carry out activities associated with employment or, in the case of children, age-appropriate activities. The data bearing on this issue present a more complicated picture, because the same level of hearing loss can result in a wide spectrum of disability level, depending on such diverse factors as duration and age of onset of hearing loss, availability and quality of habilitation or rehabilitation services, education, age, gender, psychological adjustment, presence of other comorbid conditions, and social and environmental support. Thus, there is a great variability in functional status for any given level of hearing loss.

The committee evaluated the fifth edition of the American Medical Association's *Guides to the Evaluation of Permanent Impairment* (American Medical Association, 2001). These guides, used in many workers' compensation procedures for disability determination, represent a more traditional quantitative approach to evaluating impairment and disability. The chapter on philosophy, purpose, and appropriate use of the *Guides* in the fifth edition explains: "The *Guides* continues to define impairment as 'a loss, loss of use, or derangement of any body part, organ system, or organ function.'" (p. 2). The chapter also states (pp. 4-5):

> The whole person impairment percentages listed in the *Guides* estimate the impact of the impairment on the individual's overall ability to perform activities of daily living, *excluding work*. . . . The medical judgment used to determine the original impairment percentages could not account for the diversity or complexity of work but could account for daily activities of most people. Work is not included in the clinical judgment for impairment percentages for several reasons: (1) work in-

volves many simple and complex activities; (2) work is highly individualized, making generalizations inaccurate; (3) impairment percentages are unchanged for stable conditions, but work and occupations change; and (4) impairments interact with such other factors as the worker's age, education, and prior work experience to determine the extent of work disability.

The section on disability in this chapter of the *Guides* discusses the evolving definitions of the term, and then states (p. 8):

The *Guides* continues to define disability as an alteration of an individual's capacity to meet personal, social, or occupational demands or statutory or regulatory requirements because of an impairment. An individual can have a disability in performing a specific work activity but not have a disability in any other social role.

It also states (p. 8):

The impairment evaluation, however, is only one aspect of disability determination. A disability determination also includes information about the individual's skills, education, job history, adaptability, age, and environmental requirements and modifications. Assessing these factors can provide a more realistic picture of the effects of the impairment on the ability to perform complex work and social activities. If adaptations can be made to the environment, the individual may not be disabled from performing that activity.

On the whole, the AMA *Guides* are in agreement with the current belief that impairment is only one of several factors determining an individual's ability to perform in daily life and the workplace and, consequently, that many factors beyond medical impairment criteria should be considered in determining whether any individual has a disability in a given situation. Table 1-2 illustrates the definitions of impairment and disability used in several systems.

In contrast to this approach, SSA currently uses "disability" or "disabled" as a term that applies to those who are deemed eligible for disability benefits as a result of the formal determination process. The agency uses the terms to describe the relationship of the person to the criteria for its programs, not necessarily as a description of his or her personal functional status.

The SSA disability determination process follows a path starting with a medical model, embodied in the listings of impairments, through Step 3 of the decision process. The listed medical conditions are assumed to produce impairments so severe that individuals are disabled by the mere presence of the condition, as determined by clinical diagnostic markers. For persons whose conditions meet or equal the listings and who are not engaged in SGA, SSA does not require that functional capacity be evalu-

TABLE 1-2 Definitions of Impairment and Disability

Organization	Impairment
American Medical Association *Guides to the Evaluation of Permanent Impairment* (5th ed., 2001)	A loss, loss of use, or derangement of any body part, organ system, or organ function.
World Health Organization (1999)	Problems in body function or structure as a significant deviation or loss. Impairments of structure can involve an anomaly, defect, loss, or other significant deviation in body structures.
Social Security Administration (1995)	An anatomical, physiological, or psychological abnormality that can be shown by medically acceptable clinical and laboratory diagnostic techniques.
State workers' compensation law (typical)	Permanent impairment "is any anatomic or functional loss after maximal medical improvement has been achieved and which abnormality or loss, medically, is considered stable or nonprogressive at the time of evaluation. Permanent impairment is a basic consideration in the evaluation of permanent disability and is a contributing factor to, but not necessarily an indication of, the entire extent of permanent disability (*Idaho Code* section 72-422).

SOURCE: American Medical Association (2001, p. 3).

Disability	Physicians' Role	Comments
An alteration of an individual's capacity to meet personal, social, or occupational demands because of an impairment.	Determine impairment, provide medical information to assist in disability determination.	An impaired individual may or may not have a disability.
Activity limitation (formerly disability) is a difficulty in the performance, accomplishment, or completion of an activity at the level of the person. Difficulty encompasses all of the ways in which the doing of the activity may be affected.	Not specifically defined; assumed to be one of the decision makers in determining disability through impairment assessment.	Emphasis is on the importance of functional abilities and defining context-related activity limitations.
The inability to engage in any substantial, gainful activity by reason of any medically determinable physical or mental impairment(s), which can be expected to result in death or which has lasted or can be expected to last for a continuous period of not less than 12 months.	Determine impairment, may assist with the disability determination as a consultative examiner.	Physicians and nonphysicians need to work together to define situational disabilities.
"Temporary disability" means a decrease in wage-earning capacity due to injury or occupational disease during a period of recovery (*Idaho Code* section 72-102[10]). "Permanent disability" results when the actual or presumed ability to engage in gainful activity is reduced or absent because of permanent impairment and no fundamental or marked change in the future can be reasonably expected (*Idaho Code* Section 72-423).	"Evaluation (rating) of permanent impairment" is a medical appraisal of the nature and extent of the injury or disease as it affects an injured employee's personal efficiency in the activities of daily living, such as self-care, communication, normal living postures, ambulation, elevation, traveling, and nonspecialized activities of bodily members (*Idaho Code* section 72-424).	Purpose is to provide sure and certain relief to those who become injured by accident or suffer effects of disease from exposure to hazards arising out of and in the course of employment.

ated to determine eligibility for benefits. This "screening in" at Step 3 is important to the SSA as a way to minimize the number of claimants for whom Step 4 and 5 consideration of vocational factors, an expensive and time-consuming process, must be performed. The criteria are purposely set high, since the additional steps will give all claimants not meeting the listing criteria an opportunity to be found eligible for benefits.

For those whose conditions do not meet or equal the medical listings, SSA switches in Steps 4 and 5 to a more complex model, performing an evaluation of functional capacity in relation to the work environment (based on a model of physical work demands). The process evaluates the claimant's ability first to perform in recent relevant employment (Step 4) and then to perform any work in the U.S. economy (Step 5). The vocational grids mentioned earlier are used as decision aids when the impairment is in the ability to perform physical labor, but for other work, the guidance is sparse at best. The decision maker considers the claimant's age, education, and work experience as well as, by inference, transferable skills. At this time, SSA prescribes no formal tests or evaluation protocols (beyond the Residual Functional Capacity form completed by a physician) to determine what the claimant actually can do; no formal method for determining what disability might result from an individual's impairments in the living and work environments; nor any assessment of the mitigating effects of environmental accommodations or assistive technology. Also there also is normally no face-to-face meeting between the claimant and the decision maker in the initial determination process, although this may change if some current pilot programs are successful. Vocational experts may be brought in to aid the decision making. In practice, the claimant's age is important in this evaluation; most older claimants, especially those over age 55, are not expected to learn new skills to find a job in a new line of work.

A recent report by the Social Security Advisory Board (2003) discussed in depth several difficulties with the SSA's current approach. It noted that (Social Security Advisory Board, 2003, p. 7):

> The core definition of disability for the Social Security program adopted fifty years ago was inability to do substantial work by reason of a physical or mental impairment. That core definition itself remains unchanged, but the context in which it operates has changed a great deal, and its validity, both as an administratively feasible definition and as an appropriate standard of benefit eligibility, is increasingly subject to challenge.

The report discussed several issues that are problematic, including the following (p. 17):

> The concept of disability has both medical and functional components. The world of work has a wide variety of tasks that require a range of

physical and intellectual functional capacities. . . Therefore a given medical condition may or may not be "disabling" depending on the specific functional capacities and how they interact with the educational and vocational profile of the affected individual. A medical condition that precludes highly exertional physical activity may be "totally" disabling for an older individual with little education and an unskilled work history and not disabling for another individual who is highly skilled and educated.

In a theoretical sense, accurately determining disability for Social Security disability benefits would require that each individual be evaluated to determine how their medical condition limits their functional capacity and then how these limitations interact with each individual's age, work history, and education. The end result would be a decision whether the medical impact on the individual's functional capacities makes work feasible.

The report acknowledged that the volume of claims has always made such individual evaluations of all claimants impracticable, but noted also (p. 7):

[T]he proportion of initial allowances based strictly on medical factors has declined from around 93 percent in the early years of the program to 82 percent in 1983 and to a 2000 level of 58 percent. By the end of the appeals process, the proportion of allowances made on strictly medical factors is around 40 percent, and because of coding deficiencies, possibly even lower.[6]

As noted above, individualized assessments of vocational disability require knowledge of the specific demands of jobs. The committee reviewed some of the job taxonomies now available and considered the reviews conducted by a previous NRC committee on visual impairments (National Research Council, 2002), but we could not identify a database of job demands that would be usable for SSA disability determination at this time. The Disability Research Institute, a research consortium under contract to the SSA, has reached a similar conclusion. A recent technical report (Heinemann et al., 2002) from their project on job demands reviewed several systems and taxonomies that could serve as information sources for SSA in determining the job demands of various occupations. It stated (Heinemann et al., 2002, p. 42):

In summary, there are several reasons for conducting a separate study for generating job demand variables for SSA's use in disability determinations. Some of the important reasons are: (a) Existing job analysis sys-

---

[6]For hearing impairment, the percentage of awardees meeting the listings is still in the 90+ percent range, except for children and working age adults over age 55.

tems do not sufficiently address the needs of SSA in assessing the RFC of claimants for the purpose of determining disability, (b) with the exception of O*NET, the available job analysis inventories (and their derived job demand variables) may not adequately reflect the fast changing world of work, especially the dot-com industry; while O*NET is a new system, its serious deficiencies in meeting the needs of SSA are well known . . . and (c) recent advances in measurement technology . . . allow for a more precise assessment and simultaneous calibration of jobs and job demand variables on a common metric.

These issues are among the ones that the committee sought to address in its approach to the determination of disability for people with hearing loss.

The Study Process

The committee performed an extensive literature review of topics relevant to the study tasks, with individual committee members reviewing the literature in their fields of special expertise. Two papers were commissioned, one on assistive listening devices and one on the literature relating hearing test performance to job performance. Data were obtained from government and other sources when appropriate.

The committee debated the criteria it should impose for accepting evidence for consideration in its work. First, it was agreed that any evidence used should be available in the open published (including on-line) literature, so that readers could examine it themselves if they wished to. We preferred to use evidence published in peer-reviewed journals but allowed other evidence as well, if we were able to determine that the work had been rigorously performed. These sources included book chapters, medical texts, papers presented at scientific and professional conferences, technical reports, and government publications. (For demographic and epidemiological data, the best sources were usually government reports.) Other evidence, such as that from unrefereed journals or advocacy groups, was evaluated very carefully before being accepted with caution.

The committee held a public forum in January 2003 to allow members of the public and representatives of service and advocacy groups to provide information. About 80 organizations working with deaf and hard-of-hearing people were sent invitations to nominate forum speakers, and seven speakers subsequently participated. Each speaker was asked to respond to a set of prepared questions, to encourage them to focus their remarks on issues relevant to the committee's tasks. All of the organizations were invited to have their representatives attend as guests as well. There was time at the forum for open discussion and questions from guests. Appendix C includes lists of the organizations invited to nominate speakers, the speakers, and the registered guests.

Guide to the Report

The remainder of this report is divided into six chapters. In Chapter 2 we review the basic mechanisms of hearing and the functioning of the human auditory system and describe the types of hearing loss and their causes. In Chapter 3 we review the testing of adult hearing and of the auditory system, beginning with a description of a standard otological exam and then turning to audiological testing. The chapter reviews current tests and test theory and describes and evaluates the tests now mandated by the SSA for hearing disability determination and other tests that were considered for possible use as replacements or augmentations of those tests. We also discuss test conditions and protocols. In Chapter 4, we present our conclusions on the testing of adults and our recommendations for tests and testing procedures. Chapter 5 is devoted to a discussion of technological aids that can mitigate the effects of hearing loss: hearing aids, prostheses such as cochlear implants, and assistive listening devices. We review the state of the art for each type of device, discussing what is known about how well each can improve the functioning of people with hearing loss. In Chapter 6, we discuss what is known of the effects of hearing loss on everyday life, work performance, and psychosocial adjustment. We evaluate the strengths and weaknesses of some instruments used to measure these effects and review some psychometric issues involved in their design and interpretation. Finally, Chapter 7 addresses hearing loss in children. The chapter reviews the effects of hearing loss on children's speech, language, and educational development and the special requirements and challenges of the development of hearing tests for children. We review and evaluate current tests and present conclusions and recommendations for testing children's hearing, speech, and language competence for SSA disability determination.

Four appendixes provide additional information. Appendix A consists of two glossaries of SSA and technical terms. Appendix B describes the standards of the American National Standards Institute pertaining to bioacoustics that are referenced in the report. Appendix C lists the organizations and speakers who were invited to the committee's public forum. Appendix D consists of biographical sketches of committee members and staff.

2

Basics of Sound, the Ear, and Hearing

In this chapter we review basic information about sound and about how the human auditory system performs the process called hearing. We describe some fundamental auditory functions that humans perform in their everyday lives, as well as some environmental variables that may complicate the hearing task. We also discuss the types of hearing loss or disorder that can occur and their causes.

INTRODUCTION TO SOUND[1]

Hearing allows one to identify and recognize objects in the world based on the sound they produce, and hearing makes communication using sound possible. Sound is derived from objects that vibrate producing pressure variations in a sound-transmitting medium, such as air. A pressure wave is propagated outward from the vibrating source. When the pressure wave encounters another object, the vibration can be imparted to that object and the pressure wave will propagate in the medium of the object. The sound wave may also be reflected from the object or it may diffract around the object. Thus, a sound wave propagating outward from a vibrating object can reach the eardrum of a listener causing the eardrum to vibrate and initiate the process of hearing.

---

[1]Most of the description of sound, the auditory system, and auditory perception is derived from Yost (2000).

Sound waves can be mathematically described in two ways, that is, in two domains. In the time domain, sound is described as a sequence of pressure changes (oscillations) that occur over time. In other words, the time-domain description of a sound wave specifies how the sound pressure increases and decreases over time. In the frequency domain, the spectrum defines sound in terms of the tonal components that make up the sound. A tonal sound has a time-domain description in which sound pressure changes as a regular (sinusoidal) function of time. If one knows the tonal components of sound as defined in the frequency domain, one can calculate the time-domain description of the sound. Using the same analytic tools, the frequency domain representation of a sound can also be calculated from the time-domain description. Thus, the time and frequency domain descriptions of sound are two different ways of measuring the same thing (i.e., the time and frequency domains are functional equivalents). Thus, one can describe sound as temporal fluctuations in pressure, or one can describe sounds in terms of the frequency components that compose the sound.

Largely because tonal (sinusoidal) sounds are the bases of the frequency domain description of sound, a great deal of the study of hearing has dealt with tonal sounds. However, everyday sounds are complex sounds, which are made up of many tonal frequency components. A common complex sound used to study hearing is noise. Noise contains all possible frequency components, and the amplitude of the noise varies randomly over time. A noise is said to be "white noise" if it contains all frequency components each at the same average sound level.

A sound waveform has three basic physical attributes: frequency, amplitude, and temporal variation. Frequency refers to the number of times per second that the vibratory pattern (in the time domain) oscillates. Amplitude refers to sound pressure. There are many aspects to the temporal variation of sound, such as sound duration. Sound pressure is proportional to sound intensity (in units of power or energy), so sound magnitude can be measured in units of pressure, power, and energy. The common measure of sound level is the decibel (dB), in which the decibel is the logarithm of the ratio of two sound intensities or two sound pressures. Frequency is measured in units of hertz (Hz), cycles per second. Measures of time are expressed in various temporal units or can be translated into phase measured in angular degrees. Below are some definitions of terms and measures used to describe sound.

• Sound pressure (p): sound pressure is equal to the force (F) produced by the vibrating object divided by the area (Ar) over which that force is being applied: $p = F/Ar$.

• DekaPascals or daPa; the Système International unit of pressure. One daPa = 100 dynes per cm^2, and one atmosphere = 10132.5 daPa.

• Sound intensity (I): sound intensity is a measure of power. Sound intensity equals sound pressure squared divided by the density (p_o) of the sound-transmitting medium (e.g., air) times the speed of sound (c): I = $p^2/p_o c$. Energy is a measure of the ability to do work and is equal to power times the duration of the sound, or E = PT, where P is power and T is time (duration) in seconds.

• Decibel (dB): dB = $10^* \log_{10}(I/I_{ref})$ or $20^* \log_{10}(p/p_{ref})$, where I is sound intensity, p is sound pressure, ref is a referent intensity or pressure, and $\log_{10}$ is the logarithm to the base 10. When p_{ref} is 20 micropascals, then the decibel measure is expressed as dB SPL (sound pressure level).

• Hertz (Hz): hertz is the measure of vibratory frequency in which "n" cycles per second of periodic oscillation is "n" Hz.

• Phase (angular degrees): one cycle of a periodic change in sound pressure can be expressed in terms of completing the 360 degrees of a circle. Thus, half a cycle is 180 degrees, and so on. Thus, time (t) within a cycle can be expressed in terms of phase (θ, expressed in degrees), θ = $360^o(t)(f)$, where f = frequency in Hz, and t = time in seconds.

• Tone (a simple sound): a tone is a sound whose amplitude changes as a sinusoidal function of time: $A \sin(2 \pi f t + \theta)$, where sin is the trigonometric sin function, A = peak amplitude, f = frequency in Hz, t = time in seconds, and θ = starting phase in degrees.

• Complex sound: any sound that contains more than one frequency component.

• Spectrum: the description of the frequency components of sound; amplitude spectrum describes the amplitude of each frequency component; phase spectrum describes the phase of each frequency component.

• Noise: a complex sound that contains all frequency components, and whose instantaneous amplitude varies randomly.

• White noise: a noise in which all of the frequency components have the same average level.

The term "noise" can refer to any sound that may be unwanted or may interfere with the detection of a target or signal sound. In some contexts, a speech sound may be the signal or target sound, and another speech sound or a mixture of other speech sounds may be presented as a "noise" to interfere with the auditory processing of the target speech sound. Often a mixture of speech sounds is referred to as "speech babble."

The Auditory System

The ear is a very efficient transducer (i.e., a device that changes energy from one form to another), changing sound pressure in the air into a

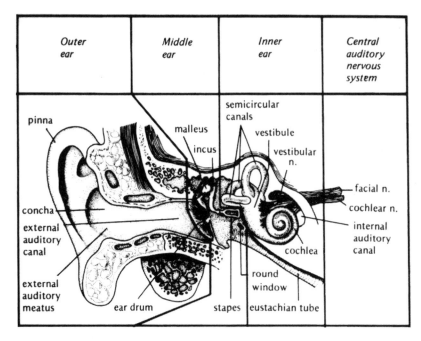

Outer ear	Middle ear	Inner ear	Central auditory nervous system

FIGURE 2-1 The anatomy of the auditory system. From Yost (2000, p. 66). Reprinted with permission of author.

neural-electrical signal that is translated by the brain as speech, music, noise, etc. The external ear, middle ear, inner ear, brainstem, and brain each have a specific role in this transformation process (see Figure 2-1).

The external ear includes the pinna, which helps capture sound in the environment. The external ear canal channels sound to the tympanic membrane (eardrum), which separates the external and middle ear. The tympanic membrane and the three middle ear bones, or ossicles (malleus, incus, and stapes), assist in the transfer of sound pressure in air into the fluid- and tissue-filled inner ear. When pressure is transferred from air to a denser medium, such as the inner ear environment, most of the pressure is reflected away. Thus, the inner ear offers impedance to conducting sound pressure to the fluid and tissue of the inner ear. The transfer of pressure in this case is referred to as admittance, while impedance is the restriction of the transfer of pressure. The term "acoustic immittance" is used to describe the transfer process within the middle ear: the word "immittance" combines the words impedance and admittance (im + mittance). As a result of this impedance, there is as much as a 35 dB loss in the transmission of sound pressure to the inner ear. The outer ear, tympanic membrane, and ossicles interact when a sound is present to focus the sound pressure into the inner ear so that most of that 35 dB impedance loss is overcome. Thus, the fluids and tissues of the inner ear vibrate in response to sound in a very efficient manner.

Sound waves are normally transmitted through the ossicular chain of the middle ear to the stapes footplate. The footplate rocks in the oval window of the inner ear, setting the fluids of the inner ear in motion, with the parameters of that motion being dependent on the intensity, frequency, and temporal properties of the signal. The inner ear contains both the vestibular system (underlying the sense of balance and equilibrium) and the cochlea (underlying the sense of hearing). The cochlea has three separate fluid compartments; two contain perilymph (scala tympani and scala vestibuli), similar to the body's extracellular fluid, and the other, scala media, contains endolymph, which is similar to intracellular fluids.

The scala media contains the sensorineural hair cells that are stimulated by changes in fluid and tissue vibration. There are two types of hair cells: inner and outer. Inner hair cells are the auditory biotransducers translating sound vibration into neural discharges. The shearing (a type of bending) of the hairs (stereocilia) of the inner hair cells caused by these vibrations induces a neural-electrical potential that activates a neural response in auditory nerve fibers of the eighth cranial nerve that neurally connect the hair cells to the brainstem. The outer hair cells serve a different purpose. When their stereocilia are sheared, the size of the outer hair cells changes due to a biomechanical alteration. The rapid change in outer hair cell size (especially its length) alters the biomechanical coupling within the cochlea.

The structures of the cochlea vibrate in response to sound with a particular vibratory pattern. This vibratory pattern (the traveling wave) allows the inner hair cells and their connections to the auditory nerve to send signals to the brainstem and brain about the sound's vibration and its frequency content. That is, the traveling wave motion of cochlear vibration helps sort out the frequency content of any sound, so that information about the frequency components of sound is coded in the neural responses being sent to the brainstem and brain.

The fact that the different frequencies of sound are coded by different auditory nerve fibers is referred to as the place theory of frequency processing, and the auditory nerve is said to be "tonotopically" organized in that each nerve fiber carries information to the brainstem and brain about a narrow range of frequencies. In addition, the temporal pattern of neural responses of the auditory nerve fibers responds to the temporal pattern of oscillations of the incoming sound as long as the temporal variations are less than about 5000 Hz.

In general, the more intense the sound is, the greater the number of neural discharges that are being sent by the auditory nerve to the brainstem and brain. Thus, the cochlea sends neural information to the brainstem and brain via the auditory nerve about the three physical properties of sound: frequency, temporal variation, and level. The biomechanical response of the cochlea is very sensitive to sound, is highly frequency selective, and behaves in a nonlinear manner. A great deal of this sensitivity, frequency selectivity, and nonlinearity is a function of the motility of the outer hair cells.

There are two major consequences of the nonlinear function of the cochlea: (1) neural output is a compressive function of sound level. This means that, at low sound levels, there is a one-to-one relationship between increases in sound level and increases in neural output; however, at higher sound levels, the rate at which the neural output increases with increases in sound level is lower. (2) The cochlea and auditory nerve produce distortion products. For instance, if the sound input contains two frequencies, f1 and f2, distortion products at frequencies equal to 2f1, 2f2, f2-f1, and 2f1-f2 may be produced by the nonlinear function of the cochlea. The distortion product 2f1-f2 (the cubic-difference tone) may be especially strong and this cubic-difference distortion product is used in several measures of auditory function.

At 60 dB SPL the bones of the skull begin to vibrate, bypassing the middle ear system. This direct vibration of the skull can cause the cochlea to vibrate and, thus, the hair cells to shear and to start the process of hearing. This is a very inefficient way of hearing, in that this way of exciting the auditory nervous system represents at least a 60 dB hearing loss.

There are many neural centers in the brainstem and in the brain that process the information provided by the auditory nerve. The primary centers in the auditory brainstem in order of their anatomical location from the cochlea to the cortex are: cochlear nucleus, olivary complex, lateral lemniscus, inferior colliculus, and medial geniculate. The outer, middle, and inner ears along with the auditory nerve make up the peripheral auditory system, and the brainstem and brain constitute the central auditory nervous system. Together the peripheral and central nervous systems are responsible for hearing and auditory perception.

AUDITORY PERCEPTION

In the workplace, hearing may allow a worker to:

1. Communicate using human speech (e.g., communicate with a supervisor who is giving oral instructions);
2. Process information-bearing sounds (e.g., respond to an auditory warning);

3. Locate the spatial position of a sound source (e.g., locate the position of a car based on the sound it produces).

There is a wealth of basic knowledge about how the auditory system allows for communication based on sound, informative sound processing, and sound localization. Listeners can detect the presence of a sound; discriminate changes in frequency, level, and time; recognize different speech sounds; localize the source of a sound; and identify and recognize different sound sources.

The auditory system must often accomplish these workplace tasks when there are many sources producing sound at about the same time, so that the sound from one source may interfere with the ability to "hear" the sound from another source. The interfering sound may make it difficult to detect another sound, to discriminate among different sounds, or to identify a particular sound. A hearing loss may make it difficult to perform one or all of these tasks even in the absence of interfering sounds but especially in the presence of interfering sounds.

Sound Detection

The healthy, young auditory system can detect tones in quiet with frequencies ranging from approximately 20 to 20000 Hz. Figure 2-2 displays the standardized average thresholds for detecting tonal sounds of different frequencies when the sounds are approximately 500 milliseconds (ms) in duration. The sounds to be detected can be presented over calibrated headphones (minimal audible pressure, MAP, measures) or from a loudspeaker in a calibrated free-field environment (minimal audible field, MAF, measures). The headphones can be circumaural, that is, with a headphone cushion that fits around the pinna and the earphone speaker resting against the outside of the outer ear canal, or they can be insert earphones whose earphone loudspeaker fits within the outer ear canal. The thresholds are expressed in terms of decibels of SPL, where zero (0) dB SPL means that the sound pressure level is 20 micropascals (i.e., the referent sound pressure (p_{ref}) is 20 micropascals). Upper limits of hearing, indicating the maximum SPL that the auditory system can tolerate, are also indicated in Figure 2-2. Thus, the dynamic range of hearing covers approximately 130 dB in the frequency region in which the human auditory system is most sensitive (between 500 and 4000 Hz). The thresholds for detecting a tonal sound increase as the duration of the sound to be detected decreases at durations shorter than 500 ms, but remain approximately constant as the duration increases above 500 ms.

The detection of tones as characterized by the data of Figure 2-2 is the basis for the primary measure of hearing loss or impairment, the audio-

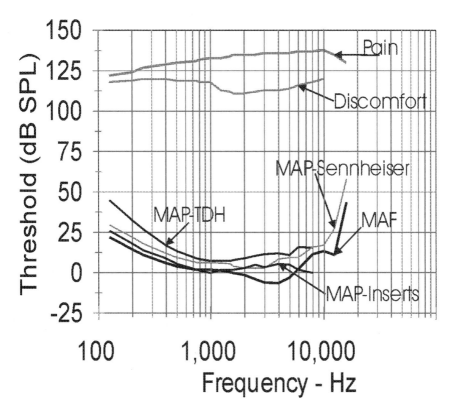

FIGURE 2-2 The thresholds (in dB SPL) of detecting tones and for discomfort and pain are shown as a function of tonal frequency. The MAP thresholds for Sennheiser and TDH are thresholds for two types of circumaural headphones.

gram. The audiogram is a plot of the thresholds of hearing referenced to the appropriate MAP or MAF thresholds shown in the figure. Thus, a person with no hearing loss at all will have a flat audiogram at zero dB HL (dB HL means decibels of hearing level, in which the reference decibel values are the appropriate MAP or MAF dB SPL values shown in Figure 2-2). A person with a 40 dB hearing loss would be said to have a threshold of 40 dB HL. If the tone being detected is 500 Hz, the threshold for detecting the tone in terms of SPL would be 50 dB SPL, since according to Figure 2-2, the threshold for detecting a 500 Hz tone is 10 dB SPL. Thus, the 40 dB hearing loss (40 dB HL) plus the 10 dB SPL threshold yields a threshold of 50 dB SPL.

In many cases, the average threshold (either in dB SPL or dB HL) for several different frequencies may be obtained to provide an estimate of overall auditory sensitivity or overall hearing loss. In this case, the threshold is referred to as a pure-tone average (PTA) threshold, in which the frequencies used for the threshold averaging are listed in abbreviated form; for example, a PTA threshold obtained at 500 Hz (.5 kHz), 1000 Hz (1 kHz), and 2000 Hz (2 kHz) would be listed as PTA 512, or sometimes PTA (512).

Many of the measurements made in hearing and the equipment used to make these measurements have been standardized by the American National Standards Institute (ANSI, see references). ANSI standards represent documents that have been reviewed by the ANSI process so that the standards represent a consensus of the best and most accurate data, method, or equipment needed to address a particular practical problem or need. Appendix B is a list of the major ANSI standards that are mentioned in this report, with descriptions of each standard. For instance, ANSI S3.6-1996 provides specifications for how audiometers, which are used by audiologists to measure the audiogram, should be built, as well as the standard thresholds of hearing used in the calculation of dB HL. A sample of an audiogram can be seen in Chapter 3.

As the intensity of a tone increases, so does its subjective loudness. Loudness is a subjective indication of the magnitude of sound. One measure of loudness level is the phon. A phon is the subjective loudness of a test sound that is judged equally loud to a standard sound. The standard sound is a 1000 Hz tonal sound presented at some SPL.

For instance, if a test sound is judged to be equally loud to the 1000 Hz standard sound presented at 40 dB SPL, the test sound is said to have a loudness of 40 phons. A sound that has a loudness of 40 phons is usually judged to be very quiet. A standardized method for determining the loudness of complex sounds in phons has also been developed (American National Standards Institute, 2003). The perceived loudness of sound will double for about every 10 dB increase in sound level (e.g., a 60 dB SPL sound may be subjectively twice as loud as a 50 dB SPL sound). People with a hearing loss experience discomfort at about the same SPL as people without hearing loss. Because people with hearing loss have elevated thresholds but have the same upper limit of audibility as people with normal hearing, the change in loudness grows more rapidly as a function of increasing sound level above threshold for a person with a hearing loss than for a person without a hearing loss. This rapid growth of loudness is referred to as loudness recruitment, and it is experienced by almost all people with sensorineural hearing loss.

As the frequency of a sound changes, so does its subjective pitch. Pitch is the subjective attribute of sound that allows one to determine if the sound is high or low along a single perceptual dimension. The pitch of a test sound can be determined by the frequency of a tonal sound that is judged to be subjectively equal in pitch to the test sound. For instance, a test sound is said to have a pitch of 400 Hz if it is judged equal in pitch to a 400 Hz tone. In addition to being measured in hertz, pitch can also be measured using the 12-note or other musical scale.

While loudness is highly correlated with sound intensity and pitch with frequency, loudness and pitch are subjective attributes of sound that may be correlated with each of the physical attributes of sound: level, frequency, and temporal properties. So for instance, a change in sound frequency may result not only in a change in pitch, but also in a change in loudness.

The presence of another sound (masking sound) presented at the same time as a tone that is to be detected (signal tone) may increase the threshold of the signal tone above that measured in quiet. In this case, the signal tone is being *masked* by the other sound. Most masking occurs (i.e., thresholds are increased the most) when the masking sound contains the same frequency components as the signal tone. For instance, less masking occurs when a 300 Hz masker masks a 1000 Hz signal than when the masker and signal are both 1000 Hz. Thus, there is a region of frequencies near that of the signal frequency (a band of frequencies with the center of the band being the frequency of the signal) that are critical for masking the signal, and the width of the critical band increases as the frequency of the signal increases. For instance, for a 1000 Hz signal, as long as the masker contains frequencies between approximately 936 and 1069 Hz (a 133-Hz-wide critical band, with 1000 Hz in the geometric center of the band), the masker will be effective in masking the 1000 Hz signal. Maskers with frequencies higher than 1069 Hz or lower than 936 Hz will be less effective in masking the 1000 Hz signal. Thus, a white noise filtered so that the noise contains frequency components between 936 and 1069 Hz will be maximally effective in masking a 1000 Hz tonal signal. If the noise has a bandwidth that is narrower than the critical band, the signal is easier to detect, but if the bandwidth is wider than the critical band, then there is no change in signal detection performance.

For listeners with normal hearing, when the power of the noise in the critical band is equal to the power of the tonal signal, then the signal is usually at its masked threshold. Over a considerable range of frequency, level, and duration, and when the signal and masker occur at the same time, each decibel increase in the level of a masking sound requires approximately a decibel increase in signal level in order for the signal to remain just detectable in the presence of the masker. That is, the signal-to-noise (S/N) ratio required for signal detection remains relatively constant over a large range of frequency, overall level, and duration.

People with hearing loss often have wider critical bands than people with normal hearing, which means that the signal can be masked by sounds with frequencies farther from the signal frequency. The wider critical band obtained for people with hearing loss is usually found for signals whose frequency content is in the spectral region of their loss. This means that people with hearing loss often require a more intense sound to detect a signal masked by other sounds, especially when the signal contains frequencies that the person with a hearing loss has difficulty detecting in quiet.

The description of masking provided above applies to situations in which the masker and signal are presented at the same time. Masking can occur when the signal is turned off before the masker is turned on (backward masking) and when the masker is turned off before the signal is turned on (forward masking). Less masking occurs for forward and backward masking than for simultaneous masking. There is very little if any masking (i.e., the threshold for detecting a sound is the same as it was in quiet) if the masker and signal are separated by more than about 250 ms. Since people with hearing loss often have difficulty sorting out the temporal properties of sound, they can experience elevated forward and backward masked thresholds, compared with those measured for people with normal hearing.

Thus, a young otologically healthy person in the workplace can detect a signal sound over the frequency range of 20 to 20000 Hz, but the level of the signal sound required for detection depends on such variables as the frequency of the sound, the duration of the sound, and the nature of any other sound that may be present at or near the same time as the signal sound that may mask the signal sound. Masking means the detection threshold of a signal sound has been elevated by the presence of the masking sound. Loudness and pitch refer to subjective attributes of sound that are highly correlated with sound level and frequency, respectively. Sounds that are spectrally similar are more likely to mask each other than are sounds that are not spectrally similar. Signals are most difficult to detect when a masker and signal occur at the same time, but masking can occur when the signals and maskers do not temporally overlap. All of these measures of auditory perception can be adversely affected if a person has a hearing loss.

Sound Discrimination

Over a range of frequencies (approximately 500 to 4000 Hz) and levels (approximately 35 to 80 dB SPL) in which humans are most sensitive, listeners can discriminate a change of about one decibel in sound level and about a half of a percent change in tonal frequency. For instance, a 50 dB SPL sound can be just discriminated from a 51 dB SPL sound, and a 2000 Hz tone can be just discriminated from a 2010 Hz tone. A hearing loss can lead to elevated level and frequency difference thresholds, making it difficult for the person with a hearing loss to discern the small differences in level and frequency that often accompany changes in the speech waveform.

Long-duration sounds require a larger change in duration for duration discrimination than do shorter duration sounds, although the exact relationship between duration and duration discrimination depends on many factors. Listeners can discriminate a sound whose overall level fluctuates (the sound is amplitude modulated) from a sound whose overall level is steady over time, when the rate of amplitude fluctuation is less than about 50 cycles per second. A sound that is amplitude modulated consists of a carrier sound that has its level varied by a different function, called the modulator. Thus, the level of the carrier sound increases and decreases over time in a manner determined by the modulator.

All of these measures of sound discrimination do not change appreciably as a function of the presence of masking sounds as long as the signal sound is readily detectable. Many people with hearing loss, especially the elderly, have difficulty processing the temporal structure of sounds. These people usually have high temporal difference thresholds, and they require slow rates of amplitude fluctuation to discriminate a fluctuating sound from a steady sound. Thus, people with such losses may not be able to follow some of the rapid fluctuations in sound intensity that are present in many everyday sounds, such as speech and music.

Thus, in the workplace, very small changes in sound level, frequency, and duration can be discriminated even when some masking sounds also exist. As long as the level of a sound does not vary too rapidly, listeners in the workplace should be able to determine that the sound is fluctuating in level (in loudness). People with a hearing loss often perform less well in these auditory discrimination tasks than people with normal hearing.

Sound Identification

Almost all of the research on sound identification has involved speech sounds. The recognition or intelligibility of speech sounds has been studied for a wide range of conditions. These conditions include both alterations of the speech sounds (e.g., whether there is a masking sound present) and aspects of the requirements of the listening task (e.g., the extent to which memory is required). In many speech recognition tasks, listeners are asked to identify phonemes (e.g., vowels), words, nonsense words, or sentences. The recognition task can be open set, in which the listeners are not aware of the set of speech utterances that will be presented, or closed set, in which the speech utterances are known (i.e., come from a list of words or sentences that the listener is aware of). Masking sounds are usually white noise, speech spectrum noise, or other speech sounds.

Speech recognition or identification is usually measured in one of two ways: the percentage of utterances correctly identified or the level of some stimulus parameter (e.g., the level of a masking noise) yielding a particular percentage-correct speech identification value (e.g., 50 percent correct identification). The speech recognition threshold (SRT) is the level of the speech signal expressed in dB required for a criterion level of performance (e.g., 50 percent correct identification). The term "signal-to-noise ratio" (S/N ratio) is used for the ratio of the speech signal level to masker level (S/N ratio is usually expressed in decibels, and as such S/N ratio is the decibel difference between the level of the speech signal and the masker), when noise is used to mask the ability of listeners to recognize speech and when the levels of the speech and masker are expressed in decibels. In some tasks, another sound (e.g., a brief acoustic click) may be embedded in the speech sound and the detection of the click is used as a measure of how salient different parts of the utterance may be (e.g., if the click is not readily detected, then it may be inferred that the information temporally surrounding the click was crucial for speech processing).

Intelligibility of speech processed in quiet by listeners with normal hearing is somewhat resistant to many forms of physical alterations. Speech can be filtered (allowing only selected frequencies to be presented), speeded up or slowed down, clipped in amplitude, etc., and still be intelligible in a quiet listening environment. However, speech is susceptible to masking or interference from other competing sounds, especially other speech sounds. Several different methods have been proposed to determine the intelligibility of speech in the presence of competing sounds. The articulation index (AI, now called speech intelligibility index, SII), which was devised at Bell Laboratories for developing the telephone system in the 1930s and 1940s, is one method that is currently used (see American National Standards Institute, 2002) to estimate speech intelligibility for situations in which the physical properties (e.g., the spectrum) of the speech and interfering sounds are known. One rule of thumb for listeners with normal hearing is that for a broadband masking stimulus such as a white noise, approximately 50 percent intelligibility occurs when only the speech and noise information is provided and the overall levels of the speech words or syllables and noise are about equal (i.e., when the S/N ratio is zero dB). However, many conditions can alter the relationship between S/N ratio and performance. Listeners with hearing loss often have much more difficulty in recognizing speech that is altered, and their S/N ratio is usually greater than zero dB.

Many different speech tasks and speech utterance lists have been developed to assess the ability of listeners, especially those with hearing losses, to process speech. These tests allow one to determine more precisely how different components of speech (e.g., vowels versus consonants) are processed or the extent to which familiarity with words influences speech intelligibility. There are many variables that might make it easy or hard to recognize a speech utterance. Speech tests are usually designed to determine if only one or maybe a small number of variables affect the ability of the subject or patient to recognize speech. For instance, many speech tests are intended to determine how much difficulty a person with a high-frequency hearing loss might have in recognizing speech. If the speech test consists of words that the patient is not familiar with, then poor performance on the test might indicate a difficulty with vocabulary rather than a hearing loss. Using test words in a language in which the patient is not fluent could also confound the assessment of hearing loss. Thus, many different speech recognition tests have been developed for the purpose of assessing hearing loss, to help ensure that the results are valid indicators of the relationship between speech recognition and hearing loss. Additional description of several speech intelligibility tests is provided in Chapters 3 and 7.

Processing speech in the workplace can be compromised when competing sounds are present. Sound reproduction systems do not have to be high fidelity to provide for acceptable speech intelligibility in the absence of competing sounds for people with normal hearing, but for people with hearing loss, such high fidelity may be essential for speech communication. However, the higher the fidelity of the reproduction system, the better speech recognition is likely to be when interfering sound sources are present. Hearing loss can lead to a significant loss of speech recognition even with high-quality amplification systems.

Sound Localization

Sound itself has no spatial dimensions, but the source of a sound can be located in three spatial dimensions as a function of the auditory system's ability to process the sound emanating from a sound source. These dimensions are azimuth—the direction from the listener in the horizontal plane (see Figure 2-3); elevation—the vertical or up-down dimension; and range—distance or the near-far dimension. A different set of cues is used by the auditory system to locate sound sources in each spatial dimension. Sounds from sources located off-center in the azimuth direction arrive at one ear before they arrive at the other ear, and the sound at the near ear is more intense than the sound at the far ear. Thus, interaural differences of time and level are the two cues used for azimuthal (directional) sound localization; interaural time is the major cue for locating low-frequency (below 1500 Hz) sound sources, and interaural

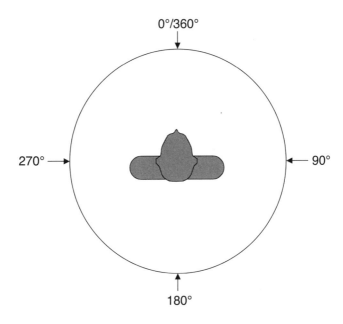

FIGURE 2-3 Azimuth: Overhead view of the listener.

level is the main cue at high frequencies. The interaural level difference results from the fact that the head and body provide an acoustic "shadow" for the ear farther away from the sound source. This "head shadow" produces large interaural level differences when the sound is opposite one ear and is high frequency. Human listeners can discriminate a change in sound source location of about 1-3° angle.

As sound travels from its source to the outer ears of a listener, it passes over and around (is diffracted by) many parts of the body, especially the pinna. These body parts attenuate and slow down the sound wave in a manner that is specific to the frequency of the sound and to the relationship between the location of the sound source and the body, especially the relative vertical location of the source. The head-related transfer function (HRTF) describes the spectral changes that a sound undergoes between the sound source and the outer ear canal. High-frequency sounds are attenuated in a frequency-specific manner that is dependent on the vertical location of the sound source relative to the body. That is, different HRTFs are produced for different vertical sound source locations. In particular, there are spectral regions of low amplitude (spectral notches or valleys) whose spectral loci are vertical-location-specific. Thus, these spectral notches in the HRTF can be a cue for vertical location. The spectral cues associated with the HRTF are probably also used to help discriminate sounds that come from in front of a listener from those that come from behind. For instance, a sound coming from directly in front of a listener will provide the same interaural time and level differences as a sound coming from directly behind. Spectral cues derived from the HRTF can assist in reducing front-back localization errors.

Faraway sounds are usually softer than near sounds, and this loudness cue can be used to determine the distance of a sound source, assuming the listener has some knowledge about the nature of the source (i.e., some knowledge about how intense the sound is at the source). If there is any reflective surface (e.g., the ground), then the reflection from a near sound source is almost as intense as the sound that arrives at the ears directly from the source, whereas for a faraway sound the reflected to direct sound level ratio is lower. Thus, the ratio of reflected to direct sound level can be a cue for sound source distance perception, and distance perception is poorer in conditions in which there are no reflections.

Locating sound sources can be more difficult for people with hearing loss. This is especially true for listeners with unilateral hearing loss. If a single hearing aid or cochlear prosthesis is used, it may provide only limited assistance for sound localization, since binaural processing is required to locate sounds in the horizontal plane. However, fitting each ear with a hearing aid or cochlear prosthesis does not always assist the patient in sound localization. In most cases, the two aids or prostheses do not preserve all of the acoustic information required by the auditory system to localize a sound source.

In reverberant spaces, such as a room, the sound waveform reflects off the many surfaces, resulting in a complex pattern of sound arriving at the ears of a listener. Listeners are usually not confused about the nature of the actual sound source, including its location, in many reverberant spaces, presumably because the auditory system processes the first sound arriving at the ears and inhibits the information from later-arriving reflected sounds. Since the sound from the source will arrive at the listener before that from any longer-path reflection, auditory processing of the direct sound takes precedence over that of the reflected sound, usually allowing for accurate sound processing even in fairly reverberant environments. Another aspect of sound reflections is that the sound in a reflective space remains in the space after the sound production ends, due to the sound continuing to reflect off the many surfaces. The reverberation time is the time (measured in seconds) that it takes the level of this reverberant or reflected sound to decay by a specified number of decibels, which is usually 60 dB. Rooms that are large and reflective have long reverberation times. People with hearing losses often perform very poorly in reverberant spaces, and the poor performance may persist even when they use a hearing aid or cochlear prosthesis. That is, people with hearing loss have difficulty recognizing speech signals when the reverberation time is long, especially if the acoustic environment is also noisy.

The detection of a signal sound source at one spatial location in the presence of a masking sound source at another spatial location is improved when the signal and masking sound sources are further apart. That is, the ability to detect a masked signal can be enhanced if the masking sound source is spatially separated from the signal sound source. The improvement in detection threshold as a function of spatial separation is referred to as the spatial masking-level difference. Thus, a variable that could affect speech recognition is the spatial separation of the test signal and other sound sources in the listening environment. Patients fitted with two hearing aids can sometimes take advantage of detecting sounds based on their spatial separation, whereas this becomes more difficult if the patient only uses one hearing aid.

Listening systems that make full use of the spectral information contained in HRTFs of individual listeners can produce sound over headphones that provides a percept as if the sound was emanating from an actual sound source located at some point in space (e.g., in a room). Systems that use HRTF technology can produce a virtual auditory environment for headphone-delivered sounds. Such HRTF-based systems can be used for testing and experimentation, eliminating the need to have specialized calibrated rooms for presenting sounds from different locations.

Thus, in the workplace, listeners can determine the location of sound sources located in all three spatial dimensions. The ability to detect a signal source can be improved if potential masking sound sources are spatially separated from the signal sound source. Having a hearing loss can compromise a person's ability to locate sounds, and hearing aids may not assist him or her in locating sound sources.

Sound Source Determination

Colin Cherry (1953) pointed out that even at a noisy cocktail party, the human listener is remarkably good at determining many of the sources of sounds (different people speaking or singing, clanging glasses, music from a stereo loudspeaker, a slammed door, etc.), even when most of the sounds from these sources are occurring at approximately the same time. Bregman (1990) referred to this cocktail party effect as "auditory scene analysis." Since the sounds from many simultaneously presented sound sources arrive at the ears of a listener as a single sound field, it is the auditory system that must determine the various sound sources—that is, determine the auditory scene. Little is known about how the auditory system accomplishes the task of auditory scene analysis, but several potential cues and neural processing strategies have been suggested as ways in which the sources of many sounds can be processed and segregated in a complex, multisource acoustic environment. People with hearing loss often remark that they have problems in noisy situations, such as at a cocktail party, implying that they are not able to determine the auditory scene as well as people without hearing loss.

Thus, listeners with normal hearing can use many potential cues to determine many of the sources of sounds in the workplace, even when the sounds from the sources overlap in time and perhaps in space.

CAUSES OF HEARING LOSS

In general, hearing loss can be caused by heredity (genetics), aging (presbycusis), loud sound exposure, diseases and infections, trauma (accidents), or ototoxic drugs (drugs and chemicals that are poisonous to auditory structures). Hearing loss can categorized into the following ranges based on PTAs (PTA 512):

- slight (16-25 dB hearing loss)
- mild (26-40 dB hearing loss)
- moderate (41-55 dB hearing loss)
- moderately severe (56-70 dB hearing loss)
- severe (71-90 dB hearing loss)
- profound (greater than 90 dB hearing loss)

The loss can be caused by damage to any part of the auditory pathway. Three major types of hearing loss have been defined: conductive, sensorineural, and mixed. Conductive hearing loss refers to damage to the conductive system of the ear—that is, the ear canal, tympanic membrane (eardrum), and ossicles (middle ear bones)—and can include fluid filling the middle ear space. Sensorineural hearing loss indicates a problem in the inner ear, auditory nerve, or higher auditory centers in the brainstem and temporal lobe. Mixed hearing loss designates that the hearing loss has both a conductive and sensorineural component. Treatments for hearing loss involve surgery, hearing aids of various types, cochlear prostheses, medication, and various forms of habilitation and rehabilitation.

Conductive Hearing Loss

If a problem arises in the external or middle ear, a conductive hearing loss occurs that is largely due to the outer and middle ear's no longer being able to overcome the loss in sound transmission from the outer to the inner ear. Many conductive hearing losses, due to such causes as a perforation in the tympanic membrane, loss of ossicular continuity, or increased stiffness of the ossicular chain, can be repaired surgically, restoring the conductive hearing loss. During an acute ear infection, fluid can accumulate in the middle ear, resulting in a temporary conductive hearing loss. If the ear develops chronic otorrhea (drainage of purulent fluid), an infected skin cyst (cholesteatoma) may be the cause. A conductive hearing loss without ear pain is the usual course of this disease, but medical attention must be sought to prevent extensive damage to the ossicles and inner ear. Such conductive losses can produce up to a 60 dB hearing loss.

Sensorineural Hearing Loss

Sensorineural hearing loss is caused by problems associated with the neural transduction of sound. Diseases and disorders that damage the cochlea and auditory nerve result in a sensorineural hearing loss. In the past, sensorineural hearing loss was referred to as "nerve deafness"; however, in most instances of sensorineural hearing loss, the auditory nerve is intact and an impairment in the hair cells within the inner ear results in the hearing loss. Loss of hair cells and the neurotrophic factors that they produce eventually lead to nerve cell loss. Because the hair cells and auditory nerve complex relay information in a frequency-specific manner to the brainstem and brain, loss of hair cells in a particular part of the cochlea will cause hearing loss in a particular frequency region. Hair cell damage at the base of the cochlea near the stapes causes high-frequency hearing loss, while hair cell loss away from the base (near the apex) leads to low-frequency hearing loss. Sensorineural hearing losses due to cochlear damage can occur at any frequency and can range from mild to profound.

Presbycusis and noise exposure are the most common causes of adult hearing loss. Both result in an initial high-frequency sensorineural deficit, caused by damage to hair cells at the base of the cochlea. In presbycusis, other cells in the inner ear are also affected in many cases; these include the nerve cells that innervate the hair cells and cells in the structure known as the stria vascularis. In individuals with these conditions, other parts of the inner ear still function, allowing for the normal perception of low-frequency sounds. The primary difficulty for such a person lies in an inability to distinguish high-frequency sounds, such as the consonants of speech that are crucial for human communication. As the conditions progress, middle- and low-frequency hearing can also deteriorate. Traditional acoustic amplification (hearing aids) is often ineffective at making speech sounds understandable to individuals with high-frequency hearing loss when the loss becomes severe (Ching, Dillon, and Byrne, 1998; Hogan and Turner, 1998). In individuals who have profound sensorineural hearing loss across the frequency range, hearing aids may not be as effective in improving hearing as a cochlear implant. Infections (viral or bacterial), disorders such as Meniere's disease and autoimmune inner ear disease, hereditary disorders, trauma, and ototoxic drugs are other causes of sensorineural hearing loss.

Acoustic trauma can be a significant problem in the workplace. If the level of sound is intense, especially if the sound lasts for a long time, listeners exposed to such intense sounds may experience either a temporary or a permanent threshold shift—that is, their threshold for detecting sound is either temporarily or permanently elevated above that measured in quiet and before the exposure. A temporary threshold shift (TTS) can recover to normal detection threshold after a few minutes to a few days, depending on the parameters of the exposing sound and their relationship to those of the sound to be detected. Permanent threshold shifts (PTS) never recover and therefore indicate a permanent hearing loss that can range from mild to severe.

There is a trade-off between sound level and duration in terms of producing TTS and PTS. The greater the level or the longer the duration of the exposing sound, the greater the threshold shift and the longer it takes to recover from TTS. Most TTS occurs at frequencies the same or slightly higher than the frequency of the exposing sound. The Occupational Safety and Health Administration (OSHA) and the National Institute of Occupational Safety and Health provide regulations and guidance (e.g., Occupational Safety and Health Administration, 2002) for occupational noise exposure to mitigate its effects in the workplace.

Etiology of Severe to Profound Hearing Loss

It is estimated that 1 person in 1,000 has a severe to profound hearing loss. The number with bilateral (both ears) profound deafness is lower. Loss of hearing has a significant impact on the development of speech and spoken language skills, which are dependent on the age of onset of deafness. Children born with bilateral profound hearing loss or who acquire profound loss before the acquisition of speech and spoken language (approximately age 2 years) are identified as prelingually deafened. Children and adults deafened at any age after developing speech and spoken language are referred to as postlingually deafened.

Children

High-risk factors for congenital hearing loss include a family history of congenital hearing loss or delayed-onset sensory hearing loss of childhood, physical findings (birthweight less than 1,500 grams, craniofacial anomalies, the variable physical signs of Waardenburg's syndrome), and maternal prenatal infections (cytomegalovirus, syphilis, rubella, herpes).

Prelingual deafness can also arise from severe vital function depression at birth when Apgar scores are in the 0 to 3 range at five minutes. Hyperbilirubinemia severe enough to require exchange transfusion; treatment of postnatal infection with ototoxic drugs, such as gentamicin, tobramycin, kanamycin, and streptomycin; systemic infections including meningitis, congenital syphilis, mumps, and measles all can result in bilateral profound deafness. Closed head trauma and neurodegenerative diseases including Tay-Sachs disease, neurofibromatosis, Gaucher's disease, Niemann-Pick disease, and myoclonic epilepsy are rare additional etiologies of deafness that manifest themselves in childhood.

Genetic causes for prelingual and postlingual deafness are thought to account for 50 percent of the sensorineural hearing loss in childhood. The remainder are either environmental (about 25 percent) or sporadic idiopathic (about 25 percent). Genetic hearing loss can be congenital or delayed, progressive or stable, unilateral or bilateral, syndromic or nonsyndromic. The majority of genetic hearing losses are thought to be recessive (about 75 percent); 20 percent are attributable to dominant genes and a small percentage are X-linked disorders. Autosomal dominant disorders include Waardenburg's syndrome (20 percent associated with hearing loss); Stickler's syndrome (sensorineural or mixed hearing loss, 15 percent); branchiootorenal syndrome; Treacher Collins syndrome (sensorineural or mixed hearing loss); neurofibromatosis II; and dominant progressive hearing loss. Autosomal recessive disorders associated with sensorineural hearing loss are Pendred's syndrome, Usher syndrome, and Jervell and Lange-Nielsen syndrome. Sex-linked syndromes associated with sensorineural hearing loss are Norie's syndrome, otopalatodigital syndrome, Wildervaank's syndrome, and Alport's syndrome. Most hereditary hearing loss in early childhood is "nonsyndromic," that is, there are no other apparent abnormalities. While mutations in any of dozens of genes can cause hearing loss, a gene that controls the production of a protein called connexin 26 is responsible for a large proportion of such cases, with studies on various populations reporting differing prevalences (Dahl et al., 2001; Erbe, Harris, Runge-Samuelson, Flanary, and Wackym, 2004; Gurtler et al., 2003; Nance, 2003).

Recently a condition termed "auditory neuropathy" (Starr, Picton, Sininger, Hood, and Berlin, 1996) has been identified in individuals with severe to profound hearing loss. Patients with this condition typically show severely distorted or absent auditory brainstem response (explained in Chapter 3) with recordings showing prominent cochlear microphonic (CM) components, and normal otoacoustic emissions. The otoacoustic emissions and CM findings in patients with auditory neuropathy usually indicate that the cochlear hair cells, at least the outer hair cells, are functioning normally while the abnormal auditory brainstem response is indicative of disease in the inner hair cells, auditory nerve, or brainstem. Some theorize that the disorder is a specific neuropathy of the auditory nerve; thus the name of the disorder (Starr et al., 1996; Starr, Picton, and Kim, 2001). Starr et al. (2001) have found indirect evidence of peripheral nerve involvement based on sural nerve biopsy or nerve conduction velocity measures. More recently, they have documented specific neuropathy of the auditory nerve in a patient with well-documented clinical signs of auditory neuropathy on audiological tests (Starr et al., 2003). Such histological findings (fair to good hair cell populations along with poor ganglion cell and nerve fiber survival) have been reported previously (Hallpike, Harriman, and Wells, 1980; Merchant et al., 2001; Spoendlin, 1974; see Nadol, 2001, for a review of these pathologies in humans). However, others suggest that there is a "general lack of anatomic foundation for the label" (Rapin and Gravel, 2003, p. 707) because of difficulty in documenting specific peripheral neuropathy in patients, especially at the level of the auditory nerve.

When auditory neuropathy exists, neither the auditory brainstem response nor the otoacoustic emissions can be used to determine the degree of hearing loss. The degree of hearing loss in patients with this condition can be anywhere from none to profound (Sininger and Oba, 2001). The hearing loss of patients with auditory neuropathy can fluctuate dramatically and rapidly, sometimes within a single day (Sininger and Oba, 2001). In rare cases, increases in core temperature from fever can bring on severe to profound hearing loss that will return to prefever levels as the condition resolves (Starr et al., 1998). Recent publications report that cochlear implants have been effective in individuals displaying signs of auditory neuropathy (Peterson et al., 2003; Shallop, Peterson, Facer, Fabry, and Driscoll, 2001). This finding could be due to electrical synchronization of the neural response, or it may suggest that the etiology of profound deafness could be located in the inner hair cells.

An excellent review of sensorineural hearing loss in children can be found in a chapter by Brookhouser (1993).

Adults

Although many diseases and disorders can induce hearing loss, relatively few result in profound sensorineural deafness. Infections, immune-mediated disorders, trauma, idiopathic and hereditary disorders, and oto-toxic agents are the most common etiologies of bilateral profound hearing loss in adults.

The most common infections associated with profound hearing loss are bacterial and viral meningitis. Neural syphilis can produce progressive bilateral fluctuating hearing loss and spells of vertigo. If not treated with long-term antibiotics and steroids, profound hearing loss can occur. Even with treatment, some individuals continue to lose hearing.

Idiopathic disorders of cochlear otosclerosis and Meniere's disease can produce profound bilateral hearing loss infrequently. Immune-mediated bilateral sensorineural hearing loss has recently been recognized as a cause of profound deafness. A history of rapid progressive hearing loss in both ears over weeks to months is the hallmark of this disease (McCabe, 1979). Fluctuation of hearing and spells of vertigo may occur. Other autoimmune disorders, such as Cogan's syndrome, Wegener's granulomatosis, and systemic lupus, also can result in profound hearing loss.

Aminoglycoside antibiotics have long been associated with ototoxic-ity. These drugs concentrate in perilymph and have a longer half-life in this fluid than in blood. In renal failure their levels are elevated. Aminoglycosides are directly toxic to outer hair cells, but they can also affect ganglion cells. Ototoxicity has been observed within the "safe" limits of nephrotoxicity. The effects can be observed even after discontinuing the drug. The agents associated with the highest degree of toxicity of the inner ear include kanamycin, tobramycin, amikacin, neomycin, and dihydrostreptimycin. (Some families may have a genetic disposition to developing deafness with these drugs.) The only treatment is to discontinue the drug. Antimetabolites such as Cisplatin and nitrogen mustard are also ototoxic. The risk to hearing is related to the amount of a given dose rather than cumulative amount.

TINNITUS AND HYPERACUSIS

Ear disorders cause many different symptoms, including hearing loss, tinnitus, pain, otorrhea (ear drainage), facial nerve paralysis, vertigo, and disequilibrium. Most of these symptoms are only tangentially relevant to the work of the committee, which is limited to the effects of hearing loss. In contrast, tinnitus and a related symptom, hyperacusis, may be considered by some to be "hearing impairments," although neither tinnitus nor hyperacusis is mentioned in the current SSA regulations covering hearing impairment. We therefore offer a brief discussion in this section, concluding that most people with tinnitus or hyperacusis are not disabled (as that term is defined by SSA) and that the tests audiologists and otolaryngologists use to detect and measure abnormal function of the ear cannot separate people with tinnitus or hyperacusis who are disabled from those who are not disabled. For these reasons, these symptoms are not discussed in detail in later chapters, and we make no recommendations for procedures SSA might use in evaluating claims for disability based on tinnitus or hyperacusis. More extensive discussions are available in books edited by Tyler (2000) and Snow (2004), and in an earlier NRC report (National Research Council, 1982).

Tinnitus

Tinnitus is a sensation that often is associated with suffering, which may occasionally be severe enough to preclude work. Sensation and suffering are separate aspects of tinnitus and should not be confused.

Tinnitus sensation is the perception of sound when there is no external acoustic stimulus, and it can be either objective or subjective. Objective tinnitus occurs in rare cases when there is an internal acoustic stimulus. For example, turbulent blood flow in an artery close to the ear can make a pulsing sound that is audible not only to the person whose ear is affected, but also to a physician applying a stethoscope to the patient's head. Subjective tinnitus almost always occurs when there is no acoustic stimulus at all, and only one person can hear the sound. People with subjective tinnitus typically describe their sensations as ringing, buzzing, humming, whistling, or hissing sounds. Most people with tinnitus also have hearing loss that is measurable by audiometry; however, many people with hearing loss do not have tinnitus, and no objective audiological or medical test has been shown to predict whether a person with hearing loss will have subjective tinnitus. In other words, the ears of people with hearing loss and subjective tinnitus are not different, as far as we know, from the ears of people with hearing loss alone.

When asked to match their tinnitus sensations to tones presented from an audiometer, most people select tones that are close to the frequencies they have difficulty hearing. The intensity of an external tone matched in loudness to a person's tinnitus is usually less than 10 dB above that person's threshold for the tone. Although there is no objective test that can demonstrate whether a person has tinnitus or not, tinnitus matching results that are repeatable and consistent with the patterns described above can sometimes offer evidence that corroborates a person's claim to have tinnitus. However, tinnitus matching tests are not well standardized or widely used. Most importantly, they can at best describe tinnitus sensation and say nothing about tinnitus suffering.

The distribution of tinnitus suffering can be described as a pyramid. At its broad base are the majority of people with tinnitus, who find that it does not interfere significantly with their daily lives and never seek medical attention. The next level includes those who visit a physician, but only to find out whether their tinnitus is a sign of some serious medical problem. A smaller group of people with tinnitus complain of substantial difficulty with activities of daily life, especially sleep disturbance, trouble concentrating, emotional problems (anxiety, depression, etc.), and trouble understanding speech (Tyler and Baker, 1983). Since most people with tinnitus also have audiometrically measurable hearing loss, it is difficult to know whether tinnitus per se interferes with speech understanding. As stated by Stouffer and Tyler (1990), "it seems likely that patients confuse the effects of tinnitus on speech understanding with the effects of hearing loss on speech understanding." At the narrow top of the pyramid are a very few persons who are severely disabled; cases of suicide have been reported, but almost exclusively in people who have many other risk factors for suicide, such as male sex, advanced age, social isolation, and especially depression (Lewis, Stephens, and McKenna, 1994).

Tinnitus sensation (as measured in the audiology booth using matching tests) and tinnitus suffering (as assessed by self-report) are uncorrelated (Baskill and Coles, 1999). Tinnitus sufferers differ from nonsufferers not in the pitch or loudness of the sounds they hear, but in the nature of their reaction, coping, and adjustment to tinnitus sensations. Patients who go to specialized tinnitus treatment clinics are very frequently found to meet formal psychiatric criteria for diagnosis of major depressive disorder, and about half of these have a history of major depression or anxiety disorder prior to the onset of tinnitus (Sullivan et al., 1988; Zoger, Svedlund, and Holgers, 2002).

Audiologists and otolaryngologists can provide useful information regarding the existence, perceptual qualities, and causation of tinnitus, but a person's claim to be disabled by tinnitus might best be supported by psychiatric or psychological evidence, as well as by corroborative reports of employers, coworkers, family, and others; audiologists and otolaryngologists cannot provide objective evidence to support or refute such a claim. We note in passing that the American Medical Association's *Guides to the Evaluation of Permanent Impairment* (American Medical Association, 2001) permit physicians to add up to 5 percent to a person's "binaural hearing impairment" score if that person has tinnitus that interferes with activities of daily living. This could increase a person's "whole person impairment" by no more than 2 percent, unless that person also had impairments in other domains (such as the "mental and behavioral" domain).

Most people with tinnitus do not choose to be treated, in large part because no treatment has been demonstrated to permanently eliminate tinnitus sensation (Dobie, 1999). Masking therapy (the covering up of tinnitus with external sound) can temporarily reduce or eliminate tinnitus sensation while the masking noise is present. Tinnitus suffering is frequently addressed through psychological counseling and antidepressant or antianxiety drugs (Snow, 2004).

Hyperacusis

The word "hyperacusis" has sometimes been used to refer to "an exceptionally acute sense of hearing" (Dorland, 1974), but it is doubtful that there are actually people who hear so well that their thresholds are distinctly separate from, and better than, the normal distribution of hearing thresholds in young healthy adults. More commonly, clinicians use the term to refer to a relatively rare condition of abnormal intolerance of even moderately loud sounds, such as conversation, traffic, and music (the terms "hyperacusis" and "phonophobia" are often used interchangeably), usually accompanied by avoidance behavior (e.g., wearing earplugs at all times, staying at home, severing social relationships). People who complain of intolerance to everyday sounds usually have bothersome tinnitus as well, but they represent less than 1 percent of tinnitus patients at one national center (Vernon and Meikle, 2000). There is no widely used criterion for the diagnosis of hyperacusis, although some clinicians have used "loudness discomfort levels" (LDLs) for this purpose. People with normal hearing, and most people with hearing loss, report that they can tolerate tones up to 90-105 dB HL in the audiometry booth, while most patients who complain of severe sound intolerance have LDLs below 85 dB HL (Hazell, Sheldrake, and Graham, 2002). Most of these patients have required treatment for psychological problems prior to the onset of hyperacusis (Hazell and Sheldrake, 1991). Treatment of hyperacusis has usually consisted of desensitization to gradually increasing sound levels or treatment of underlying psychiatric disorders.

No objective audiological or medical test can distinguish people who complain of hyperacusis from other people. It is far from clear that hyperacusis should even be considered an ear disorder. As in the case of tinnitus, the best evidence supporting or refuting claims of disability based on hyperacusis is likely to come from psychiatrists and psychologists and from lay persons who can corroborate the claimed disability.

SUMMARY

Adults and children depend on hearing for their ability to function in work, school, and other daily activities, to be able to communicate using speech, and to better process information about objects in their environments. Using hearing to function in the world means detecting, discriminating, localizing, and identifying sound produced by the many sound sources that constantly surround one. There are many causes of damage to the auditory system that result in a hearing loss that reduces one's ability to detect, discriminate, localize, or identify sound. These losses can adversely effect an adult's ability to work and a child's ability to process sound.

3

Assessment of the Auditory System and Its Functions

In this chapter we discuss the methods used to assess the functioning of the adult claimant's auditory system and hearing functions. We begin with an overview of the otolaryngological examination (for adults and children), describing the features of a "standard" examination based on best professional practices, and make some recommendations on how and when the examination should be performed. We then describe audiological tests and review current knowledge of audiological testing for adults, with special reference to the tests that are now prescribed by the Social Security Administration (SSA) for use in determining disability due to auditory impairment and to other tests that might be suitable for this purpose (testing of children is discussed in Chapter 7). Our conclusions and recommendations for Social Security disability determination are presented in Chapter 4.

STANDARD OTOLARYNGOLOGICAL EXAMINATION

SSA regulations as presented in the Blue Book (Social Security Administration, 2003) require, as part of the disability determination process, "medical evidence about the nature and severity of an individual's impairments(s)" from either a claimant's own physician or a consultative examiner (CE). Medical reports from either the treating physician or the CE should include (Social Security Administration, 2003, p. 11):

- Medical history;

- Clinical findings (such as the results of physical or mental status examinations);
  - Laboratory findings (such as blood pressure, x-rays);
  - Diagnosis;
  - Treatment prescribed with response and prognosis;
  - A statement providing an opinion about what the claimant can still do despite his or her impairment(s), based on the medical source's findings on the above factors. This statement should describe, but is not limited to, the individual's ability to perform work-related activities such as . . . hearing. . . . For a child, the statement should describe his or her functional limitations in learning, . . . communicating.

SSA regulations also require that hearing tests "should be preceded by an otolaryngologic examination." In contrast, the committee recommends that the otolaryngological examination should follow the audiological examination (but by no more than 6 months), because a physician cannot provide a competent report, including the six elements listed above, without recent audiometric data. The appropriate source for the otolaryngological examination is an otolaryngologist certified by the American Board of Otolaryngology. Otolaryngologists specialize in disorders of the ear, nose, throat, and related structures of the head and neck and have completed at least five years of residency training following receipt of the M.D. or D.O. (doctor of osteopathy) degree.

Medical History

The elements of the medical history in an examination performed to provide medical evidence for SSA program eligibility are identical to those included in a routine medical examination. There are, however, some areas of emphasis worthy of mention.

Chief Complaint and Present Illness: The claimant's chief otological complaint may not be hearing loss; it may be tinnitus, vertigo, otalgia, or otorrhea. For each significant otological symptom, but especially for hearing loss, the physician should inquire about:

- The nature of the symptom—Are hearing difficulties noticed in one ear or both? For what types of sounds?
  - Severity
  - Chronology—Onset? Change over time? Fluctuation?
  - Exacerbating and/or ameliorating factors, such as background noise
  - Effects on activities of daily living—ordinary conversation, telephone use, work.

Review of Systems: Review of organ systems will occasionally reveal problems in other systems that are relevant to otological diagnosis (e.g., eye symptoms in Cogan's syndrome). Review of systems is more likely to be helpful in cases of hearing loss with onset in childhood or in cases demonstrating rapid progression or fluctuation of hearing loss.

Past Medical History: A history of mumps or measles (or of maternal rubella or cytomegalovirus) can be relevant if hearing loss began in childhood. Head injury often causes hearing loss. Most ototoxic drugs are given in the context of hospitalization for severe infections (aminoglycosides) or cancer (cisplatin and carboplatin). A history of previous otological treatment, especially ear surgery, is always relevant.

Social History: A discussion of family and marital status includes communication difficulties with the claimant's spouse or partner, relatives, and other persons. The claimant's educational and occupational history will assist in understanding both the difficulties experienced in the workplace and the knowledge, skills, and abilities that might be useful in other jobs. Previous hazardous noise exposure may be uncovered in a discussion of both work history (including military service) and recreational activities (e.g., shooting, woodworking). If there has been significant noise exposure in the past 72 hours, audiometry should be deferred.

Family History: Hearing loss or deafness prior to age 60 or ear surgery in a close relative may suggest a hereditary disorder.

Clinical Findings (Physical Examination)

Informal Observation of Communication: The otolaryngologist can usually directly observe the claimant's ability to hear and understand in a communication environment similar to some workplaces: one-to-one conversation in a relatively quiet room. It is neither necessary nor desirable to do this separately from the process of obtaining a history and performing a physical examination. Instead, the claimant's ability to hear and understand can be assessed based on informal conversation during history taking, ear examination, etc. If the claimant has either hearing aids or a cochlear implant, these should be used during as much of the interview and examination as possible. During this process, the examiner can note whether the claimant does poorly under certain conditions (e.g., inability to see the examiner's face, increased distance from the examiner, presence of background noise, removal of hearing aids) and whether the claimant's behavior is consistent. Any obvious language or cognitive problems should be noted.

Otoscopy: Observation and palpation of the auricle, followed by pneumatic otoscopy, will usually suffice to detect outer ear and middle ear abnormalities that may contribute to diagnosis. When conductive or mixed hearing loss is present, the ears should usually be examined by otomicroscopy.

Tuning Fork Tests (optional): Audiometric tests usually provide unambiguous evidence of the type of hearing loss (conductive, sensorineural, or mixed). Nevertheless, tuning fork tests (most often, Weber and Rinne tests using the 512 Hz fork) can sometimes provide a useful cross-check on the validity of the audiometric data. This is especially true if insert earphones are not used, because collapsing ear canals can cause apparent (but spurious) conductive hearing loss, which will be absent on tuning fork testing.

Head and Neck Examination: In the presence of chronic otitis media, examination of the neck, nasal cavities, and pharynx may disclose relevant findings. In congenital hearing loss, examination of the face, neck, oral cavity, and eyes may contribute to the identification of a hereditary or acquired syndrome. With these exceptions, head and neck examination is rarely helpful.

Cranial Nerves (optional): The functions of the third through twelfth cranial nerves are usually tested as part of a complete otological examination, especially if there is asymmetrical hearing loss.

Balance and Cerebellar Tests (optional): When the claimant's complaints include vertigo, unsteadiness, or lightheadedness, the otological examination usually includes observation of the claimant's gait; standing balance will be addressed with eyes open and closed. Tests of fine motor coordination and ability to determine the spatial position of body parts without vision are often used to assess cerebellar function.

Laboratory Findings

In most cases, the only relevant "laboratory findings" are the results of the audiological examination. In some cases of asymmetrical hearing loss, imaging tests are necessary before a firm diagnosis can be made. In rare cases of rapidly progressive or fluctuating hearing loss, blood tests for infection, immunological disorders, or other systemic disorders can be helpful. Tests of vestibular function may assist diagnosis when there are symptoms of dizziness or unsteadiness. For stable or slowly progressive symmetrical hearing loss without vestibular symptoms, laboratory tests (other than audiometry) are rarely useful in diagnosis or prognosis.

Diagnosis

The nature of the hearing loss (sensorineural, conductive, or mixed) is usually apparent from the audiometric data. The cause(s) are not always certain, but the physician should state an opinion about causation to a "reasonable medical certainty." In other words, the physician should identify a cause only if it is more likely than not that it contributed to the patient's hearing loss.

Treatment Prescribed with Response and Prognosis

In many cases (especially when the hearing loss is conductive or mixed), medical or surgical treatment is advised. For most people applying for Social Security Disability Insurance or Supplemental Security Income because of hearing loss, medical treatment is no longer an issue. Hearing aids or cochlear implants may be advised. Prognosis (including expected response to recommended medical, surgical, or prosthetic intervention) is essential, because of the SSA standard of an "impairment which can be expected to last for a continuous period of at least twelve months." Hearing impairment that has not been present and stable for at least 6 months will rarely meet this standard.

What the Claimant Can Still Do

Information collected during the history-taking and physical examination is combined with audiometric data and information obtained from previous medical and audiometric records to support an opinion regarding the claimant's ability to hear and understand in a variety of communication settings.

Children

The history and physical examination described above is typical not only for adults, but also for children of school age. Some parts of the physical examination (e.g., tuning fork tests and assessment of ability to communicate) will not be feasible in very young children, who may require additional evaluations before a determination of causation and prognosis can be made. These additional evaluations may include: medical genetics, ophthalmology, pediatric neurology, and speech-language pathology.

ASSESSMENT OF AUDITORY FUNCTION

The basic audiometric test battery recommended by the committee includes assessment of pure-tone thresholds by air conduction and bone conduction, speech recognition thresholds, suprathreshold speech recognition in quiet and noise, and acoustic immittance measures. This protocol will enable the determination of the degree of hearing loss, the site of lesion in the auditory periphery, and the capacity of the individual to understand speech in typical listening environments. Many of the stimuli and procedures for conducting the routine assessment have been standardized for English-speaking adults. Modifications to this test battery are necessary for assessment of children and non-English speakers. Additional electrophysiological measures of auditory function include otoacoustic emissions (OAEs) and auditory evoked potentials (AEPs), which may be performed in place of, or in addition to, the routine audiometric measures. These tests are particularly useful for assessment of infants and young children, as well as individuals who are difficult to test. To ensure accuracy of test results, the test environment must be controlled and the test equipment must be calibrated as described in Chapter 4.

Pure-Tone Threshold Audiometry

Hearing sensitivity is measured separately in each ear for pure-tone signals, which are single-frequency tones generated electronically and transduced through an earphone or bone conduction vibrator. The "gold standard" of hearing sensitivity is the pure-tone audiogram, shown in Figure 3-1. The audiogram displays a listener's detection thresholds (in dB hearing level [ANSI S3.6-1996] (American National Standards Institute, 1996) for pure-tone signals at octave frequency intervals within the range of 250-8000 Hz, in both ears. This frequency range encompasses the spectrum of speech sounds. Consequently, an average of pure-tone detection thresholds corresponds with the average threshold for speech (Fletcher, 1950). Hearing thresholds may also be assessed at selected interoctave frequencies (e.g., 3000 and 6000 Hz), particularly in cases of suspected noise-induced hearing loss.

The standard method for measuring the pure-tone detection threshold is the modified Hughson-Westlake technique (American National Standards Institute, 1997; American Speech-Language-Hearing Association, 1978; Carhart and Jerger, 1959). This is a single-stimulus technique that combines ascending and descending methods of limits. Stimulus duration is 1-2 seconds, and the signal may be steady-state or pulsed (Mineau and Schlauch, 1997). The operational definition of threshold is the lowest level at which a listener detects a signal for 50 percent of the ascending runs. Pure-tone thresholds are assessed in the air conduction mode (250-8000 Hz) and the bone conduction mode (250-4000 Hz). The preferred earphones for air conduction threshold assessment are insert earphones to prevent ear canal collapse and ostensible high-frequency conductive hearing loss that may occur with supra-aural earphones

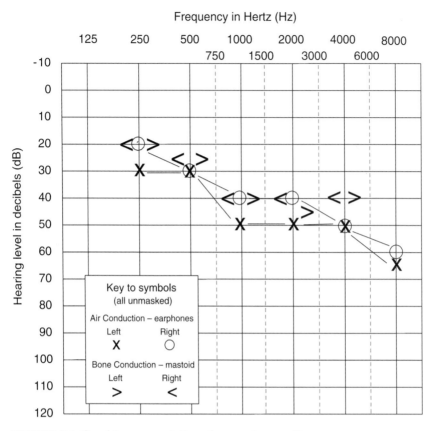

FIGURE 3-1 Graphic representation of a pure-tone audiogram.

(Clemis, Ballad, and Killion, 1986). However, supra-aural earphones are acceptable for routine clinical use.

Measurement of pure-tone detection thresholds is essential for determination of the degree of hearing loss, and it forms the basis of disability determination for SSA. A classification scheme for degree of hearing loss, shown in Table 3-1, is based on the mean air conduction pure-tone thresholds at 500, 1000, and 2000 Hz (PTA 512) (Clarke, 1981; Goodman, 1965). (PTA 512 is the pure-tone average implied in the text of this report that deals with adult hearing, unless a different frequency set is specified.) This classification scheme is appropriate if the thresholds do not vary dramatically across audiometric frequency. In the event of widely varying thresholds, the degree of hearing loss should be described separately for frequencies with minimum hearing loss and maximum hearing loss.

TABLE 3-1 Categories of Degrees of Hearing Loss, Based on Air
Conduction Pure-Tone Average at 500, 1000, and 2000 Hz

Degree of Hearing Loss Category	Pure-Tone Average Range
Normal hearing sensitivity	–10 dB HL to 15 dB HL
Slight hearing loss	16 dB HL to 25 dB HL
Mild hearing loss	26 dB HL to 40 dB HL
Moderate hearing loss	41 dB HL to 55 dB HL
Moderately severe hearing loss	56 dB HL to 70 dB HL
Severe hearing loss	71 dB HL to 90 dB HL
Profound hearing loss	91 dB HL to equipment limits

SOURCE: Clarke (1981).

In particular, hearing loss in adults is often more severe in the higher
frequencies than in the lower frequencies.

This severity scale classification scheme attempts to describe the average communicative effect of a hearing loss without the use of a hearing
aid. Individuals with normal hearing experience no significant difficulty
hearing faint speech or speech in moderate noise levels. The category
included in Table 3-1 of "slight" hearing loss has been applied tradition-
ally to children, who experience detrimental effects of this degree of
hearing loss for developing normal speech and language. Recent reports
suggest the slight hearing loss category is appropriate for adults as well,
because many adults with PTAs in this range complain of difficulty hearing
faint speech in noise and may seek amplification (Martin and Champlin,
2000).

Those with mild hearing losses experience difficulty hearing faint
speech or speech from a distance, even in quiet. Moderate hearing loss is
associated with frequent difficulty with normal speech (Bess and Humes,
2003); conversational speech may be heard only at close range. Individuals with a moderate-to-severe hearing loss may detect the presence of
conversational speech, but are often unable to understand conversational
speech without amplification, due to insufficient audibility. In addition,
most energy in speech is concentrated in the lower frequencies and then
decreases in the higher frequencies, coinciding with the frequency region
corresponding to the most hearing loss in adults. Thus, higher frequency
speech information will often be inaudible for individuals with an average hearing loss in the moderate range or even the mild range. Because
most consonant phonemes in speech are composed of weak, high-
frequency energy, individuals with such high-frequency hearing losses

may have considerable difficulty understanding speech accurately although they are able to detect the presence of speech.

In addition to the loss of audibility, hearing impairment in the mild to moderately severe range is often accompanied by distortion of the acoustic signal. The detailed spectral, temporal, and intensive characteristics of the speech signal are processed differently in the impaired auditory system from in the normal auditory system. This is thought to result in considerable difficulty understanding a spoken message, particularly in challenging listening environments that include noise and reverberation (Plomp, 1986; Plomp and Duquesnoy, 1980).

Individuals with a severe hearing loss (71-90 dB HL PTA in the better ear) who do not use a hearing aid cannot detect the presence of conversational speech and may hear only shouted speech. These individuals may derive limited benefit from a hearing aid, depending on their previous experience with amplification.

A profound hearing loss typically is associated with extremely limited capacity to receive speech in the auditory mode. Individuals with a profound hearing loss may hear very loud or amplified sounds, but they often cannot benefit from a hearing aid for understanding speech. Hearing is not the primary communication channel for people with a profound hearing loss who do not use hearing aids or cochlear implants. Because of their limited ability to receive spoken language in the auditory-only mode, people with severe or profound hearing losses are candidates for admission to schools for the deaf, where numerous accommodations and other special services are available. For example, the application information for the National Technical Institute for the Deaf specifically states that the only audiological criterion for admission is a PTA score of 70 dB HL or greater in the better ear.

Speech Audiometry

Speech audiometry encompasses a range of measures that include assessment of speech thresholds, suprathreshold speech recognition in quiet, and suprathreshold speech recognition in noise. Although suprathreshold speech recognition measures are usually obtained for an auditory-only presentation mode (unisensory), they may also be obtained for an auditory + visual presentation mode (bisensory). Stimuli may be recorded or live, but only recorded stimuli can undergo standardization procedures. Recorded speech stimuli are routed through a speech audiometer to ensure accurate signal presentation levels. Standards governing the calibration of the speech signal through the speech audiometer

(American National Standards Institute, 1996) provide the RETSPL for speech signals.[1]

Speech Thresholds

The pure-tone examination assesses an individual's detection thresholds for tones that encompass the range of speech sounds, from 250 to 8000 Hz. Validity of these pure-tone thresholds can be established by verifying that these thresholds actually reflect the ability to detect speech. To that end, a threshold level for speech is obtained to assess the validity of the pure-tone audiogram. Two types of speech thresholds may be measured: the speech detection threshold (SDT) and the speech recognition threshold (SRT). The SDT is the lowest intensity level for 50 percent detection of the speech signal. The SDT normally is obtained at a level that is 8-9 dB lower than the speech recognition threshold. The SRT is the minimum hearing level of a speech signal at which a listener correctly repeats 50 percent of the spoken message.

Usually the speech signals are spondee words,[2] but they may be sentences. The SRT obtained with spondees corresponds with the three-frequency PTA (500, 1000, 2000 Hz) in individuals with normal hearing or reasonably flat audiograms, and with a two-frequency PTA (an average of the best two thresholds obtained between 500 and 2000 Hz) in individuals with sloping or rising audiometric configurations (Carhart, 1971; Fletcher, 1950), if the speech signal is calibrated according to the RETSPLs for speech (American National Standards Institute, 1996). The SRT is also useful for predicting the audibility of conversational speech

---

[1]At present, recommended procedures for recordings of speech materials are available in an appendix to the ANSI S3.6 standard. These recommended procedures specify that recordings shall provide a 1000 Hz calibration tone or a weighted random noise at the beginning of the recording, at the same level as the speech materials on the recording. In addition, the international standard, IEC 60645, indicates that speech level should be expressed as the equivalent continuous sound pressure level determined by integration over the duration of the speech signals with frequency weighting C. This indicates that specified levels of the speech stimulus are based on average levels. Some recorded speech recognition materials do not conform to these standard recording and calibration procedures. For example, the Veterans Administration recordings of speech materials use a calibration tone that reflects the peaks of the carrier phrase for each test on the recording. Normative data obtained with each speech test are therefore appropriate as a reference only if the test is presented using identical procedures for calibration and test level. In order to present a standardized test, the tester should be well informed about the correct calibration procedures and presentation levels for particular speech materials.

[2]Spondee words are two-syllable words with equal emphasis on both syllables, for example, "milkman" and "sidewalk."

and the need for amplification (Hodgson and Skinner, 1981). Standard audiometric practice includes measurement of the SRT; the SDT is reserved for cases in which an SRT cannot be measured.

Several standard methods for measurement of SRT produce reliable threshold estimates with recorded speech materials. The method recommended by the American Speech-Language-Hearing Association (ASHA) is a descending technique in which the number of spondee words presented at each step is equivalent to the step size, for either 2-dB or 5-dB step sizes (American Speech-Language-Hearing Association, 1988; Tillman and Olsen, 1973). This technique is both reliable and valid (Beattie, Forrester, and Ruby, 1977; Wall, Davis, and Myers, 1984; Wilson, Morgan, and Dirks, 1973).

Measurement of speech recognition thresholds is useful for corroborating the validity of the pure-tone thresholds and is routinely conducted by most audiologists (Martin, Champlin, and Chambers, 1998). In addition, an estimate of the audibility of conversational speech without amplification can be made directly from the SRT. For example, a score in the better ear that approximates the level of average conversational speech (45-50 dB HL) indicates that everyday speech is minimally audible to the listener, and a score that exceeds 50 dB HL indicates that virtually all unamplified speech signals are inaudible to the listener unless the talker speaks loudly or approaches the listener more closely than the typical 1.0 meter distance of casual conversation. This information is useful for determining hearing aid needs and may be used to substantiate a claim for functional hearing impairment disability. Current SSA guidance prescribes testing of SRT (Social Security Administration, 2003, p. 24).

Suprathreshold Speech Recognition

Suprathreshold measures expressed as percentage-correct speech recognition scores indicate the clarity with which an individual receives and understands a spoken message. Although speech recognition scores are correlated with pure-tone thresholds, the correlation is typically not high enough to accurately predict one from the other for an individual, so speech recognition must be measured directly.

Most speech recognition tests are presented at levels well above the listener's detection threshold to estimate maximum potential performance. These measures are used for multiple purposes: diagnosing the auditory site of a lesion, assessing potential benefit with amplification, assessing candidacy for a cochlear implant, and assessing everyday speech understanding.

SSA requires testing of "speech discrimination in quiet at a test presentation level sufficient to ascertain maximum discrimination ability"

(Social Security Administration, 2003, p. 24). The committee notes, however, that it is difficult to determine if maximum discrimination ability is assessed unless a complete performance-intensity function is obtained. Moreover, performance at the presentation levels needed to measure maximum performance does not necessarily reflect recognition of speech at typical conversational levels. Listener performance on speech recognition tests generally is not correlated with performance on self-assessment measures of hearing disability. The reason for this lack of agreement may be related to the wider range of listening conditions sampled on self-assessment tools than in the clinical setting, the influence of emotional reactions and personality variables on individual responses to the questionnaires, or the high presentation level of traditional speech tests that does not simulate everyday listening levels.

Assessment of suprathreshold speech recognition performance is relevant for SSA disability determination as an indicator of everyday speech understanding or as a potential indicator of speech understanding ability in specific listening conditions. While few studies have demonstrated the correlation between performance on specific speech recognition tests and performance on hearing-critical tasks in the workplace, theoretically there is face validity in utilizing speech recognition tests to predict communication skills on particular everyday tasks.

For example, a speech recognition test presented in quiet with few contextual cues and no visual cues is expected to predict speech understanding over the telephone. Performance on a speech recognition test presented in moderate noise levels probably correlates with on-the job communication in a typical noisy environment, such as a busy office. The closer the correspondence between the test method (stimulus materials, response mode, signal level, and presence of background noise) and everyday listening situations, the better the predictive value of the clinical test for actual communication performance in the employment setting ought to be.

Open-Set Tests

Monosyllabic Words. A variety of speech materials have been developed and evaluated for assessment of suprathreshold speech recognition. Monosyllabic word tests with free recall (referred to as open-set[3]) chal-

---

[3]A speech recognition test is considered to be "open-set" if the listener is required to give a free recall response without any specific response set. A speech test is "closed set" or "closed message" if the listener must choose from a limited set of known response alternatives.

lenge a listener's ability to recognize discrete phonemes while deriving meaning from the stimulus. They are presented routinely in quiet by the vast majority of audiologists (Martin et al., 1998). Each standardized test involves presenting full lists of the recorded materials (usually 50 words) at the presentation level used in the standardization procedure. Performance is quantified by a percentage-correct score.

Examples of open-set monosyllabic word lists that have been standardized on a normal-hearing sample include Central Institute for the Deaf Test W-22 (CID W-22) (Hirsh et al., 1952), Northwestern University Auditory Test No. 6 original recordings (NU6) (Tillman and Carhart, 1966), and NU6 Veterans Administration (VA) compact disc recordings (Wilson, Zizz, Shanks, and Causey, 1990). The NU6 test has also been standardized with a sample of listeners with hearing loss (Tillman and Carhart, 1966). The standardization reports of these tests indicate the psychometric functions (performance versus intensity) and the interlist equivalence of the recorded tests. In addition, the variability of percentage-correct scores on open-set speech recognition tests is determined by the number of stimulus items in the test and the test score, as described by the binomial probability theorem (Thornton and Raffin, 1978). The application of this statistical principle indicates that the standard deviation of a test score is inversely proportional to the square root of the number of test items and is larger as the test score approaches 50 percent correct. Hence, one method to reduce variability in speech recognition testing is by presenting a larger number of items in the test.

We note several limitations of open-set monosyllabic word testing in quiet, as the single metric of speech understanding performance, for purposes of SSA disability determination. First, the monosyllabic word stimuli do not represent speech used in everyday communication because they do not contain contextual cues. Second, most recorded and standardized monosyllabic speech recognition tests contain only three or four equivalent lists; this number may not be sufficient for a full evaluation. Third, presentation of the stimuli in quiet does not represent the environment in some workplaces, which may be degraded by a background of steady-state noise or the speech of coworkers.

Two paradigms have been used to assess monosyllabic word recognition performance in noise. The first is presentation of the stimuli in a fixed noise level, using either broadband noise or a competing message (Wilson et al., 1990) and determining the percentage-correct score at several fixed stimulus levels. For listeners with normal hearing, the psychometric functions so determined are shifted toward higher signal levels in both broadband noise and competing message conditions relative to the functions in quiet. The signal-to-noise (S/N) ratio at which listeners achieve a 50 percent correct score can be derived from these psychometric functions. For example, Wilson et al. (1990) assessed performance with fixed noise levels of 60 dB SPL and varied speech levels in 4-dB steps between 52 and 88 dB SPL for the broadband noise condition, and between 40 and 76 dB SPL for the competing message condition. For listeners with normal hearing, 50 percent correct scores were obtained in broadband noise at a S/N ratio of +11 dB and in competing-message noise at a S/N ratio of -4dB with the VA recording of NU6 (Wilson et al., 1990).

The second paradigm adaptively varies the level of a background competition following each response, to measure the S/N ratio at which a listener achieves a criterion level of performance (Dirks, Morgan, and Dubno, 1982). The procedure is repeated at four signal presentation levels that span the range of average-to-loud conversational speech and amplified speech (60-96 dB SPL). Performance data indicate that most listeners with hearing loss require more favorable S/N ratios than those required by listeners with normal hearing to achieve 50 percent recognition performance, although this varies somewhat with signal presentation level. In both procedures, the normative performance data are specific to the recorded stimuli, noise, presentation levels, and calibration procedures reported.

One emerging issue in assessing monosyllabic word recognition is the role of cognitive and linguistic capabilities that influence activation and selection of a target word from long-term memory. The neighborhood activation model of lexical processing suggests that words are recognized in relation to other phonemically similar words (Luce and Pisoni, 1998). Three factors in particular appear to affect speech recognition performance: the number of phonemically similar words for a target word ("neighborhood density"), the average frequency of occurrence of words that are phonemically similar ("neighborhood frequency"), and the frequency of occurrence of a particular word in the language ("word frequency"). Studies indicate that these structural factors between words influence monosyllabic word recognition performance of listeners with normal hearing and with hearing loss when the words are presented in both quiet and noise (Dirks, Takayanagi, Moshfegh, Noffsinger, and Fausti, 2001). A test based on these principles, the Lexical Neighborhood Test (LNT) (Kirk, Pisoni, and Osberger, 1995), has been developed for assessment of children, but no comparable test is available for evaluation of adults.

Sentence Tests. Speech recognition tests that incorporate the use of everyday sentences are desirable for estimating the level of performance in daily communication situations. However, everyday sentences inherently contain contextual cues for identification of individual words. Thus, a concern with the use of these materials is the extent to which syntactic, semantic, and lexical contextual cues (see Appendix A for definitions) influence overall performance, and the interaction of these factors with a listener's knowledge of the language. Such an interaction might mean, for example, that standardization on subjects who are native speakers of the test language would yield norms that are inappropriate for nonnative speakers. A second issue is the method of scoring sentence recognition performance, although most contemporary sentence tests assess accuracy based on recognition of keywords. A third issue is whether the test has been standardized in quiet, noise, or both environmental conditions. For SSA disability determination, a sentence test standardized in both quiet and noise would be particularly valuable in estimating functional hearing ability for many job-related tasks.

Sentence recognition tests that have been developed for presentation in quiet include the CID everyday sentences (Silverman and Hirsh, 1955) and the City University of New York (CUNY) Sentences (Boothroyd, Hanin, and Hnath, 1985). Recorded versions of both of these materials are available. The CID everyday sentences contain 10 lists of sentences with 50 keywords per list. Individuals with mild or moderate hearing losses obtain excellent scores on this test; as a consequence, these materials are used most often in assessment of listeners with profound hearing loss (Owens, Kessler, Raggio, and Schubert, 1985; Tyler et al., 1985). The CUNY Sentences (Boothroyd, Hanin, and Hnath, 1985a) are a popular corpus of everyday sentences that are used for assessment of individuals with profound hearing loss. Data reporting listeners' psychometric performance and test-retest reliability on these two tests are not available.

Several sentence recognition tests in noise have been developed. The Speech Perception in Noise (SPIN) test (Kalikow, Stevens, and Elliott, 1977) assesses a listener's recognition of keywords embedded in sentences with controlled word predictability: half of the sentences on each list include semantic contextual cues (high-probability sentences) and the other half are semantically neutral (low-probability sentences). The identical keywords are used in high-probability and low-probability sentences appearing in different lists. The revised version of this test (R-SPIN) (Bilger, Nuetzel, Rabinowitz, and Rzeczkowski, 1984) has been standardized with a background of multitalker babble at a signal to babble (S/B) ratio[4] of +8 dB. Calibration tones are equivalent in root-mean-square (rms) level to the average levels of the sentences and the babble. The eight sentence lists are equivalent, and test-retest reliability is high among lis-

---

[4]When the background noise is speech babble, the term S/B or signal-to-babble ratio may be used with the same meaning as S/N or signal-to-noise ratio.

teners with hearing loss (Bilger et al., 1984). Scores on the low-probability items reflect a listener's ability to recognize the acoustic and phonetic characteristics of the speech signal; scores on the high-probability items indicate the extent to which a listener can utilize semantic contextual cues in addition to acoustic or phonetic information.

The Connected Speech Test (CST) (Cox, Alexander, and Gilmore, 1987; Cox, Alexander, Gilmore, and Pusakulich, 1988) presents pairs of equivalent passages containing keywords used for scoring. A competing speech babble is presented during the test at two S/B ratios. Percentage-correct scores are derived for each passage and are transformed to rational arcsine units (rau) (Studebaker, 1985). Assessment of listeners with normal hearing and with hearing loss on this test demonstrates that it has high content validity, good sensitivity, and a large number of equivalent forms.

An abbreviated test of speech in noise (SIN test) (Etymotic Research, 1993) presents high- and low-level sentences to listeners at four S/B ratios. A percentage-correct score is calculated from the 25 keywords appearing in the five sentences for each condition. In addition, the S/B ratio corresponding to a 50 percent correct score can be derived. The original SIN test did not contain equivalent lists, and its level of difficulty was inadequate for listeners with normal hearing and hearing loss (Bentler, 2000). Revisions to the SIN test (R-SIN) (Cox, Gray, and Alexander, 2001) have improved the equivalence of the different lists and the sensitivity of the test for identifying changes in performance, but it requires a longer administration time.

The QuickSIN test was developed recently by Etymotic Research, Inc. (Etymotic Research, 2001) to assess the S/N ratio loss in a one-minute test. The test consists of one list of six sentences with five keywords per sentence and a background noise of four-talker babble. The test is presented at six prerecorded S/N ratios (25, 20, 15, 10, 5, and 0). Raw test results are reported as the S/N ratio at which the listener achieves a 50 percent correct score (the SNR-50), which is then compared to the normal SNR-50 to derive the S/N ratio loss. This loss reflects the increase in S/N ratio required by the listener with hearing loss to achieve a 50 percent correct score, relative to listeners with normal hearing. S/N ratio loss scores are categorized according to degree of severity: normal to near-normal (S/N ratio loss = 0-2 dB); mild (S/N ratio loss = 2-7 dB); moderate (S/N ratio loss = 7-15 dB); and severe (S/N ratio loss > 15 dB). The QuickSIN test is used primarily as an aid to selecting appropriate amplification and as a guide to counseling individuals regarding the potential benefit of different amplification options. The validity and reliability of the QuickSIN test for listeners with normal hearing or with hearing loss have not been reported in the literature.

The Hearing in Noise Test (HINT) (Nilsson, Soli, and Sullivan, 1994) assesses a listener's recognition of everyday sentences in quiet and noise. The standardized HINT employs an adaptive technique for adjusting stimulus level based on the accuracy of the listener's recall of short, individual sentences, to measure the sentence SRT. Reliability of threshold estimates with the HINT presented in quiet has been demonstrated, with a standard deviation of difference scores of 1.39 dB (Nilsson et al., 1994). The standardized HINT also involves measurement of the sentence SRT in speech spectrum noise presented at a fixed level of 72 dBA.[5] An adaptive procedure is used to estimate the S/N ratio for a criterion level of performance. For the HINT measured in noise, the mean S/N ratio for listeners with normal hearing is -2.92 dB; this value indicates that people with normal hearing correctly repeat 50 percent of the sentences at a speech level that is less intense than the fixed noise level. A higher S/N ratio on this measure indicates that a listener requires a higher signal level to achieve 50 percent correct recognition, thus reflecting poorer performance. The repeatability of the sentence SRT in noise is high (Nilsson et al., 1994). The sentence SRT in noise demonstrates a listener's ability to understand speech in noisy environments, such as when operating a vacuum cleaner or attending a small party. Thus, it is viewed as an alternate procedure to other speech recognition measures in noise.

Although the HINT test was developed as a measure of SRT in quiet and in noise, the stimulus materials are often presented at a suprathreshold level to assess a percentage-correct score in quiet or in noise at fixed speech and noise levels. While this application of the HINT may be appealing, there are no data on the interlist equivalence of the HINT, test-retest reliability, or psychometric functions for listeners with normal hearing and with hearing loss at suprathreshold levels. Such data would be important for standardizing the HINT for suprathreshold presentation.

Closed-Set Tests

A wide range of closed-message speech recognition tests—in which the items are limited to a set known to the listener—have been developed over the years. In these tests, a target stimulus is presented and the listener's task is to select the stimulus from a closed set of choices. The number of choices dictates the guess rate for a particular test (e.g., 25 percent guess rate for a four-choice response alternative, 17 percent guess

---

[5]dBA refers to a reading obtained from a sound-level meter using the A-weighting scale, which reduces the importance of the low frequencies; it is used for many noise measurements.

rate for a six-choice response alternative). Individual performance is higher on a closed-set speech recognition test than on an open-set test for the same speech stimuli.

Closed-message tests are available with a wide range of stimulus items. Nonsense syllable tests present single syllables in a consonant-vowel or vowel-consonant format. Because the stimuli are not meaningful lexical items, listener performance is thought to reflect perception of the acoustic cues of speech rather than knowledge of the language. The Nonsense Syllable Test developed by researchers at the City University of New York (CUNY NST) (Resnick, Dubno, Hoffnung, and Levitt, 1975) is an example of a standardized, closed-set test that uses nonsense syllables. This test has excellent interlist equivalence and test-retest reliability (Dubno and Dirks, 1982). It permits assessment of the specific consonant phonemes that a listener with hearing loss can identify as well the frequency of occurrence of particular consonant confusions (Dubno, Dirks, and Langhofer, 1982).

Monosyllabic words have also been used as the stimuli for closed-message tests. One example is the California Consonant Test (Owens and Schubert, 1977), which was developed to reveal the perceptual problems in speech recognition of individuals with high-frequency sensorineural hearing losses. The test assesses an individual's ability to identify monosyllabic words with initial or final fricatives, sibilants, and plosives; these phonemes are often difficult to perceive for individuals with high-frequency sensorineural hearing loss. The response alternatives are chosen to be highly confusable with the target stimuli, so this test may reveal subtle difficulties in speech perception among individuals with selective high-frequency hearing loss that are not revealed on standard open-set monosyllabic word tests.

The Synthetic Sentence Identification test (SSI) (Speaks and Jerger, 1965) is an example of a closed-set sentence test. The sentence-length stimuli for this test were chosen to follow an approximation to the syntactic order of words in sentences, although the sentences are not meaningful. Listeners are asked to select each sentence they hear from a list of 10 sentences. This test is presented with a competing message either in the stimulus ear or the opposite ear, at varying S/N ratios. Abnormally poor performance on this test provides a diagnostic indication of the side and site of a retrocochlear lesion.

Listener Performance on Speech Recognition Tests

The performance of listeners with hearing loss on speech recognition tests is affected by the degree of hearing loss, the configuration of hearing loss, the site of the lesion, the listener's knowledge of the language, the speech recognition materials, the speech presentation level, and the listening environment (quiet or noise). Individuals with normal hearing sensitivity or conductive hearing loss generally exhibit excellent performance (90-100 percent correct) on monosyllabic word tests and sentence tests presented in quiet. Listeners with sensorineural hearing loss show a range of scores, from 0 to 100 percent correct.

Individual performance on a variety of speech recognition measures can be predicted with ANSI standards, including the articulation index (AI) (American National Standards Institute, 1969) and the speech intelligibility index (SII) (American National Standards Institute, 2002b). These predictions are based on the audibility of the speech signal, the relative intensities of the speech signal and background noise (the S/N ratio) in different frequency bands, and the importance of different frequency bands for accurate performance on a particular speech recognition test. According to both the AI and the SII, predicted performance generally is inversely proportional to the degree of hearing loss, for individuals with hearing loss attributed to cochlear lesions. People with hearing loss primarily affecting the high frequencies may demonstrate poor speech recognition scores at conversational speech levels, especially in noise (Suter, 1985), an observation attributed to the importance of high-frequency consonant information for understanding speech and the direct masking of low frequency cues by background noise. AI/SII predictions, however, do not always completely predict actual performance for listeners with hearing loss, particularly in noise (Dirks, Bell, Rossman, and Kincaid, 1986). For example, SII overpredicted average recognition scores for the low-probability items of the SPIN test and for the Nonsense Syllable Test by approximately 17-18 percent at +8 dB S/N ratio in a group of older listeners with hearing loss (Hargus and Gordon-Salant, 1995).

Speech Recognition with Auditory and Visual Cues

The preceding section discussed assessment of speech recognition for signals presented in the auditory modality without amplification. There are circumstances in which it is desirable to assess recognition of speech presented in both auditory and visual modalities. This type of presentation simulates a face-to-face conversation, permitting the receiver to take advantage of visual cues from the face to aid perception. A comparison of performance in the auditory modality to performance in the combined auditory and visual modalities indicates the magnitude of benefit the receiver obtains from speech-reading in addition to acoustic information.

One key issue in assessing auditory + visual speech reception is the use of standardized materials. The importance of audio recordings of speech materials for assessing speech recognition in the auditory modality was discussed previously. Similarly, video recordings are essential for assessing speech recognition when visual cues are presented, because there is wide variability in the extent to which different talkers provide visible speech cues through lip and jaw movement and expressive facial movements (which may be obscured by such things as facial hair). Tests for adults include the Iowa Sentence Test (Tyler, Preece, and Tye-Murray, 1986) and the CUNY Sentences (Boothroyd et al., 1985). The CUNY Sentences are topic-related sentences consisting of 6 lists of 12 sentences each. Performance is scored for keywords correct per list. Performance reliability estimates are predicted from the binomial probability theorem based on 25 independent items per list (Boothroyd, Hnath-Chisolm, Hanin, and Kishon-Rabin, 1988). Audiotape, videotape, and video laser disk recordings are available from the authors. The Iowa Sentence Test also uses everyday sentences as the stimulus materials. This test has been recorded on video laser disk, although equipment for playback of laser disks is no longer available for purchase. Presentation of these audiovisual materials involves routing the visual speech signal through a video monitor under controlled lighting and distance conditions. The auditory signal is routed through an audiometer for control of signal level. Normative data have not been published describing validity, reliability, or performance-intensity functions in combined auditory + visual modalities for these materials.

The appendix of the ANSI standard for the speech intelligibility index (American National Standards Institute, 2002b) suggests a method for calculating the audiovisual SII, S_{av}, to approximate performance of listeners who are not specifically trained in speech-reading under optimal viewing conditions. The prediction uses the formula

$$S_{av} = b + cS,$$

where S is the audio-only calculated SII, and b and c are constants. For S ≤ 0.2, b and c are 0.1 and 1.5, respectively. For S > 0.2, b and c are 0.25 and 0.75, respectively. Using values from the transfer functions derived for the NU6 Auditec audio recording (Schum, Matthews, and Lee, 1991; Studebaker, Sherbecoe, and Gilmore, 1993), a value of S = 0.3 is associated with an NU6 score of approximately 50 percent correct and an auditory + visual S_{av} = 0.475, yielding a predicted NU6 score of 80 percent correct. When S = 0.2, the NU6 score would be expected to be about 20 percent, but with the addition of vision S_{av} = 0.4, and the predicted NU6 score would be about 65-70 percent correct.

Actual auditory + visual performance may be substantially different from these estimated predictions, although data comparing predicted to actual performance are not available. A number of factors influence a person's unaided speech-reading performance, including familiarity with the talker (Lloyd and Price, 1971), visual acuity (Hardick, Oyer, and Irion, 1970), knowledge of the language, live versus recorded materials, and degree of hearing loss (Erber, 1979). For example, word recognition performance improves 19-28 percent for individuals with severe hearing loss with the addition of visual cues, but improves only 1-15 percent for individuals with profound hearing loss (Erber, 1975). Although reception of everyday sentences is usually optimal for audition + vision conditions (Tye-Murray, 1998), some individuals with severe or profound hearing losses may exhibit very poor performance (10 percent correct) for recognition of everyday sentences presented with auditory + visual cues (Sims and Hirsh, 1982). These unaided performance levels do not reflect the combined benefit of speech-reading and use of amplification or a cochlear implant in suitable candidates.

Multicultural and Multilingual Issues in Evaluation of Speech Recognition

U.S. society is becoming increasingly multicultural and multilingual. Individuals seeking audiometric evaluation may have no knowledge of the English language or may have limited fluency in English. Presentation of a standardized English speech recognition test to these individuals is problematic for several reasons. First, a lack of familiarity with the vocabulary is known to reduce performance on a speech recognition test. As a result, nonnative speakers of English obtain lower scores on English speech recognition tests than do native speakers of the language (Gat and Keith, 1978). Second, listeners whose first language is not English perceive individual consonant and vowel phonemes differently than native speakers of English (Danhauer, Crawford, and Edgerton, 1984). Finally, nonnative speakers derive less meaning from sentence-length materials than native speakers of English, in part because of differences between the overall rhythmic pattern of English and that of many other languages. For bilingual speakers, the age of second language acquisition is an important factor influencing proficiency in English. This is particularly apparent on speech recognition tests in noise: nonnative adult speakers of English who learned English before age 6 perform better in noise than adult listeners who learned the language after puberty, even though all listeners achieve nearly perfect performance in quiet (Mayo, Florentine, and Buus, 1997).

Despite these obstacles, it remains desirable to evaluate a listener's speech recognition performance during an audiometric assessment. A number of alternative materials and methods have been recommended for evaluating nonnative speakers of English. The preferred strategy is to present a speech recognition test for which recordings are available in

TABLE 3-2 Speech Recognition Materials Available in Languages Other Than English

Test Type/Language	Source
Bisyllables	
Spanish	Auditec of St. Louis
Luganda	Nsamba, 1979
Monosyllabic Words	
Spanish	Auditec of St. Louis
Russian	Aleksandrovsky, et al., 1998
Hearing in Noise Test (HINT)	
Spanish	Cochlear Corporation, 2002
French	Laroche, et al., University of Ottowa, 2002
Mandarin	Wong, University of Hong Kong, 2002
Cantonese	Wong, University of Hong Kong, 2002
Japanese	Kubi, Osaka University, 2002
Picture Identification	
Spanish	VA recordings: McCullough and Wilson, 1998
Trisyllabic Words (for SRT)	
Spanish	Auditec of St. Louis
Bisyllabic Words (for word recognition)	
Spanish	Auditec of St. Louis
Synthetic Sentence Identification (SSI) Test	
Spanish	Auditec of St. Louis

NOTE: Entries are publications, vendors, or contact names for obtaining each set of materials.

the listener's native language. A listing of speech recognition tests that have recordings available in languages other than English is shown in Table 3-2. Lists of Spanish bisyllabic words tend to yield performance scores by Spanish speakers that are comparable to English monosyllabic word recognition scores by native speakers of English (Weislander and Hodgson, 1989). Listener responses can be scored phonetically with reasonable accuracy even if the audiologist is unfamiliar with the test language (Cakiroglu and Danhauer, 1992; Cokely and Yager, 1993). Alternatively, a closed-set, picture-pointing task can be used for test administration in a language unfamiliar to the audiologist. This method removes any potential bias or scoring error. Tests that incorporate picture-pointing tasks on paper and computer are available in Spanish and Russian (Aleksandrovsky, McCullough, and Wilson, 1998; Comstock and Martin, 1984; McCullough, Wilson, Birck, and Anderson, 1994; Spitzer, 1980).

　　There are many languages for which there are no recorded versions of speech recognition tests. One recommendation is to assess the speech recognition threshold using digit pairs in place of spondee words, because new language learners acquire knowledge of digits relatively early, and audiologists can easily score the responses (Ramkissoon, Proctor, Lansing, and Bilger, 2002). This digit-SRT test can be administered to listeners from any language, and results appear to be valid, based on high correlations between digit-SRTs and the PTA measured for nonnative English speakers (Ramkissoon et al., 2002). A comparable test for assessing suprathreshold speech recognition in listeners with various linguistic backgrounds has not been developed.

Acoustic Immittance Measures

Acoustic immittance measures are a series of electrophysiologic tests that assess the integrity of the middle ear system and the structures comprising the acoustic reflex pathway. Acoustic immittance measures are administered routinely as part of the standard audiometric evaluation (Martin et al., 1998), using commercially available acoustic immittance systems calibrated according to ANSI standards (American National Standards Institute, 2002a). Interpretation of the acoustic immittance test results, in conjunction with the audiogram, aids in determining the site of the lesion associated with a hearing loss. The three basic subtests of the acoustic immittance battery are tympanometry, acoustic reflex thresholds, and acoustic reflex adaptation.

Tympanometry

Tympanometry is an assessment of the ease of acoustic energy transfer (acoustic admittance) through the middle ear system, as a function of air pressure. In the normal middle ear system, energy transfer of the middle ear, as measured at the plane of the tympanic membrane, is maximal at atmospheric pressure (0 dekaPascals, or daPa) and is minimal at air pressures that produce a stiffening of the middle ear system (air pressures remote from 0 daPa, such as +200 daPa or –200 daPa).

Tympanometry is performed by presenting a probe tone to the ear canal and measuring the acoustic admittance (in mmhos, an expression of the ease of energy flow that has a reciprocal relationship with impedance as measured in acoustic ohms) of this tone, as the air pressure presented to the sealed ear canal varies from positive to negative (usually in the range +200 daPa to -400 daPa). The standard probe tone frequency is 226 Hz, although many additional probe frequencies can be presented. The resulting tympanogram is a pressure-admittance function that depicts the admittance characteristics of the tympanic membrane and middle ear system of the test ear. Three parameters of the tympanogram can be quantified: peak admittance (Peak Y), tympanometric width (TW), and equiva-

TABLE 3-3 Norms for Peak Admittance (Y), Tympanometric Width (TW), and Equivalent Volume (V_{ec})

Age Group	Y (mmho)	TW (daPa)	V_{ec} (cm^3)
Adults			
Mean	0.79	77	1.36
90th percentile range	0.30–1.70	51–114	0.9–2.0
Children			
Mean	0.52	114	0.58
90th percentile range	0.25–1.05	80–159	0.3–0.9

SOURCE: Margolis and Hunter (1999).

lent volume (V_{ec}) (American Speech-Language-Hearing Association, 1990). Normal values for each of these parameters are shown in Table 3-3.

Peak admittance is the admittance value observed at the peak point on the tympanogram, in mmhos. Abnormally low values indicate a stiffening pathology of the middle ear, including otitis media with effusion and otosclerosis. Excessively high peak admittance values are consistent with a hypermobile middle ear system, such as ossicular discontinuity or scarring of the tympanic membrane.

Tympanometric width is the pressure interval on the tympanogram corresponding to a 50 percent reduction relative to the peak height. It is an indication of the shape of the tympanogram. A flat tympanogram, often associated with otitis media with effusion, produces an abnormally wide TW.

Equivalent volume is an indication of the volume of the external auditory canal. It is obtained at a pressure that minimizes the admittance of the middle ear (e.g., +200 daPa or -400 daPa). Thus, the height of the tympanogram at one of these values is the equivalent volume of the external auditory canal. Most acoustic admittance systems provide the V_{ec} in a printout accompanying the tympanogram. Abnormally high V_{ec} coupled with a flat tympanogram is observed in cases of a perforation of the tympanic membrane.

In summary, abnormal tympanograms are observed for a variety of pathological conditions affecting the tympanic membrane and middle ear, including otitis media with effusion, otosclerosis, ossicular discontinuity, tympanic membrane perforation, and a scarred (monomeric) tympanic membrane. A normal tympanogram indicates the presence of a normally functioning middle ear system, either with or without normal hearing.

Acoustic Reflex Thresholds

The acoustic reflex is a contraction of the stapedius muscle of the middle ear in response to loud sound. The pathways for this reflex ascend from the peripheral auditory system to the brainstem and then descend both ipsilaterally and contralaterally, so presentation of a loud sound in one ear results in bilateral contraction of the stapedius muscles. This contraction stiffens the middle ear system, causing a reduction in the transfer of low-frequency energy.

The clinical procedure for assessing the acoustic reflex threshold involves presenting a low-frequency probe tone (i.e., 226 Hz) to one ear, presenting high-intensity signals to the same or the other (contralateral) ear, and monitoring a decrease in the acoustic admittance of the probe tone in response to the presentation of the high-level signal. The minimum stimulus level that results in an observable decrease in acoustic admittance is defined as the acoustic reflex threshold. Acoustic reflex thresholds are usually measured from 500-2000 Hz, in both ipsilateral and contralateral modes, for each ear.

In listeners with normal hearing, the acoustic reflex threshold is elicited at levels approximating 85 dB HL (+/- 10 dB). The acoustic reflex is absent if the signal doesn't reach the cochlea with sufficient intensity, if there is damage affecting any of the structures along the acoustic reflex pathway, or if there is a stiff middle ear system in the probe ear. Examples of conditions in which the acoustic reflex is absent include conductive hearing loss of 25 dB HL or greater in the stimulus ear, conductive hearing loss of 10 dB HL or greater in the probe ear, sensorineural hearing loss exceeding 75 dB HL in the stimulus ear, a lesion of the facial nerve in the probe ear, and a lesion in the auditory brainstem affecting the crossing pathway of the acoustic reflex arc. The acoustic reflex may also be absent with a lesion of the vestibulocochlear nerve in the stimulus ear, depending on the extent of the lesion. The acoustic reflex is expected to be present in cases of mild, moderate, or moderately severe sensorineural hearing loss associated with a cochlear lesion. The acoustic reflex threshold generally increases as a function of pure-tone threshold in these cases (Silman and Gelfand, 1981).

Otoacoustic Emissions

Otoacoustic emissions (OAEs) are noninvasive, objective measures of cochlear functioning. The cochlea contains two distinct types of sensory hair cells, outer and inner hair cells. When the inner hair cell senses vibration (sound), it will send the information by releasing neurotransmitters at its base to initiate activity in the primary auditory nerve. The outer hair cell also will sense sound as vibration, but it does not send information to the central nervous system. Rather, the role of the outer hair cell is to amplify the vibration at specific regions of the cochlea by actually expanding and contracting in response to sound (Brownell, Bader, Bertrand, and de Ribaupierre, 1985; Russell and Sellick, 1978). This added vibration is imparted to adjacent inner hair cells, thereby increasing the overall sensitivity of the auditory system to weak sounds. Otoacoustic emissions are produced when some of the energy from the outer hair cells is propagated through the fluids in the cochlea back to the middle ear and tympanic membrane to create a sound wave in the external ear canal (Kemp, 1986).

OAEs are highly dependent on the outer hair cells (Schrott, Puel, and Rebillard, 1991), which are generally more vulnerable to disease and damage than inner hair cells. Therefore when OAEs are normal, it is presumed that the inner hair cells are functioning normally as well. Consequently, when an OAE is recorded, one can usually assume that hearing thresholds are 30-40 dB HL or better. In addition, frequency regions of normal and abnormal outer hair cell function can be predicted by patterns of OAE response. In this way the OAE can aid in objective measures of hearing (but see caveat below).

Two basic types of OAE are used clinically and both are acceptable for use in infants, children, and adults. Each type requires a small probe to be placed into the ear canal. The probe contains one or two sound production devices (transducers) as well as a microphone to record the emission itself. The transient-evoked OAE generally uses a click stimulus, but occasionally a tone burst is used. The response is spread over about 10 ms time due to travel time in the inner ear. Responses from many stimuli are averaged to reduce noise. Several types of statistical measures are used to determine the presence of a reliable response.

The other type of OAE used clinically is the distortion-product OAE, which is measured in response to two tones. The interaction of the two tones produces distortion, creating a third tone at a frequency predictable from the eliciting tones. A computer presents the primary tones and analyzes the microphone output for the presence of the distortion product. For a thorough review of clinical applications of both types of OAEs, see Prieve and Fitzgerald (2002).

It is important to keep in mind that an OAE can be present in narrow regions of good outer hair cell function and should be interpreted in a frequency-specific manner. As such, the OAE can help to fill in information from specific frequency regions. Caution should be used in overinterpretation of very narrow, low-amplitude regions of OAE, which can be spurious noise. Also, OAEs are not strong in low-frequency regions (1000 Hz and below) in infants and toddlers due to physiological noise, and thus absent OAEs in low-frequency regions should not be given great weight in interpretation.

OAE presence indicates good hair cell function and generally indicates that the hearing thresholds should be better than 30-40 dB. OAEs, however, cannot be used to determine exact hearing thresholds. In contrast, the absence of an OAE can be due to a variety of causes, from middle ear dysfunction to sensorineural disorders producing hearing loss of any degree. The absence of an OAE alone should not be interpreted as indication of significant hearing loss. There are conditions in which the presence of an OAE alone does not ensure normal hearing sensitivity. Disease that spares the cochlea and impairs function in the auditory nerve or low brainstem (for example acoustic neuroma or auditory neuropathy) can also cause significant hearing loss. The OAE therefore should not be tested in isolation but must be included in a battery of tests for accurate interpretation. Nevertheless, measurement of OAEs provides a quick, noninvasive view of the functioning of the inner ear. Because of the value of these measures, the evaluation of OAEs is routine in many diagnostic audiology settings.

Auditory Evoked Potentials

Auditory evoked potentials (AEPs) are recordings of neural activity evoked by sound. The AEP is collected using surface electrodes placed on the scalp and near the ear. Computer-generated sounds are presented to subjects via earphones, and each presentation triggers a synchronized recording of neural activity. The responses to many stimuli are averaged in a manner time-locked to the stimulus to reduce the contribution of nonauditory generators, such as random muscle or brain activity.

AEPs occur within fractions of a second following stimulation. The earliest activity, known as the auditory brainstem response or ABR, has a latency of 0-20 ms depending on the age of the subject and the nature of the sounds used to elicit the response. This response is generated in the auditory nerve and brainstem auditory pathway. Other evoked potentials include the middle latency response (MLR), generated in the thalamus and primary auditory cortex, with a latency of 20-100 ms, and the late cortical response (LCR), generated in the auditory cortex and association areas, with a latency of 100-250 ms. While all of these AEPs can be used to predict hearing threshold levels, the one used most commonly in the United States is the ABR. In contrast, most of the audiology literature from other parts of the world supports the use of late responses for threshold estimation in adults (Coles and Mason, 1984; Hone, Norman, Keogh, and Kelly, 2003; Hyde, Alberti, Matsumoto, and Yao-Li, 1986; Tsui, Wong, and Wong, 2002). Most recently, a variation of standard evoked potential technique, referred to as auditory steady-state response (ASSR), has been used successfully to predict frequency-specific hearing thresholds.

The ABR is a recording of activity generated in the auditory nerve and subsequent brainstem auditory pathways. Short-duration sounds are presented to the ear through earphones. These generate a series of neural impulses in the brainstem auditory pathway.

The ABR requires that the electrode-recorded activity be averaged following presentation of hundreds of stimuli. A computer time-locks the recording of neural activity to the onset of stimuli and creates an average neural response. The averaging process allows the minute (nanovolt level) changes in electrical potentials in the brainstem that occur in response to sound to be distinguished from other electrical activity in the brain and muscles of the head and neck.

The ABR, when elicited by clearly audible stimuli, produces a consistent series of peaks labeled with Roman numerals I-V. In infants, only peaks I, III, and V are visible. As the stimulus level approaches the threshold of hearing, ABR peaks diminish in amplitude and number and increase in latency (see Figure 3-2). The lowest stimulus level that will produce a visually detectable ABR is termed the ABR threshold. The ABR threshold in most instances is a very good indicator of the hearing threshold that would be determined by standard audiometric techniques (Sininger, Abdala, and Cone-Wesson, 1997; Stapells, Gravel, and Martin, 1995). In the absence of neurological disease, the ABR threshold can be used to accurately predict audiometric thresholds. This is a standard technique used to predict degree and configuration of hearing loss in infants under 6 months of age and in uncooperative toddlers. It can also be used to predict hearing thresholds in adult patients who cannot or will not respond to standard audiometric testing procedures. ABRs should not be used in isolation; rather, they should be part of a test battery including otoacoustic emissions, middle ear assessment, and some observation of behavior in response to sound (see Chapter 7). In addition, when the auditory nerve or low brainstem is specifically impaired, the ABR threshold may not be an accurate indicator of hearing threshold (Sininger and Oba, 2001).

The stimuli used for ABR testing are of different types. Clicks are broadband stimuli that are particularly good for eliciting an ABR because they excite many cochlear elements and neurons almost simultaneously. ABR thresholds determined using click stimuli correspond closely to the average hearing levels of an audiogram (Sininger and Abdala, 1998). Frequency-specific tone bursts (short-duration tones created with slow rising onset and offset ramps) are the best ABR stimuli for the purpose of determining the degree and configuration of hearing loss and for predicting the specific thresholds on an audiogram. Figure 3-2 shows a typical ABR

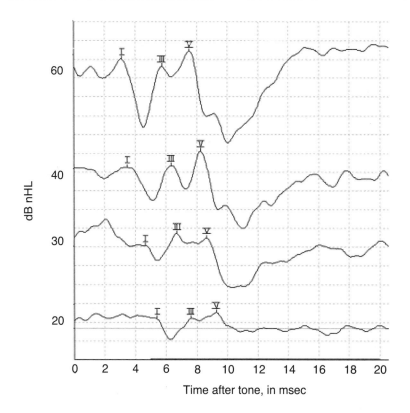

FIGURE 3-2 Infant auditory brainstem response to 4000 Hz tone burst.

intensity series recorded from an infant with normal hearing in response to 4000 Hz tone bursts. Generally, tone bursts in the frequency range between 500 and 4000 Hz provide adequate information for accurate prediction of the hearing thresholds in subjects of any age.

Subjects must cooperate for the ABR evaluation by reclining and remaining nearly motionless in a darkened, sound-treated room during the test. Infants generally are tested during natural sleep; toddlers may need mild sedation for a competent evaluation. Older children and adults are tested in a quiet dark environment while reclined and are encouraged to sleep during the evaluation. The test requires that a minimum of three electrodes be attached to the scalp after mild skin abrasion for adequate connection. The subject is asked to wear headphones or use foam insert plugs connected to transducers. A full evaluation may take 15 minutes to 2 hours, depending on results and degree of cooperation. ABRs can be elicited with bone-conducted stimuli when needed for differential diagnosis of conductive hearing loss or evaluation of ears with closed ear canals (Lasky and Yang, 1986; Stuart, Yang, and Green, 1994; Yang and Stuart, 1990; Yang, Rupert, and Moushegian, 1987).

The auditory steady-state response (ASSR), previously known as the steady-state evoked potential (SSEP), is another way of objectively assessing frequency-specific responses. In simple terms, this technique uses pure-tone (carrier) stimuli that are modulated at an appropriate amplitude with another tone at an appropriate modulation frequency. For infants and children, the appropriate modulation frequency range is about 80-100 Hz. Long segments of these stimuli are presented and ongoing electroencephalographic activity is sampled and analyzed in the frequency domain. When the neural activity shows a preference for the modulation frequency over other frequencies in the analysis, it is assumed that the auditory system is responding to the carrier frequency. A response is determined statistically by highly coherent phase in repeated measurements at the target frequency, or by significantly greater amplitude of modulation spectral components than surrounding frequencies, or both.

ASSR detection is completely automated. In addition, it can be quite fast as a clinical measure. Picton has shown (Picton et al., 1998), by using a variety of modulation frequencies, that up to four stimuli can be tested in each ear simultaneously. This technique has been shown to be of value in assessing aided hearing thresholds in the sound field (Picton et al., 1998). Hearing thresholds have been estimated to be within about 10-15 dB of thresholds obtained by standard audiometric techniques in adults with normal hearing and hearing loss using the multifrequency ASSR (Dimitrijevic et al., 2002).

One reservation about the use of ASSR for measurement of hearing is the lack of good data on infants and children (Stapells et al., 1995). Rickards et al. (1994) have found that normally hearing infants may not have a reliable response below about 40 dB. This would make it impossible to distinguish between mild hearing loss and normal hearing, a distinction that is critically important for determination of amplification needs. Perez-Abalo and colleagues (2001) have shown that, although they were able to determine hearing loss in the severe and profound range, in general, there was only fair agreement between ASSR thresholds and hearing levels in children with hearing loss. Her data also show that ASSR was unable to determine hearing levels below 40 to 50 dB nHL in the children at any frequency. At this time it would be not be prudent to recommend the use of ASSR to determine hearing loss in infants and young children, especially those with mild and moderate hearing loss.

Assessment When Exaggerated Hearing Loss Is Suspected

On occasion, an individual may feign a hearing loss or exaggerate one during routine audiometric assessment for financial compensation, to gain attention, or to acquire some form of special treatment. The terms "pseudohypacusis" and "malingering" may be used to describe these cases. Pseudohypacusis refers to a hearing loss without an organic basis; malingering describes cases of willful simulation of a hearing loss. Regardless of the motivation for pseudohypacusis, the audiologist's responsibilities are to determine whether an individual is providing accurate thresholds and, if not, to estimate the true audiometric thresholds.

Some behavioral signs of pseudohypacusis include exaggerated behavior during a case history interview or report of a hearing loss that is inconsistent with an individual's apparent communication ability. Routine pure-tone and speech audiometry often reveal inconsistencies that are indicative of pseudohypacusis: poor agreement between repeated thresholds measured at one frequency (> 5 dB), poor agreement between average pure-tone thresholds and the speech recognition thresholds (> 6 dB), exaggerated inconsistency between average pure-tone thresholds measured with a descending procedure and speech recognition thresholds measured with an ascending procedure (> 10 dB) (Schlauch, Arnce, Olson, Sanchez, and Doyle, 1996), absence of a "shadow" threshold curve in the poorer ear in cases of a profound unilateral hearing loss, excellent speech recognition scores at relatively low presentation levels (20 dB above admitted threshold), and no response to unmasked bone conduction stimuli with bone conduction oscillator placement on the poorer ear.

In addition, acoustic reflex thresholds may be elicited at levels that are lower (better) than admitted behavioral pure-tone thresholds, confirming the presence of pseudohypacusis.

Pseudohypacusis frequently is resolved with reinstruction and repeated assessment of pure-tone thresholds using an ascending technique on the same day or on another day. Other behavioral techniques that can be used to estimate pure-tone thresholds with reasonable accuracy and without the need for special equipment are the Stenger test for cases of unilateral hearing loss (Newby, 1964) and the Sensorineural Acuity Level (SAL) test (Rintelmann and Harford, 1963). A simple technique is to count pulses of variable intensity (Ross, 1964), that is, to ask listeners to count a series of beeps. This technique is particularly useful for children.

For individuals whose exaggerated auditory thresholds do not resolve with these or other special behavioral techniques (e.g., Bekesy tracking, Jerger and Herer, 1961; delayed auditory feedback, Ruhm and Cooper, 1964), the ABR is the technique that will be chosen by most audiologists in the United States to estimate hearing sensitivity. Cortical

evoked potentials, also known as late potentials, can also be used successfully in the objective assessment of hearing for adults (Coles and Mason,
1984; Hone et al., 2003; Hyde et al., 1986; Tsui et al., 2002). A discussion of
techniques for management of pseudohypacusis can be found in a review
chapter by Snyder (2001).

Multiple Conditions

Patients may present with a variety of disabling conditions, in addition to the hearing loss, that may interfere with routine testing procedures. For example, a severe neurological or motor problem that prevents
an individual from providing a time-locked behavioral response requires
modification of the standard paradigm in order to obtain an accurate
measure of threshold. Any behavioral response that is under the listener's
control may be used to signify signal detection, such as a finger motion,
an eyeblink, or a directed eye gaze. Loss of visual acuity as the sole additional disabling condition generally has no effect on routine audiometric
assessment procedures. However, this condition would negatively impact performance on measures that combine auditory and visual presentation of stimuli. Individuals with mental retardation or developmental
disabilities may have difficulty responding to abstract pure-tone signals
with a standard behavioral response. Techniques used for children of an
equivalent developmental age may be applied with these persons. When
modified procedures do not produce reliable thresholds (pure tone or
speech) or suprathreshold speech recognition scores, then assessment with
electrophysiological techniques such as ABR is often utilized.

4

Testing Adult Hearing: Conclusions and Recommendations

KEY ISSUES

The committee was charged to answer several questions, which are addressed here as they pertain to adults. A few of these questions, dealing with nonspeech sounds, objective/physiological tests, and improving reliability, are relatively easy and are discussed first. The remaining questions involve issues of predictive validity—Can a particular result on a hearing test predict inability to work?—and are both complex and difficult; much of this section is devoted to a discussion of what is known and what is not yet known about these issues.

Nonspeech Sounds

Perception of nonspeech sounds is important in the workplace because many workers need to be able to detect, discriminate, recognize, and localize nonspeech sounds. However, there are no tests of discrimination and localization abilities of nonspeech sounds in routine clinical use today, and the committee therefore can make only recommendations for research in this area (see Research Recommendations 4-9 and 4-10). In contrast, the ability to detect nonspeech sounds such as warning signals can be predicted using procedures that take into account the intensity and frequency content of the signal and background noise, as well as the puretone thresholds (the audiogram) of the worker, with or without a hearing protection device (International Organization for Standardization, 1986).

Because jobs vary so greatly with regard to the need to hear warning signals (in many cases, accommodations such as visual warning signals can be substituted), and because the spectrum and level of specific warning signals would need to be known to predict signal audibility, the committee does not recommend their inclusion in the Social Security Administration (SSA) medical listings of Step 3. Rather, these issues are best dealt with in Steps 4 and 5 of the SSA process, when expert opinion on specific work conditions can be obtained.

Objective Tests

As described in Chapter 3, objective (physiological) tests, such as evoked potentials and otoacoustic emissions, are extremely useful for determining what part of the auditory system is affected in a person with hearing loss, and for testing persons who cannot or will not cooperate in behavioral testing. Nevertheless, in almost all cooperative adults, behavioral tests produce the best evidence of hearing abilities. For uncooperative adults, frequency-specific evoked potential threshold tests, while much more time-consuming than behavioral audiometry, provide good evidence of hearing loss, but only to the extent that they are known to correlate with pure-tone audiometry. These statements represent conventional wisdom in the international audiology community, and we are unaware of any data or even opinion to the contrary.

Improving Reliability

Current Step 3 procedures in adults require speech discrimination testing (which we refer to as speech recognition testing), but they do not specify several important variables: the word list used, recording versus live voice, the number of test words, the level of presentation, and whether people who use hearing aids or cochlear implants are tested with or without their devices. All of these variables affect the difficulty and the variability of speech tests. Recommended guidelines for speech testing used by SSA in Step 3 should control each of these variables to improve the reliability of speech testing.

Predictive Validity

The committee's key task, a very difficult one, is to recommend standardized hearing tests that optimally predict the inability to work, taking into account issues of hearing aids, cochlear implants, non-English-speaking claimants, nonauditory deficits, and the hearing demands of different workplaces. This task can be approached as a problem in diagnostic test accuracy (Swets, 1988). For any given test and cutoff (such as 40 percent correct on a test of word recognition, as in the current medical listings), a claimant will fall into one of four groups:

True positive (TP): test score is below cutoff and the claimant is in fact disabled.
False positive (FP): test score is below cutoff but the claimant can work.
True negative (TN): test score is above cutoff and the claimant can work.
False negative (FN): test score is above cutoff but the claimant is in fact disabled.

Obviously, TPs and TNs are accurate and desirable outcomes, and FPs and FNs represent undesirable errors. In general, the fewer errors the better, but what should be recommended if two tests (or two cutoffs) produce similar numbers of total errors but different proportions of FPs and FNs? For example, assume that for one group of 1,000 claimants the 40 percent cutoff on the speech test produced 20 FPs and 50 FNs. Assume further that a 60 percent cutoff produced 50 FPs and 20 FNs (because every additional TP reduces the number of FNs by one, an equivalent description of this hypothetical example would be that changing the cutoff from 40 to 60 percent produced marginal increases of 30 TPs and 30 FPs).

It would be impossible to choose one cutoff over the other based only on the total number of errors, but if one type of error were more undesirable than the other, one would pick the cutoff that minimized the more costly error. The costs of an FP error at Step 3 of the SSA disability process include reduced productivity from an individual who could be employed as well as the cost of SSA benefits. FN costs include the hardship of the wrongly denied claimant, although these costs can be reduced in Steps 4 and 5 of the process, in which a claimant denied in Step 3 may still be found to be disabled. If one test (e.g., word recognition) produced fewer of both types of errors than another (e.g., a sentence test), the choice of tests would be easy, but choosing the optimal cutoff would still involve a trade-off in which it is impossible to reduce one type of error without increasing the other. It is difficult to recommend optimal tests and cutoffs without specifying the relative costs of FP and FN errors; this would require a value judgment that is beyond the purview of the committee.

Regardless of the relative costs of FP and FN errors, if the "diagnosis" of a claimant for SSA is indeed "inability to engage in any substantial gainful activity," there are strong reasons, discussed in Chapter 1, to believe that this cannot be done with perfect accuracy in a process, like

SSA's Step 3, that considers only a claimant's hearing test results. This is true—even if one were to limit oneself to predicting the ability to understand speech at work—because there are three sets of variables that interact in determining how well listeners can recognize, identify, and comprehend speech, but clinical hearing tests can address only one of these sets. Hearing tests do not evaluate nonauditory variables specific to the claimant (age, education, intelligence, motivation, native language, cognitive problems, etc.), nor do they evaluate the variable communication demands of different workplaces. The spectrum of communication demand in the workplace is nearly infinite, but a few examples illustrate the broad range of possibilities:

1. Jobs in which accommodations for deaf and hard-of-hearing persons (e.g., email, instant messaging, and occasional use of interpreters) make it possible for them to function without ever needing to use speech communication;

2. Jobs that require only occasional unhurried conversation, face-to-face in a quiet office, talking with familiar persons about familiar subjects, with the opportunity to ask for repeats and clarifications;

3. Jobs that require frequent conversation with strangers about unfamiliar topics, often without the aid of vision (for example, on the telephone);

4. Jobs that sometimes require rapid high-stakes responses to unpredictable messages that may come from distraught strangers who speak English poorly, in noisy backgrounds without visual input (a police officer or firefighter, for example).

Job type 1 requires no hearing. There must be many such jobs: 75 percent of working-age men who describe themselves as deaf are employed (Houtenville, 2002). Job types 2, 3, and 4 all require hearing ability, but many people who could perform job type 2 would be unable, because of hearing loss or nonauditory problems, to meet the communication demands of job types 3 and 4. Job type 4 probably requires an alert, motivated, trained person who hears as well as a typical healthy young adult. Without knowing the distribution of jobs with differing levels of communication demand available to people who apply for SSA disability, and without knowing the distribution of nonauditory characteristics among claimants, it is difficult to propose a Step 3 medical listing criterion that would be likely to accurately identify people as disabled in all cases.

LIMITATIONS OF CURRENT FORMULA AND TESTING PROTOCOL

Hearing impairment in adults that qualifies for disability benefits under the existing SSA determination in Step 3 is a loss of hearing that is not restorable by a hearing aid. The current formula specifies that disability determination is met by documentation of average hearing thresholds (500, 1000, and 2000 Hz) of 90 dB hearing level (HL) or worse for air conduction stimuli and at maximal levels for bone conduction stimuli in the better ear or speech discrimination scores of 40 percent or less in the better ear. Expert testimony presented in the public forum held by the committee indicates that these criteria often fail to identify individuals who may be at risk in the workplace because of hearing loss, particularly those in hearing-critical jobs. There are several reasons for such failures:

• The existing formula for disability determination for adults doesn't take into account speech recognition performance at average conversational speech levels, which are likely to be encountered in everyday communication situations.

• The current procedure doesn't evaluate speech recognition in noise; poor speech understanding in noise could severely impair the ability to function effectively in many jobs that are dependent on oral communication.

• The current procedures and formula do not consider performance with a hearing aid or implantable device. Actual performance with these devices cannot be predicted from unaided performance. Direct measures of performance with the assistive device and appropriate weighting to the disability determination formulas should reflect the extent to which the assistive device benefits an individual with hearing loss for certain hearing-critical job tasks.

• The current protocol does not include assessment of sound localization, nor the ability to differentiate a change in an acoustic stimulus (i.e., sound discrimination). While these are fundamental hearing abilities, especially in certain hearing-critical jobs, there currently are no standard clinical methods of assessing these auditory functions. Research should be directed at this need.

• The current formula doesn't recognize that individuals with severe hearing losses (71-90 dB HL pure-tone average or PTA) cannot receive spoken communication auditorily without a hearing aid. Persons with severe hearing losses cannot detect the presence of conversational speech, nor can they accurately recognize the spoken message without a hearing aid. Many adults with severe hearing losses with early onset have not been successful hearing aid users, as described in Chapter 5, and function primarily in the deaf world. They have been educated at schools for the deaf, including postsecondary schools for the deaf. It should be noted that postsecondary schools for the deaf, including Gallaudet University and the National Technical Institute for the Deaf, have an enrollment criterion of average hearing loss exceeding 70 dB HL. Employment data demonstrate that, on average, adults with severe and profound hearing losses (> 70 dB HL) have a lower rate of employment (Blanchfield, Feldman, Dunbar, and Gardner, 2001) and lower earnings than individuals with normal hearing (e.g., Houtenville, 2002). The committee is not aware of published data that indicate any differences in employment trends between persons with severe hearing loss and persons with profound hearing loss. Finally, Food and Drug Administration regulations state that adults with hearing losses exceeding 70 dB HL may be candidates for cochlear implants, in recognition of the limited benefit that these individuals may receive from amplification. Thus, claimants with severe hearing losses who do not wear hearing aids or cochlear implants have essentially no ability to hear or understand conversational speech in the workplace and may be placed at a significant disadvantage as a result.

GENERAL RECOMMENDATIONS

The foregoing discussion suggests that there is a fundamental contradiction between the SSA's definition of disability based on a physical impairment and the reality of highly successful performance in the workplace by some individuals with these very same impairments. The committee deliberated about whether there should be medical listings at all. One could argue "no." However, we do not recommend eliminating medical listings at this time because evidence is lacking about their current performance (i.e., the error rate inherent in Step 3 and the quality and uniformity of individual evaluations in Steps 4 and 5) and because there are clear advantages of medical listings as consistently applied criteria that are less costly than requiring all claimants to proceed directly to Steps 4 and 5.

The committee debated whether there should be changes in the current medical listings for Step 3. For example, we carefully examined the evidence for changing the PTA cutoff from 90 to 70 dB. We do not recommend a change in the PTA cutoff at this time because evidence is lacking about the accuracy of the current PTA cutoff in correctly identifying individuals with severe disability and correctly rejecting individuals without severe disability.

The committee also considered whether the speech recognition score cutoff should change from 40 to 50 percent correct, or whether the current word recognition test should be replaced with a sentence recognition test. Again, we do not recommend a change at this time because evidence is lacking about performance of the current cutoffs and tests. In summary, there remain deficiencies in knowledge about the performance of current cutoffs in the medical listings, and it is difficult to recommend changes to them without knowledge of the performance of these criteria or alternatives to the existing criteria.

In contrast to the lack of data on the ability of clinical tests to predict ability to work, considerable research evidence now exists about the effects of procedural variables on the reliability and internal validity of performance on audiological tests. As a result, the committee is in a position to recommend removing ambiguities in the standard test protocol with the goal of improving the performance of the testing process. The principal recommended change to the disability determination process, therefore, consists of clarification of the methodological procedures used for the audiological assessment, which is expected to be useful for improving the reliability and validity of the test results. Additional test measures (e.g., speech recognition in noise) are recommended as part of the audiological assessment that will provide important documentation for decision points in Steps 4 and 5 of the SSA disability determination process.

The recommendations in this chapter are a refinement of the protocol for evaluating claimants for hearing impairment disability. The principal changes proposed for the evaluation of adults include testing speech recognition in the sound field while the claimant wears his or her own hearing aid or cochlear implant, in two conditions: (1) in quiet at 70 dB sound pressure level or SPL, using two 50-word lists of the Veterans Administration (VA) recordings of Northwestern University Auditory Test No. 6 (NU6) and (2) in two noise conditions (the noise is a single competing talker) using a single 50-word list in each noise condition, with speech presented at 70 dB SPL and noise presented at +10 dB and 0 dB signal-to-noise (S/N) ratios. If the claimant does not use a hearing aid or cochlear implant, then the speech recognition tests (quiet and noise) are presented to the listener in the sound field in the unaided mode (ears uncovered). An individual claimant is tested either in the aided mode or the unaided mode, but not both. The test in noise is included to provide relevant data for decisions in Steps 4 and 5. In addition, we propose adding a series of questions to be answered using a checklist during the audiological assessment to indicate the quality of the test results. A final recommendation for the protocol is to evaluate claimants who are nonnative speakers of English with speech recognition tests in their native language, if available.

There are no revisions proposed to the criteria for significant and disabling hearing impairment; rather, the existing cutoffs would be applied to measures obtained in very specific test conditions. Moreover, the criteria vary somewhat for claimants who wear a hearing aid or cochlear implant compared with claimants who are unaided. For claimants who do not wear a hearing aid or cochlear implant, the criterion for hearing disability is a PTA in the profound range (≥ 90 dB HL) or speech recognition performance less than or equal to 40 percent correct in quiet. For those claimants who wear a hearing aid or cochlear implant, the criterion for hearing disability is aided speech recognition performance less than 40 percent correct in quiet under specified test conditions.

These changes to the protocol are expected to yield an improvement in validity and can be supported by two generic examples:

1. Under the current medical listings, many persons with severe hearing loss who are not cochlear implant users are denied eligibility because their PTA 512 is better than 90 dB HL and their speech recognition score, measured at unrealistically high presentation levels, is higher than 40 percent correct. Many of these individuals are false negatives. Specifying the presentation level of 70 dB SPL in the sound field will certainly reduce these false negatives (but will also create some new false positives, it is hoped few in number compared with the reduction in the number of false negatives).

2. Under the current medical listings, assuming most SSA personnel don't permit aided testing, virtually everyone with a cochlear implant is declared eligible. Clearly, many of these individuals are false positives because with the cochlear implant they can perform well in the workplace. Specifying aided sound field testing will certainly reduce false positives (but will also create some new false negatives, it is hoped few in number compared with the reduction in false positives).

SPECIFIC RECOMMENDATIONS

The following discussion on tests for disability determination applies to tests that may be used in Steps 2, 3, 4, or 5 of the SSA disability determination process. Any recommendations for medical listings (Step 3) are identified explicitly as such.

Otolaryngological Examination

Action Recommendation 4-1. The otolaryngological exam that is required for disability determination should be performed by an otolaryngologist certified by the American Board of Otolaryngology. The recommended examination is described in detail in Chapter 3. The committee recommends that this examination follow the audiological testing, but by no more than six months. This reversal of the order of examinations from the current SSA guidance is based on the committee's judgment that the results of audiological testing must be considered by the otolaryngologist in reaching his or her conclusions about the claimant.

Criteria for Selecting Tests for Disability Determination

The committee considered a number of different issues in developing criteria for the selection of tests to be recommended for use in disability determination. Some issues were specified by the SSA: the tests should be readily available at no additional cost to the agency, should be part of the standard of care, should yield reliable and valid data, and should provide good descriptors of human performance in the real world. The committee was steadfast to the principle that each test must have undergone rigorous testing procedures for standardization, so that the following characteristics of the test are known:

- expected performance of individuals with normal and disordered auditory systems,
- expected variability in performance,
- expected performance at particular presentation levels and through particular transducers, and
- test-retest stability.

Another highly desirable goal was to select tests for which correlations are known between performance on the test in specific conditions and actual performance in the workplace. We also sought tests that could be performed in unaided and aided listening conditions to indicate the benefit that a claimant receives from a hearing aid, cochlear implant, or other assistive listening device in real-world situations. Tests that could be performed by claimants who are nonnative speakers of English were also preferred.

Few tests examined by the committee met all of these criteria. As a result, we identified tests that met most of the principal criteria specified. We recommend use of the tests described in this section until such time as new tests are developed, or existing tests are modified, to meet all of the criteria stipulated. As acceptable tests become available, they should be considered by SSA for inclusion in the disability determination process. Specification of required standardization procedures is provided throughout this section for the benefit of individuals interested in developing tests for future use by SSA.

The Test Battery Approach

Action Recommendation 4-2. In order to capture an accurate assessment of an individual's hearing abilities on a given day, a test battery is recommended. The test battery approach permits a determination of the validity of the claimant's responses by examining intertest agreement. If SSA continues to use both pure-tone and speech testing, then more than one test in the battery can be used to determine if an individual has met the requirements for a disability based on hearing impairment. A person who may not be able to take a particular test in the battery (e.g., because of a language barrier) may still have a successful claim on the basis of performance on other component tests in the battery. The measures to be assessed in the test battery for adults are:

- pure-tone thresholds in each ear presented via air and bone conduction transducers,
- speech thresholds using earphones in each ear,
- speech recognition performance for signals presented in the sound field at average conversational levels in quiet and in noise,
- tympanometry, and
- acoustic reflex thresholds.

The latter two tests are included to rule out conductive pathology, because a conductive component to the hearing loss often can be managed medically with improvement in hearing sensitivity. In addition, acoustic reflex threshold assessment can be useful in identifying cases of feigning a severe or profound hearing loss that would be undetected by other tests in the battery. It is recommended that the entire test battery be completed before a determination of disability is formulated.

Personnel to Conduct the Testing

Action Recommendation 4-3. The test procedures required for determining a disability based on hearing impairment must be conducted by a clinical audiologist who holds state licensure (if applicable). Audiologists working in states in which no licensure exists should be certified by the American Speech-Language-Hearing Association (Certificate of Clinical Competence in Audiology, or CCC-A) or by the American Board of Audiology.

Audiologists are hearing health care professionals who identify, assess, and manage disorders of the auditory system of individuals across the life span and of individuals from diverse linguistic and cultural backgrounds. They follow a stringent code of ethics (American Speech-

Language-Hearing Association, 2002). A professional audiologist is deemed necessary because the recommended procedures include performing tests with the claimant's own hearing aid(s) or cochlear implant(s) set to their optimal adjustments. The only professional who has the requisite knowledge, training, and clinical experience to perform these and other auditory tests comprising the test battery is the clinical audiologist.

Environment and Equipment for Testing

Action Recommendation 4-4

Test Environment

Audiological assessments are conducted in controlled acoustic environments to minimize the detrimental and unpredictable effects of background noise. The environment for assessment of auditory threshold must conform to standards of the American National Standards Institute (ANSI) for limits on maximum permissible ambient noise levels (American National Standards Institute, 2003a). The presence of noise in excess of these required levels produces shifts in measured auditory thresholds, particularly for low-frequency sounds.

The reverberation characteristics of the test environment should also be controlled if sound field measures are conducted. Reverberation refers to the prolongation of sound in a room, resulting from reflections of sound at the boundaries of the room enclosure. Reverberation is quantified by the reverberation time, defined as the duration, in seconds (sec), for a signal to decay 60 dB below its steady-state value after termination. The recommended reverberation time for the audiometric environment is 0.2 sec or less (American Speech-Language-Hearing Association, 1991a). Control of both noise and reverberation can be achieved with double-walled sound-attenuating chambers.

Equipment for Testing

The principal equipment used for behavioral assessment of auditory thresholds and speech recognition is the audiometer. The audiometer generates pure-tone signals and can present speech signals that are either live voice or prerecorded. The examiner controls signal intensity, stimulus temporal characteristics, and signal transducer (earphones, bone conduction vibrator, or loudspeaker). ANSI Standard S3.6-1996 (American National Standards Institute, 1996) specifies the reference-equivalent threshold sound pressure levels (RETSPL) for signals presented via earphones and loudspeakers, as well as reference-equivalent threshold force levels (RETFL) for signals presented via bone conduction transducers. These terms (RETSPL and RETFL) refer to the sound pressure levels or force levels of explicit signals (pure tones and speech), presented via specific transducers, that correspond to the average threshold of hearing in young adult listeners with normal hearing. A full electroacoustic calibration of audiometric equipment to these reference levels (or those specified in future, revised ANSI standards) should be conducted initially with new equipment and annually thereafter (American Speech-Language-Hearing Association, 2002).

Other types of audiometric equipment are used for the electrophysiological measures described in other sections of this report. Acoustic immittance meters measure the admittance of the middle ear system and are employed in assessment of middle ear function (tympanometry and acoustic reflexes). Calibration of these devices is detailed in ANSI Standard S3.39-1987 (R2002) (American National Standard Institute, 2000b). Auditory evoked potentials (e.g., electrocochleography, auditory brainstem response or ABR—see the section later in the chapter) and otoacoustic emissions (e.g., transient-evoked otoacoustic emissions, distortion product otoacoustic emissions) can be measured with clinical instruments or more sophisticated laboratory equipment. As of this writing, there are no national standards governing the calibration of this type of equipment. However, electroacoustic equipment should be calibrated to conform to the manufacturer's specifications, when appropriate (American Speech-Language-Hearing Association, 1993). All power-line-operated instruments must also satisfy minimum ANSI safety requirements for grounding and levels of electrical stimulation (American National Standards Institute, 1993).

A stringent protocol for infection control is used for all audiometric equipment (Cohen and McCullough, 1996). In particular, any audiometric supplies that come into direct contact with the external auditory canal (such as ear tips) must be either discarded after a single use or sterilized to prevent the spread of infectious disease.

The Checklist

Action Recommendation 4-5. The committee recommends that SSA require a checklist to accompany all hearing test results obtained for adults who are filing a claim for hearing disability. The checklist should be completed by the clinical audiologist at the time of the test and submitted with other data as part of the claim for disability. (Item 5 should be completed by the audiologist or the otolaryngologist, whoever is last to examine the claimant.) Thus, any individual interested in filing a disability claim based on hearing loss must ensure that the checklist is completed at the time of the audiological examination. The checklist is an indication of the quality of the data collected to be used in the disability determination process and includes additional useful information for evaluating a claim in Steps 3, 4, and 5. Checklist items, together with the rationale for their selection, appear throughout this section. The complete checklist is presented in Box 4-1, with a notation of answers that are unacceptable and thus require retesting. If any answers are missing or not satisfactory, the examination report should not be accepted for use in disability determination.

Brief Case History

A brief case history should be obtained prior to the hearing assessment for disability determination. The case history ensures that the individual is not experiencing temporary conditions that may affect the accurate assessment of hearing acuity. Essential questions to be asked during this brief case history pertain to recent noise exposure that may produce a temporary threshold shift. It is recommended that an individual not be tested if there is a history of recent noise exposure (within 72 hours) or if hearing sensitivity is noticeably poorer on the exam day, in cases of fluctuating hearing loss. Another important issue is whether the person experiences a fluctuating hearing loss. If the hearing isn't stable, this would suggest the need for additional testing.

CHECKLIST ITEM 1: Does the claimant work in a noisy environment?

CHECKLIST ITEM 2: Is there a history of significant noise exposure in the past 72 hours?

CHECKLIST ITEM 3: Does the claimant report a fluctuating hearing loss? If so, was the claimant tested on a day when his or her hearing was noticeably poorer?

A person's performance on some auditory tasks is often a function of the age of onset of hearing loss and mode of onset (sudden versus gradual). Adults who have a recent, sudden onset of hearing loss sometimes exhibit particular difficulty on audiological measures. A checklist item is included that inquires about mode of onset and, if sudden, if it was recent. For a very recent hearing loss, a second audiogram may be advised, after the claimant has had more time to adjust to the loss.

BOX 4-1
Checklist for Disability Determination

The following questions must be answered "Yes" or "No." A response that falls in a shaded box indicates that the test results are not acceptable. The test must be repeated on another day.

Item   Response

1. Does the claimant work in a noisy environment? — Yes · No

2. Is there a history of significant noise exposure in the past 72 hours? — *Yes* · No

3. Does the claimant report a fluctuating hearing loss? If so, was the claimant tested on a day when his or her hearing was noticeably poorer? — *Yes* · No

4. Did hearing loss begin suddenly? If so, did it begin recently (in the past year)? — Yes · No

5. Is the time between the medical exam and the audiometric exam 6 months or less? — Yes · No

6. Did the audiologist obtain a speech recognition threshold with respondees? — Yes · No

7. Did the evaluation yield information indicating that the test results appear to be valid? (Judgment based on PTA-SRT agreement, communication skills during the case history, and interlist consistency of speech recognition performance.) — Yes · *No*

8. Does the claimant wear a hearing aid, cochlear implant, or other device? — Yes · No

9. If yes, was the claimant tested with the hearing aid, cochlear implant, or other device? — Yes · *No*

10. Has the claimant been using a hearing aid or cochlear implant for a sufficient duration to derive maximum benefit from it? — Yes · *No*

11. Answer both (a) and (b), based on your professional opinion:
(a) Has the claimant been tested with a reasonably optimal amplification system or coclear implant? — Yes · No
(b) Is this person a candidate for either a hearing aid or a cochlear implant at this time? — Yes · No

12. Is the claimant required to use hearing protection on the job? — Yes · No

CHECKLIST ITEM 4: Did the hearing loss begin suddenly? If so, did it begin recently (in the past year)?

CHECKLIST ITEM 5: Is the time between the medical exam and the audiometric exam 6 months or less? (To be completed by professional who is the last to examine the claimant.)

Rationale and Procedures for Pure-Tone Testing

An essential component of the test battery is an assessment of the softest sounds an individual can detect. The standard pure-tone threshold audiometric test for stimuli presented via earphones (air conduction) and via a bone oscillator (bone conduction) is required for this purpose. The test frequencies include the octave intervals from 250 to 8000 Hz for air-conducted stimuli, and from 250 to 4000 Hz for bone-conducted stimuli, with masking used as necessary to eliminate stimulus perception by the nontest ear. The resulting pure-tone audiogram will permit a determination of the degree and type of hearing loss, as well as the relationship of the hearing sensitivity between the two ears.

The pure-tone test must be conducted without the use of a hearing aid or cochlear implant (unaided). That is, any device must be removed from the claimant in order to conduct the test. Even if an individual wears a cochlear implant, it is necessary to assess hearing sensitivity bilaterally as part of the record, and because there may be some residual hearing in the unimplanted ear.

Generally, a single audiogram is required for disability determination. If an individual reports being in a noisy environment within the past 72 hours, he or she must return for testing another day when they have been free of noise exposure for at least a 72-hour period of time. This is the amount of time required for recovery from a temporary threshold shift resulting from most forms of noise exposure. However, if there is a recent history of acoustic trauma (i.e., exposure to a blast or explosion) or of the use of ototoxic drugs, then a repeat audiogram may be necessary after 3-6 months recovery time (Pahor, 1981; Segal, Harell, Shahar, and Englender, 1988). A second audiogram may also be obtained in cases of fluctuating hearing loss, recent head trauma, or very recent, possibly unstable, hearing loss, when the audiologist makes this determination.

The pure-tone audiogram is useful for predicting speech recognition performance at average conversational speech levels (60-70 dB SPL) in quiet. It is an independent measure of hearing sensitivity, regardless of an individual's use of amplification. Pure-tone threshold testing can be completed successfully regardless of an individual's native language (assuming that test instructions are given appropriately); thus it is free of possible language barriers that can impede performance on speech recognition measures. An individual's performance on a standard pure-tone threshold test may also indicate signs of feigning a hearing loss or exaggerating a true hearing loss.

Pure-tone thresholds are measured with high test-retest reliability in cooperative adults (Carhart and Jerger, 1959). The 95 percent confidence interval for a measurement of pure-tone threshold is about ± 5 dB (Brown,

1948; Robinson, 1960). Because audiometric thresholds vary over about 100 dB, the confidence interval is about 10 percent of this range. Thus, pure-tone audiometry has been considered a relatively reliable test. Its validity has been tested by many studies comparing average pure-tone thresholds (most often for 500, 1000, and 2000 Hz, referred to in this report as PTA 512) to self-report using a variety of questionnaires that assessed hearing difficulties in everyday life (reviewed by Hardick, Melnick, Hawes et al., 1980; King, Coles, Lutman, and Robinson, 1992). Correlation coefficients typically ranged from 0.5 to 0.7, representing a moderately strong relationship between pure-tone thresholds and self-report. The pure-tone audiogram has been the standard test procedure for disability determination in the past. As a consequence, a comparison can be made between previous hearing test results and current test results, to determine if there has been a significant change in hearing sensitivity over time.

As described earlier, the committee decided to recommend no change in the medical listing criteria for pure-tone audiometry: 90 dB for PTA 512. We debated not only the "cutoff" of 90 dB but also the choice of PTA 512. It is clear that people with hearing loss limited to frequencies above 2000 Hz have more trouble in difficult listening situations, such as identifying isolated words in a noisy background without being able to see the speaker, than do normal listeners (e.g., Suter, 1985). Because of this, the American Medical Association and most state workers' compensation programs use PTA 5123 (adding 3000 Hz) as the variable on which "binaural hearing impairment" and monetary compensation are based. For the same reason, in Chapter 7 we recommend that disability for children, which begins in the mild range of hearing loss, should also consider frequencies above 2000 Hz. Nevertheless, we recommend that SSA retain the use of PTA 512 for adult disability determination for several reasons:

1. As is true for the 90 dB cutoff, there are no data to show that any other pure-tone audiometric variable would perform better in predicting an inability to work.

2. Frequencies above 2000 Hz appear to be less important for people with severe to profound hearing loss than for people with mild hearing loss (Webster, 1964). The Step 3 medical listings currently are applied at the boundary between severe and profound hearing loss.

3. Most research describing the problems and auditory performance of people with severe or profound hearing loss has used PTA 512 as the relevant classifying variable (e.g., Blanchfield et al., 2001; Corthals, Vinck, De Vel, and Van Cauwenberge, 1997; Flynn, Dowell, and Clark, 1998). We know of no study showing that another frequency combination correlates better than PTA 512 with the hearing difficulties of such people.

4. The demonstration that frequencies above 2000 Hz can make a difference in difficult situations cannot be extrapolated to a conclusion that they are as important as lower frequencies across the range of listening situations in everyday life. The research cited above does not demonstrate that any other frequency combination generally correlates better than PTA 512 with self-reported hearing problems. One reason for this finding may be that many everyday listening situations permit the use of vision; visual cues are complementary to low-frequency auditory cues and somewhat redundant with high-frequency cues. Another reason is that many everyday conversations take place in relatively quiet places and involve sentences rather than isolated words; both of these factors reduce the relative importance of high-frequency auditory cues.

There are many cases in which hearing sensitivity changes over time, especially cases of presbycusis, recent ototoxicity, and continuing noise exposure. In order to present a consistent report of findings to SSA, it is strongly recommended that the time interval between the audiometric assessment and the otological evaluation be 6 months or less. However, this may not always be reasonable in certain health care settings. If the audiogram is more than 6 months old and the claimant does not meet the listings, SSA may request a new audiogram.

Rationale and Procedures for Speech Threshold Testing

A speech threshold is a required measure in the test battery for the primary purpose of cross-checking the validity of the pure-tone audiogram and indicating the person's ability to detect and recognize speech. The standard procedure is to measure a speech recognition threshold (SRT) using recorded spondees and a descending procedure (American Speech-Language-Hearing Association, 1988). A checklist item should be completed to indicate that standard test stimuli were used for assessing the speech threshold.

CHECKLIST ITEM 6: Did the audiologist obtain a speech recognition threshold with spondees?

The SRT should agree within ± 6 dB with the three-frequency PTA (500, 1000, 2000 Hz) (Wilson and Strouse, 1999) or with the Fletcher average (average of two best thresholds obtained between 500 and 2000 Hz) in cases of audiograms for which the threshold at 2000 Hz differs from the threshold at 500 Hz by 20 dB or more (Fletcher, 1950). In the event that an individual cannot repeat the spondee words at suprathreshold levels, a speech detection threshold (SDT) should be measured.

In listeners who can perform both measures, the SDT is obtained at levels that are 8-12 dB better (lower) than the SRT because the SDT requires simple detection while the SRT requires detection and recognition. Because the SDT is obtained at relatively low levels, the SDT is expected to be better than the PTA by 2 to 18 dB. However, because detection thresholds are measured in both the SDT and pure-tone thresholds, the SDT generally corresponds to the best pure-tone threshold (Campbell, 1998). The audiogram forms should indicate the procedure, SRT or SDT, that was used in the assessment.

Consistency between the speech threshold and the pure-tone thresholds indicates that the audiogram is probably valid, and that should be noted on the following checklist item. In evaluating the validity of the hearing test results, the audiologist also should consider the claimant's communication skills during the case history and the overall consistency of speech recognition performance, in relation to the pure-tone audiogram. If the test isn't valid, it should be repeated and, if still invalid, the patient should be tested using auditory evoked potentials.

CHECKLIST ITEM 7: Did the evaluation yield information indicating that the test results appear to be valid? (Judgment based on PTA-SRT agreement, communication skills during the case history, and interlist consistency of speech recognition performance.)

If a claimant is not a native speaker of English, a recommended modification of the standard procedure for measuring SRT is to present digit pairs in place of spondee words. If the claimant is unable to identify these items with a verbal or a pointing response, then a SDT should be assessed.

Criteria for Selecting a Speech Recognition Test for Disability Determination

The ability to understand conversational speech in quiet and in noise is essential to communication in a range of work settings. For SSA disability determination, it is important to assess speech recognition performance in quiet to predict the extent to which an individual can receive instructions and communicate orally with coworkers, clients, patients, supervisors, and students in quiet listening environments. Because many work environments have noise backgrounds, assessment of speech understanding performance in simulated noise conditions is also important to predict the communication function of workers in these typical situations. The preferred procedure for assessing speech recognition for disability determination would be one that replicates a typical communication interaction in the workplace, including the type of communication message, the sex of the talker, the sound pressure level of the speech signal, the acoustic characteristics of the environment (presence of noise, S/N ratio, presence of reverberation, and reverberation time), and the ability to see the speaker's face. The closer the correspondence between the stimuli and procedures of the speech recognition test and communication in the workplace, the better the clinical test ought to predict performance in the workplace. Conversely, the more the test conditions simulate the claimant's specific job, the less standard the testing will be across claimants. This could result in a problem of perceived fairness.

The ideal assessment to determine an individual's disability in the workplace would be to conduct a task analysis of the communication demands placed on the worker, determine job-specific phrases in that work setting, assess typical background noise levels and speech levels experienced by the worker in the field, and attempt to closely approximate the work setting in the clinical audiometric assessment of the individual. Although this approach is expensive, it is at the very heart of the process of identifying actual disability on an individual basis. SSA should consider developing strategies to facilitate this type of work-related disability assessment for hearing impairment. Nevertheless, at the present time there is a gap in knowledge about the relationship between the communication performance of workers in real-world communication settings and speech recognition performance on current clinical procedures, and data are urgently needed to examine this relationship. Until evidence is available establishing a close link between clinical tests and actual performance in the workplace, SSA must rely on a set of commonsense principles to use in recommending appropriate tests for evaluation. To that end, the committee developed a set of specific criteria to use in selecting clinical speech recognition tests for disability determination at the present time. These specific criteria are in addition to those described above in the section on criteria for selecting tests for disability determination.

A basic principle is that a speech recognition test is a specific recording of test materials. A speech recognition test without recorded materials is unacceptable for disability determination for adults. In addition, if more than one recording of a set of speech materials is available, only the recorded version that conforms to the specified requirements may be used in the evaluation.

The first criterion in selecting a speech recognition test is that normative data must be available for the recorded test conducted both in quiet and in noise. The rationale for this requirement is that use of the same measure for testing in quiet and in noise permits a direct assessment of the impact of the noise environment on communication.

A second criterion for the speech recognition test is that normative data must be available for the speech signals presented at SPLs representing typical speech levels encountered in communication. Specifically, normative data must be available for a typical speech level of 60-70 dB SPL in the sound field (or equivalent level in dB HL), which is within the range of everyday conversational speech levels.

A third criterion for the speech recognition test is that normative data must be available for background noise presented at typical S/N ratios encountered in daily communication. A single S/N ratio representative of work settings is difficult to quantify, as noted above. An alternative to testing performance at one "average" S/N ratio is to evaluate performance at two S/N ratios that represent a moderate noise level and a more challenging noise level, such as +10 dB and 0 dB, respectively. A moderate S/N ratio is observed in many acoustic environments in which communication takes place with a slight noise background; the more severe S/N ratio represents only the most challenging communication situations. The more severe S/N ratio (0 dB) may be important for predicting communication performance in hearing-critical jobs known to have high noise levels.

Extrapolation of data published by Wilson et al. (1990) indicates that people with normal hearing score approximately 87 percent correct (standard deviation approximately 3.8-5.0 percent) at the more favorable S/N ratio condition of +10 dB. People with normal hearing score approximately 63 percent correct (standard deviation = 8 percent) in the more severe S/N ratio condition of 0 dB, on the VA compact disc version of the VA-NU6 with a single competing talker (Wilson et al., 1990). The committee recommends that this kind of additional testing in noise should be conducted for all claimants and should be included to provide data for expert opinion in Steps 4 and 5. Determination of significant difficulty in noise should be made after consideration of normal listeners' performance in noise, which, as noted above, is often less than optimal.

At the present time, there is only one speech recognition test that meets these three basic criteria: the VA compact disc (versions 1.0 and 1.1) of the NU6 test (Tillman and Carhart, 1966), as described in the normative studies by Wilson et al. (1990) and Stoppenbach et al. (1999) (henceforth referred to as VA-NU6).[1] While some limitations are noted with this test, particularly the use of monosyllabic words and only four equivalent lists, it is the only test for which normative data are available in quiet and in competition at typical S/N ratios. This version of the NU6 is the only test

---

[1]The web site www.va.gov/621quillen/clinics/asp/products contains details and ordering information about the test. We recommend that SSA work with the VA to acquire a license for the test and to develop a mechanism for mass distribution of this material to audiologists conducting assessments for disability determination.

identified by the committee that meets the recommended criteria for SSA disability determination. It should be noted that the calibration tone for the VA-NU6 test reflects the peaks of the carrier phrase. Thus, the root-mean-square (RMS) level of each test word is slightly lower than that of the calibration tone.

The "competition" or "noise" in this test consists of sentences spoken by a single talker. The single-talker competition was chosen rather than a broadband noise competition because for this version of the VA-NU6 test, the mean speech recognition performance levels of listeners with normal hearing are within the range 50-90 percent correct, over the S/N ratios of interest. Specifically, listeners with normal hearing exhibited mean speech recognition scores of approximately 87 percent and 63 percent at +10 dB and 0 dB S/N ratios, respectively, for the single-talker competition, but only 47 percent and 8 percent, respectively, for the broadband noise competition. There was a concern that measuring the performance of listeners with hearing impairment in the broadband noise competition at typical S/N ratios where listeners with normal hearing score so low would always result in floor effects. More importantly, using a single-talker masker gives the potential to identify listeners with hearing loss who are especially disadvantaged by background noise situations that are very little trouble to many other listeners. These are the individuals who may score considerably above 40 percent in quiet but less than 40 percent in noise at the +10 dB S/N ratio. This is because they are not able to take full advantage of the periodic dips in the level of the masker. The purpose for testing in noise is to identify persons for whom working in a noisy situation is worse than one might ordinarily predict. The committee determined that a single-noise masker is a good choice for that task.

The recommended protocol includes presentation of two 50-item lists of VA-NU6 for testing in quiet. Percentage-correct scores should be derived for each of these 50-item lists and compared. In addition, a composite score based on all 100 items should be derived if the two 50-item scores are within the maximum acceptable test-retest differences, as shown in Table 4-1. This table was constructed using Thornton and Raffin's data (1978, p. 515) (n-50 column) showing maximum acceptable differences ($p > .05$) between the two 50-word scores. Comparing the two 50-word scores permits the audiologist to determine whether or not the difference between the two test scores is within the expected normal variability. If the intertest difference exceeds the table entries, the test should be considered invalid. For example, if the lower score obtained for the two tests is 20 percent, then the higher score should be 36 percent or less for the two scores to be considered valid. In addition, the combined 100-word score has better reliability than a 50-word score. For example, the 95 percent confidence interval for a score of 40 percent on a

TABLE 4-1 Maximum Acceptable Test-Retest Differences for 50-Word Test Scores

If the lower score is:	Then the difference should be no greater than:
0 percent	4 percent
2	8
4	10
6	12
8 to 12	14
14 to 20	16
22 to 60	18
62 to 70	16
72 to 78	14
80 to 82	12
84 to 86	10
88 to 90	8
92	6
94 to 96	4
98	2

SOURCE: Based on Thornton and Raffin (1978, Table 4, p. 515).

50-word list is 26 to 58 percent, but for a 100-word score, the 95 percent confidence interval is narrower, 30 to 50 percent.

The recommended protocol also involves presentation of one 50-item list of the VA-NU6 test in competing message (single-talker competition) at +10 dB S/N ratio and one 50-item list in competition at 0 dB S/N ratio. The level of the speech signal is constant at 70 dB SPL. The nominal 70 dB SPL for the VA-NU6 test is actually a frequent-peak level. The long-term RMS level is closer to 65 dB SPL, comparable to the long-term RMS level of conversational speech. All speech recognition testing is conducted in the sound field with speech and competition presented through a single loudspeaker located at 0° azimuth at a distance of 1 meter from the listener. Stimuli presented in the sound field should be calibrated according to methods specified in ANSI S3.6 (American National Standards Institute, 1996). Additional issues regarding sound field measurements, including equipment specifications, the environment, and control of extraneous variables, can be found in American Speech-Language-Hearing Association (1991b).

Other tests may be developed or modified to meet the criteria listed above, and indeed this is encouraged, especially for tests that use everyday sentences or job-related phrases. There is some concern, however, that other tests will not yield equivalent scores to the VA-NU6, and results obtained with these tests will be difficult to interpret in relation to cutoff values established for VA-NU6. To be acceptable for use in disability determination, other tests must undergo rigorous standardization procedures. These standardization procedures include demonstrating the equivalence of scores on the new test relative to the VA-NU6 version for standard presentation levels and noise levels with the same group of listeners, the equivalence of scores on different lists of the new test, the content validity, and the test-retest reliability of the new test.

In addition to these requirements for any new test, there are preferred characteristics for tests to be developed. These characteristics include stimuli that reflect everyday speech, recorded versions that are standardized on listeners with normal hearing and with hearing loss, recordings in the most common non-English languages spoken in the United States that are standardized on native speakers of those languages, evidence of reliable scores, availability of numerous equivalent lists, procedures that minimize the influence of cognitive factors, a reasonable administration time, and known psychometric properties (i.e., performance-intensity functions). It would also be valuable for test developers to derive the frequency importance function, which indicates the relative importance of individual spectral regions for a particular set of speech materials, to improve the accuracy of articulation index (AI)/speech intelligibility index (SII) calculations, as well as the transfer function for the new speech material, which is a function relating the speech intelligibility score to the SII (American National Standards Institute, 2002e). The transfer function will depend on the syntactic, semantic, linguistic, and contextual information being transmitted, as well as the characteristics of the talkers and listeners; it will be useful for comparing expected performance on the new test to expected performance on other available speech recognition tests.

Many promising tests are currently available but not yet recommended for use in disability determination. One example is the Hearing in Noise Test (HINT) (Nilsson, Soli, and Sullivan, 1994). A notable advantage of the HINT is that recordings are available in several languages, in addition to English. This test meets many of the other desired characteristics of a recommended test, but it is not easy to obtain the test without purchasing additional equipment, the cost is high, and the test was standardized as a threshold test rather than a suprathreshold test presented at typical speech levels. The scores on this sentence test that would yield performance equivalent to scores on the VA-NU6 are not known.

Another attractive test is the QSIN (Etymotic Research, 2001), which involves presentation of sentence materials at multiple S/N ratios. However, normative data are not yet available for this test.

RECOMMENDED PROTOCOL (STEPS 3, 4, AND 5)
AND MEDICAL LISTING FORMULA (STEP 3)

The broad objective of the recommended disability determination for adults is to identify individuals who are unable to perform on the job because of the limitations imposed by significant and permanent hearing loss. The basic premise in determining the criteria is that an individual who cannot hear speech at a conversational level, or who understands fewer than 40 percent of isolated words without contextual cues in a typical listening environment, has a significant hearing disability. The recommended protocol and cutoffs for disability determination are intended to reduce the likelihood of failing to identify an individual with hearing loss who cannot function in a particular workplace. The methods used to accomplish this include evaluating claimants on speech recognition tests presented in the sound field at conversational speech levels and retaining the 40 percent cutoff for speech recognition performance in this condition for the Step 3 medical listing. The testing of claimants with their own hearing aids or cochlear implants in this condition is expected to reduce the likelihood of identifying people as disabled who are able to function well in the workplace with their own devices. In addition, testing in noise is recommended for the basic protocol at two S/N ratios; this information will be useful for evaluation of a claim in Steps 4 and 5.

There is very little research-based evidence to link performance on clinical audiometric tests with actual performance in the workplace, and this is perhaps the most pressing research recommendation for the SSA. Lacking empirical evidence, the committee relied on its collective expertise to develop a set of linkages between performance on clinical tests and expected performance on work-related hearing-critical tasks, presented in Table 4-2. On the basis of this framework, clinical test results indicating that an individual cannot hear conversational-level speech (as is the case for a claimant with a severe hearing loss who doesn't use a hearing aid), or understands no more than 40 percent of isolated words in a typical listening environment with minimal contextual cues and no visual cues, should be interpreted as showing that the claimant has a significant hearing disability.

The recommended formula does not change the medical listing for hearing impairment in Step 3. Rather, it changes the procedures for assessment that should significantly impact outcomes in Step 3. The current SSA formula defines hearing disability for claimants who do not use a hearing aid or a cochlear implant as a sensorineural hearing loss of 90 dB HL or worse in the better ear, based on the air conduction PTA of 500, 1000, and 2000 Hz and bone-conduction thresholds at the limits of the test equipment. A person with these audiometric characteristics cannot detect

TABLE 4-2 Relationships Between Performance on Audiometric Tests and Performance on Work-Related Hearing-Critical Tasks

Test Type	Performance Level	Expected Performance in the Workplace
Pure tones	PTA 512 ≥ 90 dB HL	Unable to hear or understand conversational-level speech; may detect amplified sounds only.
Pure tones	PTA 512: 71-89 dB HL	Unable to hear or understand conversational-level speech; will detect amplified speech; distortion of amplified speech usually present; hearing loss sufficient to render the individual a visually oriented person; may or may not be able to understand speech with a hearing aid without visual cues.
NU6 speech test in sound field at 70 dB SPL, in quiet	0-40 percent correct	Very poor word recognition performance in quiet; unable to understand most spoken words without contextual cues and without visual cues. Severely limited ability to follow novel auditory-only words embedded in instructions in the workplace. Severely limited ability to understand individual spoken words using the telephone. Severely limited ability to understand televised or videotaped spoken words if speaker is off-camera. Severely limited ability to understand a lecture if seated at a distance (unable to see the speaker's face). Severely limited ability to follow individual words in a conversation at a meeting when the talker or topic is switching.
NU6 speech test in sound field at 70 dB SPL with noise (+10 dB S/N ratio)	0-40 percent correct	Very poor word recognition performance in moderate noise levels. Severely limited ability to follow individual spoken words while using the telephone in a typical office environment (i.e., with moderate noise, such as background of people talking, office machinery noise, phones ringing, etc.). Severe difficulty understanding individual words in unfamiliar phrases, when there are limited contextual cues and no visual cues in a typical office environment (i.e., with moderate noise, such as background of other people talking, office machinery noise, phones ringing).

Continued

TABLE 4-2 Continued

Test Type	Performance Level	Expected Performance in the Workplace
		Severe difficulty understanding shouted individual words with a background of moderate-level equipment noise.
NU6 speech test in sound field at 70 dB SPL with noise (0 dB S/N ratio)	0-40 percent correct	Very poor word recognition performance in high noise levels.
		Severely limited ability to understand individual words in unfamiliar phrases, when there are limited contextual cues and no visual cues in environments with high noise levels.
		Severe difficulty understanding shouted individual words with a background of high-level equipment noise.

conversational-level speech without amplification and, as a result, has such limited audibility without a hearing aid or cochlear implant that they could not converse in most settings without visual cues.

The committee carefully weighed lowering the PTA criterion to 70 dB HL (severe hearing loss). However, data do not currently exist on employment trends for individuals with severe hearing losses, and it is difficult to determine the specificity and sensitivity of a change in the medical listings. As a result, the committee recommends retaining the medical listing in Step 3, based on PTA, until additional data are available (see research recommendations).

An alternative criterion in the recommended hearing disability formula is a speech recognition score of less than or equal to 40 percent correct, for speech stimuli presented at an average conversational level (70 dB SPL) in the sound field at $0°$ azimuth (directly in front of the listener) in quiet. Two full lists (50 words each) of the VA-NU6 test should be presented and a composite score derived (i.e., percentage correct out of 100 items). Claimants who wear hearing aids or cochlear implants are tested only in the aided condition, using their own hearing aids or cochlear implants set to the usual settings. If the claimant does not own a hearing aid or cochlear implant, he or she should be tested unaided with both ears uncovered. Individuals who meet the recommended medical listing for speech recognition are unable to understand most isolated words in sentences spoken at an average conversational level without visual or contextual cues.

Although it is true that there are no published reports of standardization of the recommended aided testing procedure, there is considerable published research supporting the use of monosyllabic word tests presented in the sound field at an average conversational level. For example, Larson et al. (2000) evaluated 360 individuals with moderate hearing impairment using NU6 words presented in the sound field in quiet at a conversational speech level in unaided and aided conditions. Mean unaided performance was approximately 58 percent correct and mean aided performance was approximately 88 percent correct. Similarly, Flynn et al. (1998) used a comparable procedure for assessing aided performance in individuals with severe and profound hearing losses. A number of studies have also assessed the performance of cochlear implant users with NU6 words presented in the sound field at average conversational levels (Fishman, Shannon, and Slattery, 1997; Tyler, Fryauf-Bertchy, Gantz, Kelsay, and Woodworth, 1997) or with other similar monosyllabic word recognition tests (e.g., Skinner et al., 2002). Thus it appears that use of the recommended test procedures is common practice for evaluating listener performance with hearing aids or cochlear implants, and that aided performance with these devices often demonstrates improvement over unaided performance.

The criteria above apply to the use of recorded, standardized speech materials, such as the VA-NU6 test (Wilson et al., 1990). Other speech recognition tests may be used in place of the VA-NU6, but the cutoff score for the disability criterion must be adjusted to the 40 percent equivalent score of the VA-NU6, delivered at a speech presentation level of 70 dB SPL in quiet. The equivalent scores must be established in the same subjects in a research study and must appear in a peer-reviewed publication prior to adoption for SSA disability determination.

The committee recommends that the standard audiometric protocol should include speech recognition testing in noise. As in the quiet situation, claimants should be tested with their own hearing aids or cochlear implants, adjusted to the usual settings, or unaided if the claimant does not use a hearing aid or cochlear implant. The recommended test is the VA-NU6 test presented at a speech level of 70 dB SPL with a single competing talker at two S/N ratios: +10 and 0 dB. A single, full (50-item) list is sufficient for each of these conditions. Both the speech and the noise (competing talker) should be presented through a single loudspeaker in the sound field, located at 0° azimuth. The +10 dB S/N ratio is intended to capture the acoustic characteristics of typical, moderate noise environments, whereas the 0 dB S/N ratio simulates work settings characterized by high noise levels. High noise levels are found in industrial settings with heavy machinery, on the runway at airports, inside the cab of trucks, at construction sites, inside homes and offices during cleaning with machinery, and in restaurants and bars, among others.

The selection of a single-talker competition in the evaluation protocol is somewhat of a compromise. The committee sought to include a speech recognition test in noise in the SSA disability determination process that conformed to the criteria stipulated above. As noted, there was only one recorded, standardized speech recognition test at the time of this writing that satisfied these criteria: VA-NU6. Although this recording of VA-NU6 words has been standardized with both a single-talker competition and a broadband noise competition, the performance of normal-hearing listeners in the broadband noise competition was extremely limited, suggesting that this noise would not be practical for testing listeners with hearing impairment.

Nevertheless, the committee recognizes that there are some limitations inherent in the use of a single competing talker. The level of the single-talker masker will vary with time; the level will decrease during the pauses between words and during the lower level parts of speech. Speech recognition scores with a single-talker masker will generally be higher than with a steady-state masker, because listeners can take advantage of the momentary improvements in S/N ratio that occur during the dips in the noise level. However, listeners with hearing loss may not be able to take advantage of these dips as well as listeners with normal hearing for various reasons.

A second issue relates to "informational masking" or the nonenergetic masking that occurs due to the perceptual similarity between the signal and the masker. Steady-state noise creates a direct covering of the target signal through energetic masking, but a background noise consisting of talkers creates informational masking in addition to the energetic masking. Thus, some of the advantage of the single-talker masker that results from improved S/N ratios during the dips may be minimized due to informational masking. This discussion underscores the need for additional research aimed at developing speech tests in noise using background noises that simulate different listening environments consisting of talkers or steady-state noise or both, and typical S/N ratios (see Research Recommendation 4-2).

When claimants are tested in the more severe noise condition (S/N ratio = 0 dB), their performance should be compared with normative data collected under the same test conditions. It is suggested that a criterion for disability in this condition should be at least two standard deviations below mean normal performance, and it is at the discretion of the expert providing an opinion in Steps 4 and 5.

If the claimant doesn't speak English, he or she should be tested in the native language using the SSA-recommended test or an equivalent test, if available. If an acceptable speech recognition test is not available in the claimant's native language, then a determination of disability will be made exclusively on the basis of the pure-tone threshold results. This could be perceived as unfair to persons who do not speak English well, since they would lose the chance to qualify on the basis of reduced speech recognition. According to the U.S. Census Bureau (2003) approximately 18 percent of the U.S. population speaks a language other than English in the home. Communication in some work environments also takes place in languages other than English. Thus, a priority for research is the development and validation of speech recognition tests in the most common languages other than English spoken in the United States that produce performance scores that are equivalent to those obtained on tests standardized in English. Individuals who cannot be tested reliably with standard behavioral techniques for pure-tone threshold assessment should be tested with auditory evoked potentials.

If an adult claimant wears a hearing aid or a cochlear implant, this must be noted on the checklist. Any claimant who wears a hearing aid must be evaluated in the unaided mode on the pure-tone threshold test and speech threshold test (described above) in addition to aided conditions for speech recognition testing (detailed below). Similarly, a claimant who wears a cochlear implant must be evaluated under earphones without the device, for the pure-tone threshold test and speech threshold test, and while wearing the device for the speech recognition tests.

CHECKLIST ITEM 8: Does the claimant wear a hearing aid, cochlear implant, or other device?

CHECKLIST ITEM 9: If yes, was the claimant using the hearing aid, cochlear implant, or other device during the speech recognition test?

In this case, the audiologist must determine how long the individual has used this device, the daily use of the device (hours/day), and if the individual has had a sufficient adjustment period to the device. The recommended adjustment period is at least 3 months for a hearing aid and 6 months for a cochlear implant. The audiologist also must measure the electroacoustic characteristics of the hearing aid following prevailing ANSI standards (American National Standards Institute, 2002c, 2002d, 2003b, or updated versions) and determine if the hearing aid is a reasonably optimal amplification system for this individual, in relation to the pure-tone thresholds and amplification targets derived from a hearing aid prescription. If the examining audiologist determines that the hearing aid is not a reasonably optimal fit for the claimant, it should be noted in Checklist Item 11. The audiologist should not alter the device, but should proceed to aided testing with the hearing aid set to the claimant's usual settings. However, the claimant should be encouraged to have the hearing aid adjusted by the fitting audiologist or the examining audiologist, and return for additional testing after a suitable period of adjustment. We strongly recommend that claimants who wear cochlear implants be evaluated at a center that programs cochlear implant devices and manages cochlear implant patients, to ensure that the cochlear implant map is appropriate for the patient at the time of the evaluation. If the claimant is tested at a cochlear implant center, then the audiologist should assess their map (t-levels and c-levels) and determine if the cochlear implant is operating adequately for this individual. If the evaluation does not take place at a cochlear implant center, then the audiologist should not make any adjustments to the device but should proceed to behavioral measures in the sound field. Several aided behavioral tests are recommended, in addition to those specified in the standard protocol, to ensure that the device is a reasonable fit for the claimant. These behavioral measures must be conducted with the hearing aid or cochlear implant adjusted to the claimant's usual settings.

The additional testing with the claimant's own device(s) consists of measures of signal detection in the sound field. Detection thresholds in the sound field are assessed differently with the two types of devices (hearing aids and cochlear implants), in accordance with current standards of care, although speech recognition measures are assessed identically. Behavioral measures obtained in the sound field for cochlear implant users include thresholds for frequency-modulated (warble-tone) stimuli and speech recognition scores in quiet and noise using the same stimuli and noises as recommended for unaided testing. A cochlear implant generally is considered to be working correctly if the electric thresholds to FM stimuli are 35-45 dB HL (assuming that electrode impedances are low and balanced and the battery is charged).

Sound field measures for hearing aid users are speech recognition thresholds and speech recognition scores in quiet and in noise. The recommended loudspeaker arrangement for sound field testing is for both target speech and background noise to be presented at $0°$ azimuth, to accommodate variations in monaural or binaural devices. Based on the behavioral and electroacoustic measures, the audiologist should complete checklist questions pertaining to the use and adequacy of the hearing aid or cochlear implant.

If a claimant does not use a hearing aid or a cochlear implant, he or she is tested in the unaided condition only. In some cases, the individual claimant will not wear a hearing aid or cochlear implant and the audiologist may determine that he or she can benefit from a hearing aid. Such a person should be encouraged to obtain an appropriate device through the state department of vocational rehabilitation or through Medicaid, because the expense of a suitable hearing aid or cochlear implant may far exceed the resources of the claimant. If the claimant is able to obtain a suitable hearing aid or cochlear implant, then he or she should be retested for disability determination after receiving the device and having a sufficient opportunity to adjust to it. We recommend that the claimant be fully eligible to receive disability support on the basis of unaided testing until they receive and adjust to their hearing aid or cochlear implant.

> **CHECKLIST ITEM 10:** Has the claimant been using a hearing aid or cochlear implant for a sufficient duration to derive maximum benefit from it (3 months for a hearing aid and 6 months for a cochlear implant)?

> **CHECKLIST ITEM 11:** Answer both (a) and (b), based on your professional opinion:
> (a) Has the claimant been tested with a reasonably optimal amplification system or cochlear implant?
> (b) Is this person a candidate for either a hearing aid or a cochlear implant at this time?

For aided evaluation, the speech recognition criteria for disability determination are the same as those recommended for unaided assessment. Specifically, if an individual demonstrates aided performance that is 40 percent correct or poorer in quiet, then he or she qualifies for disability. If an individual does not qualify for disability on the basis of aided testing, then the claimant is not awarded benefits at Step 3 (based on meeting the medical listings), although evidence considered at Steps 4 and 5 may result in the awarding of benefits.

Some work environments are characterized by high noise levels. The Occupational Safety and Health Administration regulations require workers to use hearing protection if they work in environments with noise levels exceeding 90 dBA for an 8-hour day, to reduce the traumatic effects of noise on hearing. However, the requirement to wear hearing protection can make it more difficult for people with sensorineural hearing loss to function on the job. Knowledge about employment in industrial settings with high noise levels and the communication demands in the workplace may be useful for disability examiners and vocational experts in formulating disability decisions in Steps 4 and 5. The need to use hearing protection can make the work environment even more difficult for a worker who would benefit from hearing aids in other settings, and might affect the claimant's ability to perform a particular job.

CHECKLIST ITEM 12: Is the claimant required to use hearing protection on the job?

Table 4-3 presents a nonexhaustive set of descriptors of auditory tasks that may be encountered in the workplace. The current set of recommendations addresses many of these auditory tasks, but not all of them. Table entries include identification of those tasks addressed in the current protocol and formula, as well as those not addressed. The hearing-related tasks in the workplace that have not been addressed are those that should be evaluated in future research aimed at identifying the importance of these tasks in the workplace, as well as developing tests to measure performance on these tasks.

TABLE 4-3 Dimensions and Difficulty of Auditory Tasks in the Workplace in Relation to Clinical Tests Measured in the Standard Audiometric Protocol

Dimension	Easy	Addressed?	Difficult	Addressed?
Talker familiarity	Familiar talkers	No	Unfamiliar talkers	Yes
Phrase familiarity	Familiar job-related phrases	No	Novel phrases	Yes (assumed)
Talker gender	Adult male	No	Adult female	Yes
Speech level	Maximum level for highest score (PB-max)	No	Conversational-level speech	Yes
Background noise	Quiet	Yes	Noise	Yes
Type of noise	Modulated	Yes	Steady-state	No
Energetic vs. informational masking noise	Energetic masking (no speech content)	No	Informational masking (speech content)	Yes
Number of background talkers	Single talker	Yes	Multiple talkers	No
Signal-to-noise ratio	Favorable (+10 dB)	Yes	Challenging (0 dB)	Yes

Continued

TABLE 4-3 Continued

Dimension	Easy	Addressed?	Difficult	Addressed?
Spatial separation between target signal and background noise or speech	Large spatial separation	No	No spatial separation	Yes
Visual cues	Visual cues (in addition to auditory cues)	No	Auditory cues only	Yes
Number of talkers	One	Yes	Multiple talkers, switching	No
Location of talkers	Fixed	Yes	Variable	No
Reverberation	Short (< .2 sec RT)	Yes	Long (1.0 sec or more RT)	No
Task duration	Brief	Yes	Long (> 30 min)	No
Signal quality	Excellent	Yes	Distorted (public address systems)	No
Language familiarity	Native English	Yes	Nonnative English	Yes
Use of hearing aid	Test with hearing aid	Yes	Test without hearing aid	Yes
Use of cochlear implant	Test with cochlear implant	Yes	Test without cochlear implant	No (no measurable performance)
Signal detection		Yes		
Discrimination of sound change		No		
Localization		No		

STEP-BY-STEP PROTOCOL

Action Recommendation 4-6. Presented below is a step-by-step outline of the recommended protocol. Table 4-4 summarizes the criteria for disability based on performance on pure-tone audiometry and speech recognition tests. Box 4-1 (p. 114) presents a listing of all items required on the checklist, to be included with the results of audiometric testing.

TABLE 4-4 Summary of Criteria for Hearing Disability

Test Procedure	Unaided Testing (for person who does not wear a hearing aid or cochlear implant)	Testing with Hearing Aid or Cochlear Implant
Pure tones	PTA 512 ≥ 90 dB HL in better ear and bone conduction at limits of equipment, OR	Not applicable
Speech recognition in quiet	≤ 40 percent at 70 dB SPL in sound field	≤ 40 percent at 70 dB SPL in sound field

Protocol for Person Who Doesn't Use a Hearing Aid or Cochlear Implant

Audiologist:

1. Assess pure-tone thresholds for each ear separately by air conduction under earphones and by bone conduction. Calculate PTA based on air conduction thresholds at 500, 1000, and 2000 Hz.[2] Assess SRTs for each ear separately under earphones. Conduct tympanometry and measure acoustic reflex thresholds.

2. Assess speech recognition performance for two full 50-item lists of monosyllabic words presented at 70 dB SPL in the sound field at 0° azimuth in quiet (speech recognition test: VA-NU6 recording or other equivalent tests approved by SSA subsequent to this report). Testing is binaural with ears uncovered. Calculate and report percentage-correct scores for each list individually and for the two lists combined. If the score in quiet is 0 percent correct, it is not necessary to continue testing in noise (Step 3).

3. Assess speech recognition performance for one full 50-item list of monosyllabic words (VA-NU6) presented at 70 dB SPL in the sound field in competing message (single competing talker), at +10 dB S/N ratio. Both speech and noise are to be presented from a single loudspeaker located at 0° azimuth. Subsequently, assess speech recognition perfor-

---

[2]If for any frequency the measured threshold is greater than 110 dB or if there is no response at the limit of the audiometer, a threshold value of 110 dB should be used for calculating the PTA.

mance for one full 50-item list of monosyllabic words (VA-NU6) presented at 70 dB SPL in the sound field in competing message (single competing talker) at 0 dB S/N ratio. Both speech and noise are presented from a single loudspeaker located at 0° azimuth.

Social Security Administration:

4.   Determine if claimant qualifies on basis of medical listing:

Is PTA in the better ear ≥ 90 dB HL and bone conduction at the limits of the equipment? If yes → qualifies.
   or
Is speech recognition performance in quiet ≤ 40 percent correct?
If yes → qualifies.

If claim is denied based on Step 3 medical listing, go to Steps 4 and 5 and review speech recognition performance in noise, in relation to workplace environment.

Protocol for Person Using a Hearing Aid or Cochlear Implant

Audiologist:

1. Conduct unaided testing, as above (pure tones for each ear separately by air conduction and SRTs for each ear separately under earphones, pure tones for bone conduction, tympanometry, acoustic reflex thresholds).

2. Evaluate the electroacoustic characteristics of the hearing aid, the map of the cochlear implant, and aided/electric sound field thresholds for appropriate stimuli.

3. Assess speech recognition performance for two full 50-item lists of monosyllabic words (total = 100 words) presented in the sound field in quiet at 0° azimuth, while claimant wears the hearing aid or cochlear implant, with the device adjusted to the user's normal settings. Testing is binaural with unaided ear uncovered. The speech presentation level is 70 dB SPL. Determine and report percentage-correct recognition performance for each list separately and for the two lists combined (speech recognition test: VA-NU6 recording or equivalent). If claimant scores 0 percent, it is not necessary to continue testing in noise.

4. Assess speech recognition performance in noise (single competing talker or other noise used with additional speech recognition tests ap-

proved by SSA subsequent to this report), with speech presented at 70 dB SPL and S/N ratio = +10 and 0 dB through a single loudspeaker located at 0° azimuth, while claimant wears the hearing aid or cochlear implant, with the device adjusted to the user's normal settings. Testing is binaural (if there is an unaided ear, it should be uncovered). Determine percentage correct (speech recognition test is 50-item list of VA-NU6 recording or equivalent, using a different list in each condition from those used in 3 above).

Social Security Administration:

5. Determine if claimant qualifies for disability.

If claimant scores ≤ 40 percent correct on speech recognition test in quiet → qualifies. If claimant doesn't qualify, use data collected in noise for Steps 4 and 5 disability determination.

ADVICE AND RECOMMENDATIONS FOR STEPS 4 AND 5

Action Recommendation 4-7. The current protocol includes evaluation of speech recognition performance in noise, in addition to the existing tests of speech recognition performance in quiet and pure-tone hearing sensitivity, with the goal of assisting SSA officers in evaluating claims in Steps 4 and 5. The committee recommends that SSA should examine the claimant's speech communication tasks on the job, in relation to performance on these audiological measures. The claimant should provide information about the communication and hearing requirements on their job. For example, the following communication requirements should be determined:

1. Does the claimant work in a job in which there is auditory or speech communication, and in what language?

2. Do most oral communication interactions occur in a quiet environment?

3. Does the job require two-way speech communication on the telephone?

4. Is oral communication in a moderately noisy environment (e.g., an office with coworkers talking)?

5. Is oral communication in a highly noisy environment (e.g., a factory or a restaurant)?

6. Is oral communication critical for life-threatening conditions in high noise levels (e.g., in firefighting or during a police action)?

7. Are hearing protection devices required in the work environment?

The specific communication requirements on the job should then be linked to the auditory skills that the individual possesses by examining Table 4-2.

RECOMMENDATIONS FOR NEEDED RESEARCH

The review of procedures and materials for assessing speech recognition underscores the need for additional research in a number of topic areas, particularly for purposes of developing speech recognition tests that predict functional hearing ability in the workplace. The committee recommends that SSA collaborate with other agencies, such as the National Institutes of Health and the U.S. Department of Education, to support a number of research objectives in this area. The first set of research recommendations presented below identifies those with the highest priority according to the committee.

Research Recommendations with Highest Priority

Research Recommendation 4-1. Develop standardized speech recognition measures and procedures that correlate with functional hearing ability in the workplace. Any new speech tests must be validated as predictors of performance on everyday tasks in the workplace. Validation may include establishing the relationship between aided and unaided performance on newly developed standardized speech tests administered in controlled clinical settings, either to corresponding performance on everyday communication tasks in the workplace, or to self-report or reports of others (supervisors, family members, coworkers) about oral communication difficulties. This validation step is essential for adoption of any new speech tests for purposes of disability determination.

Research Recommendation 4-2. Develop sentence materials that permit assessment of performance in both quiet and noise. Tests that quantify performance with a metric that is readily interpreted (e.g., percentage correct) would be particularly useful. Evaluation of the test properties with selected background noises that simulate different listening environments and typical S/N ratios (e.g., Pearsons, Bennett, and Fidell, 1977) is essential for estimating everyday performance.

Research Recommendation 4-3. Evaluate recognition performance for speech materials presented at conversational speech levels in the sound field by a wide range of listeners, including those with varying degrees of hearing loss and those who use hearing aids and cochlear implants. These must also be known to quantify the effects of hearing loss and the use of assistive devices on speech understanding in conditions that simulate everyday listening.

Research Recommendation 4-4. Assess basic auditory requirements of jobs, and how they relate to auditory measures that are available. This could be done on a job-specific basis, using an occupational taxonomy like O*Net, or could be based on some set of basic hearing functions.

Research Recommendations with Secondary Priority

Research Recommendation 4-5. Develop speech recognition tests in the most common languages other than English spoken in the United States, in order to evaluate nonnative speakers of English in a comprehensive assessment protocol comparable to that used with native speakers of English. Based on reports by the U.S. Census Bureau, 2003, the most common languages are Spanish (28 million speakers) and Chinese (2 million speakers), with French, German, Tagalog, Vietnamese, Korean, Russian, Polish, and Arabic also spoken by at least half a million residents each. The psychometric properties (performance-intensity functions, performance at varying S/N ratios, etc.) of these tests in a foreign language must be evaluated, as well as the validity of response formats that can be scored by audiologists unfamiliar with the test language.

Research Recommendation 4-6. Standardize video-recorded (VCR or DVD) sentence tests presented in unisensory and bisensory modalities. These would be particularly valuable to assess the extent to which the availability of visual cues aids speech reception in everyday listening situations by individuals with significant hearing loss. Normative evaluation of the psychometric properties of the materials presented in the unisensory (auditory) and bisensory (auditory + visual) modalities must be available before such tests could be adopted for use in disability determination.

Research Recommendation 4-7. Develop and validate methods to detect and manage exaggeration of speech recognition problems during administration of the speech tests, including comparison of AI/SII predictions to the observed score in quiet.

Research Recommendation 4-8. Evaluate the accuracy of the current Step 3 medical listing for hearing impairment that qualifies for disability. The committee recommends that SSA collect and analyze longitudinal data on documented earnings on claimants who fail to win eligibility over the next several years. (Such data are already available to the SSA.) All personal identifying information would be masked and the research design would be approved by the appropriate institutional review board. People who have no significant earnings from employment could be characterized as "false negatives" and people who have significant earnings would be "true negatives." In addition, performance data for those who are granted benefits or who are medically eligible but do not receive benefits could also be tracked. For all claimants, sound field testing should be performed (with hearing aids if the claimant has them), both in quiet and in noise, as part of the new recommended protocol. SSA could then analyze which of the hearing test measures (PTA, speech recognition performance in the sound field for VA-NU6 presented in quiet, speech recognition performance in the sound field for VA-NU6 in noise at two S/N ratios) predicted the outcome (false negative versus true negative). Conceivably, two or more variables could provide independent predictive power, justifying use of a composite variable in a new medical listing. If there is just one best predictor, SSA could then find the best new cutoff score by examining the marginal changes in the FN/TN ratio as the cutoff is varied.

Research Recommendation 4-9. Develop and validate clinical tests of localization for purposes of estimating everyday performance in real-world environments while listeners are unaided or use hearing aids or cochlear implants.

Research Recommendation 4-10. Develop and validate clinical tests of auditory discrimination for evaluating the ability to detect small changes in acoustic signals necessary for hearing-critical jobs.

5

Sensory Aids, Devices, and Prostheses

In disability determination for people with hearing loss, how should the Social Security Administration (SSA) account for the potential benefits that the individual might receive from a sensory aid? In determining vision-based disability, SSA mandates testing with "best correction," but for claimants with hearing loss, currently most SSA guidance directs that they should be tested without correction. Hearing aids cannot be fitted like eyeglasses, whereby a quick refraction arrives at a prescription that provides the "best correction" almost immediately. The process of achieving the best hearing correction for an individual can be long and complicated. Prosthetic correction for hearing impairment is often not as successful as vision correction, leaving the individual with substantial residual limitations. Many individuals find that the positive benefits of the prosthesis do not outweigh the negative consequences (such as ear discomfort, feedback squeal, high cost, and stigma), and they may elect to continue without correction.

This chapter reviews the variety of devices that typically are used to ameliorate the effects of hearing loss. Wearable personal devices include hearing aids and cochlear implants, as well as auditory brainstem implants. In addition, there is a class of ancillary devices called assistive listening devices (ALDs) that may be used alone or in combination with hearing aids or implants. The chapter briefly describes the main types of devices and discusses some of the issues involved in their provision and use.

HEARING AIDS

Conventional wearable hearing aids are self-contained amplifying systems. They include a microphone to pick up sound energy, an amplifier to boost the level of the signal, and various filters and other devices that modify the sound to match it more precisely to the needs of the impaired listener. In addition, air conduction instruments include a miniature loudspeaker (called a receiver) to generate the amplified sound, which is routed into the ear canal. Bone conduction instruments deliver energy to the cochlea by vibrating the skull with a small transducer. Finally, all hearing aids require a power source (battery).

Early hearing aids were worn on the body or carried in a pocket, but these types are very seldom seen today. Current air conduction hearing aids are almost all worn at ear level, and there are several different styles.

Behind-the-ear (BTE) models fit snugly over the pinna of the external ear and deliver sound to the ear canal through a plastic tube and plug (earmold).

In-the-ear (ITE) models are manufactured with all the components inside the custom earmold. This type of hearing aid fits into the concha of the ear.

In-the-canal (ITC) models are smaller ITE versions that fit mostly into the outer end of the ear canal.

Completely-in-the-canal (CIC) models are the smallest devices and fit entirely inside the ear canal.

Bone conduction hearing aids are used only when the ear canal is not able to accommodate or tolerate the insertion of an air conduction device. Conventional bone conduction devices use a BTE-style case and incorporate a vibrator that is held against the skull using a spring headband.

Signal Processing in Hearing Aids

At the most basic level, a hearing aid simply increases the loudness of sounds presented to the impaired ear. Most hearing aids also modify sounds somewhat to attempt to compensate for specific features of the individual hearing loss. It is typical to shape the frequency response to provide more amplification for frequencies for which the hearing loss is greater: this is called selective amplification. In addition, to accommodate the reduced range of sound levels available to typical hearing-impaired listeners, many instruments provide more gain for soft environmental sounds than they do for louder sounds: this is called wide dynamic range compression (WDRC) processing. Another important feature in many modern instruments is the inclusion of a directional microphone that is able to partially suppress sounds from the back and sides of the wearer in some listening environments, on the assumption that sounds from these directions have less functional importance than sounds from in front.

Some instruments filter the signal into several bands (usually 2-4 but sometimes more) to shape the frequency response. Others use several independent channels to make compression processing more precise. Still others combine both approaches. Much of this processing can be accomplished using analog technology or digitally programmable analog (hybrid) devices. However, current trends are toward using all-digital processing in hearing aids. Digital processing is able to accomplish selective amplification, compression processing, and directional sensitivity in more complex and sophisticated ways and with greater flexibility than previously possible in analog and hybrid devices. In addition, digital processing opens the door for the development of new features, such as noise management, speech enhancement, and feedback reduction. Most of the potential advantages of digital processing have not been fully realized at this time.

Candidacy for Hearing Aids

Hearing aids should not be considered for management of hearing loss until all treatable otological problems have been addressed. Use of hearing aids and cochlear implants by children with hearing loss is considered in Chapter 7.

For adults with hearing loss, hearing aids can be useful when hearing thresholds in the better ear are poorer than about 25 dB HL. In practice, most adults do not seek amplification until their hearing loss is sufficient to cause more than occasional problems in daily life. This "low fence" differs across individuals and is influenced by auditory demands. However, if hearing loss in the better ear in the mid-frequency region is worse than about 40 dB, typical adults will experience considerable problems in everyday communication, especially when ambient noise is present. About 70 to 80 percent of adults with bilateral hearing loss prefer to wear two hearing aids. The purported advantages of two hearing aids over one include improved speech recognition in difficult listening environments, improved localization, reduced head shadow effect, and a better sense of auditory space. However, it should be noted that substantial benefit can be obtained from a single hearing aid, even in the presence of bilateral hearing loss (see, e.g., Chung and Stephens, 1986; Kobler, Rosenhall, and Hansson, 2001).

Adults with severe hearing loss (greater than 70 dB) or worse may derive limited benefit from hearing aids. Many are candidates for a cochlear implant (discussed later in this chapter).

Although current hearing aids have the potential to benefit many individuals with mild to severe hearing loss, it appears that only about 22 percent of potential hearing aid candidates choose to obtain amplification (Kochkin, 2001). Many efforts have been made to determine the reasons for the low take-up rate and methods for increasing it, but this has proved to be an intransigent problem. Issues such as high cost, low perceived benefit, stigma associated with hearing loss, and denial of hearing problems may contribute to the low acceptance rate of hearing aids. As a result of these complicating factors, many individuals do not have or use amplification despite having pure-tone thresholds that suggest that they are hearing aid candidates.

Selection and Adjustment Issues

The term "hearing aid fitting" is used to encompass the process of selecting, adjusting, and fine-tuning an appropriate hearing aid for a person with hearing loss. Although there is not a fully developed science of hearing aid selection and fitting, there are several generally recognized principles. An ideal fitting will:

1. restore audibility for sounds that are soft but audible to people with normal hearing;
2. present conversational speech at a comfortable loudness level for the listener with hearing loss;
3. allow normally loud sounds to be perceived as loud;
4. prevent any sounds from violating the loudness discomfort threshold; and
5. preserve a natural, pleasant sound quality with minimal distortion.

Simultaneous achievement of all these goals often is not possible. In these cases, compromises are necessary and the best compromises are often reached using a trial-and-error method.

In many hearing aid fittings, the amount of amplification needed at each frequency is determined on the basis of a theoretical prescription. Several prescriptive methods have been developed and can be found in the audiology literature. The most thoroughly validated method is the one developed by Byrne and Dillon (1986) entitled the National Acoustics Laboratory Revised (NALR) procedure. This procedure has become the de facto gold standard for newer procedures, which may offer additional features. The NALR method provides a gain-by-frequency prescription for a single input level (conversational speech). If a WDRC hearing aid is used, additional decisions must be made about the parameters of the compression processing. These include the number of channels of compression, the input levels at which compression is initiated, how much compression to use, and how to rapidly modify the signal for best results. Some newer procedures, for example, NAL-NL1 (Byrne, Dillon, Ching, Katsch, and Keidser, 2001), DSLi/o (Cornelisse, Seewald, and Jamieson, 1995), and Cambridge (Moore, 2000), offer guidelines for some of these decisions. Even when these guidelines are used as a starting point, trial and error may be necessary to determine the best combination of settings for the individual listener.

After a hearing aid has been selected and tentatively adjusted to the appropriate settings for the listener, it is important to determine how closely the amplification matches the theoretical goals (i.e., the prescription). This part of the fitting process is called "verification," and it can be completed in several ways. One widely used method of verification, and indeed the only method currently possible with very young children, is accomplished using a probe-tube microphone in the ear canal. The probe tube is placed in the listener's ear canal and sound measurements are made both with and without the hearing aid. The difference between the aided and unaided measurements is a measure of the effective amplification provided by the fitting overall. This quantity is compared with the prescription goals, and adjustments are made until the match is satisfactory, or as good as possible. With listeners who can respond appropriately, other methods of verification are often used instead of, or in addition to, ear canal probe tube microphone measures. These include aided thresholds, sound quality ratings, and aided speech recognition tests. After the hearing aid fitting and verification are complete, a period of accommodation and adjustment is necessary before the maximum benefit can be obtained from the hearing aids. During this period, which may last from a few weeks to a few months, follow-up appointments that allow input from the hearing care professional can be important in facilitating the best outcome. This input may take the form of problem-focused counseling, hearing aid adjustments, or group audiological rehabilitation classes, depending on the needs of the hearing aid wearer. This post-fitting component of hearing aid provision is often overlooked or minimally performed. For many clients, this probably contributes to a less-than-optimal long-term outcome.

Problems Not Solved by Hearing Aids

Even when hearing aids are fitted competently, hearing aid wearers often continue to experience a variety of problems.

Even the most sophisticated hearing aids do not restore hearing to normal. Wearers often still cannot detect soft sounds. Even sounds that are audible may not be heard clearly or comfortably. These facts are often not realized by people without hearing loss, who may expect a level of performance from the hearing aid wearer that is beyond his or her ability, even with amplification. These shortcomings add to the frustrations of adjusting to wearing hearing aids.

For many hearing aid wearers who have sensorineural hearing loss, the major concern is an inability to understand speech in a situation when background noise is present. This is generally agreed to be a physiological problem resulting from hair cell loss. Recent data suggest that temporal processing and cognitive abilities also may impact speech understanding in noise. Hearing aids often do not help substantially with this problem. Thus, communication in noise remains a major difficulty for many hearing aid wearers.

The highest possible output of the hearing aid is typically adjusted with the goal of maximizing the range and variety of sounds available to the listener without causing loudness discomfort. Sometimes this effort is not fully successful, and certain environmental sounds are experienced at unpleasant loudness levels.

Another problem is that when sound that is produced by the hearing aid leaks back out of the ear canal and reaches the hearing aid's microphone, an annoying (and embarrassing) whistling can be produced. This type of feedback loop can be created by a variety of combinations of gain, earmold fit, and external conditions (such as the proximity of a hat brim or a nearby wall).

Feedback can be especially problematic when a telephone is placed near a hearing aid, as in normal telephone use. The resulting squeal can prevent effective telephone communication while using the hearing aid. Some individuals with relatively mild hearing loss can communicate on the telephone without the hearing aid, but this is not possible for those with more severe hearing problems. An induction coil (T-coil) built into the hearing aid can solve this problem for many individuals, but these coils are sometimes not provided, or the hearing aid wearer may not know how to use the T-coil, or the telephone may not be hearing aid compatible (i.e., it does not produce a suitable magnetic field for the T-coil to use).

Finally, the hearing aid wearer's own voice may be unpleasantly loud when the device is worn due to the effects of plugging the ear canal with the earmold or hearing aid. Sometimes this problem is severe enough to prompt the user to reject the device.

Hearing Aid Fitting Outcomes in Adults

There are two basic approaches to the measurement of hearing aid fitting outcomes: the first involves measures of the hearing aid's technical merit when in situ. The second involves measures of the extent to which the amplification system as a whole is reported to have alleviated the daily life problems of the person with hearing loss and his or her family. Much early research concentrated on technical outcomes. It was assumed that subjective (real-life) outcomes would be accurately predicted from these objective data. It is now clear that this often is not the case. Real-life problems associated with hearing loss are complicated by such contextual issues as personality, lifestyle, environment, and family dynamics, and these play an important part in the ultimate success of a hearing aid fitting. Numerous studies have shown that measures of technical merit are not strongly predictive of real-life effectiveness of hearing aid fitting (e.g., Souza, Yueh, Sarubbi, and Loovis, 2000; Walden, Surr, Cord, Edwards, and Olsen, 2000). Thus, it is now recognized that real-life outcomes of a fitting must be assessed separately from the technical merit of the hearing aid. Many researchers feel that both types of data are essential for a full description of hearing aid fitting outcome.

The technical merit of a fitted hearing aid may be assessed acoustically using, for example, real-ear probe-microphone measures (e.g., Mueller, Hawkins, and Northern, 1992) or audibility measures, such as the speech intelligibility index (American National Standards Institute, 2002). An equally popular approach to exploring technical merit involves psychoacoustic data, especially speech recognition scores measured in quiet or in noise (e.g., Shanks, Wilson, Larson, and Williams, 2002).

The real-life effectiveness of a hearing aid is measured using subjective data provided by the person with hearing loss or by significant others. Numerous questionnaires have been developed and standardized specifically for the purpose of assessing hearing aid fitting outcomes, and many others have been conscripted to serve this application (see reviews in Bentler and Kramer, 2000; Noble, 1998, Tables 4.1 and 4.2).

Research on Outcomes

Although the literature is replete with data depicting technical and real-life hearing aid fitting outcomes for relatively small groups (N < 50) of participants, most of these are experimental studies and do not attempt to determine the typical outcomes of representative contemporary hearing aid fittings. There are not many studies that describe results from large groups of clinic patients originating in the United States who have been fitted with current-technology hearing aids.

Larson et al. (2000) described a carefully controlled and conducted crossover trial with 360 older adults with moderate bilateral sensorineural hearing loss. Each of three hearing aid circuits was used for three months by each subject. Outcome measures included speech recognition tests and self-report using a standardized questionnaire. When speech was presented at a conversational level, recognition of monosyllabic words in quiet improved about 30 percent (from 58 to 88 percent) with amplification. When noise was present at +7 dB signal to noise (S/N) ratio (on average), unaided sentence recognition scores were about 48 percent and aided scores averaged about 64 percent. Thus, appropriate amplification improved sentence recognition in noise about 16 percent for the typical listener. Haskell et al. (2002) reported subjective outcomes from the same investigation of 360 adults. They noted that, without hearing aids, the subjects reported experiencing communication problems in about 40 percent of quiet situations and 65 percent of noisy situations. Subjective reports of real-life benefits indicated that with hearing aids, subjects reported a 20-25 percent lower frequency of problems for speech communication in quiet and a 30 percent lower frequency for communication in noisy settings.

Humes, Wilson, Barlow, and Garner (2002) presented comparable data for 134 older adults with moderate hearing loss. In this study, sentence recognition was measured after one year of hearing aid use. Results indicated that understanding of sentences at a conversational level with a +8 dB S/N ratio increased by about 19 percent for the average hearing aid user; unaided performance scores averaged about 55 percent and aided scores were about 74 percent.

Like most reports of hearing aid outcomes, the studies by Larsen et al. (2000) and Humes et al. (2002) focused on listeners with moderate hearing loss. It is likely that individuals who seek Social Security disability benefits would have more severe hearing losses than these groups. The literature yields relatively few data reflecting the performance of people with severe and profound hearing loss who have been fitted with appropriate hearing aids.

Flynn, Dowell, and Clark (1998) reported a study employing 34 listeners with severe or profound hearing loss who wore carefully fitted hearing aids. To be eligible for this study, subjects were required to be proficient in the use of spoken English. The typical subject achieved a recognition score of 55 percent when listening to amplified monosyllabic words in quiet. Everyday sentences produced an average recognition score of 72 percent in quiet and 58 percent with a +10 dB S/N ratio. It should be emphasized that the variability across subjects was large (as usually seen in studies of listeners with hearing loss): standard deviations were on the order of 25-30 percent.

Kuk, Potts, Valente, Lee, and Picirrillo (2003) reported a study of 20 individuals with severe or profound hearing losses who were carefully fitted with high-technology hearing aids. Proficiency in spoken English was not reported to be a selection criterion in this study. For speech presented at a conversational level in quiet, subjects were able to repeat about 15 percent of amplified sentences that contained no contextual cues and about 33 percent of sentences that were high in contextual cues. These subjects reported that when they use hearing aids, they experience difficulty in real life about 25 percent of the time in quiet and about 50 percent of the time in noise.

Although the mean pure-tone thresholds of the subjects studied by Kuk et al. (2003) were only slightly poorer than those studied by Flynn et al. (1998), the aided speech recognition performance observed by Kuk et al. was notably worse than that measured by Flynn et al. Such inconsistent outcomes are not unusual in investigations of individuals with hearing loss, especially in studies with small numbers of subjects. Many listener variables, such as the ability to perceive acoustic features of sounds and to utilize contextual cues, have an impact on speech recognition scores. In addition, acoustic variables such as the particular speech test used, the presentation level, and the characteristics and level of any background noise, all strongly affect obtained recognition scores. Thus, some individuals with significant hearing loss are able to perform quite well in situations requiring speech communication, while others with similar pure-tone thresholds are almost completely unsuccessful.

COCHLEAR IMPLANTS

Profound neurosensory hearing loss is one of the most significant impediments to an individual's ability to successfully communicate with other human beings using audition and spoken language. If the hearing loss occurs prior to the development of speech and language, additional lifelong reading and spoken language deficits confront those who are profoundly deaf. Individuals with moderate to severe hearing loss experience difficulty hearing sound and, more importantly, understanding speech clearly. In the presence of competing noise or other sounds speech understanding is more impaired. In the past, the only rehabilitative assistance for people with severe to profound hearing loss was the amplification of sound by hearing aids and the use of sign language. However, hearing aids can only make sound louder without providing important speech cues to improve the discrimination or understanding of words. They also do not provide sufficient cues to assist hearing in background noise.

The development of the cochlear implant has radically altered the habilitation and rehabilitation of profoundly deaf children and adults. The past 25 years of basic science and clinical research have shown that cochlear implants are safe and effective in improving speech perception in both children and adults. The introduction of this technology into clinical practice over the past 10 years has generated renewed interest in the etiology and the methods of assessment of individuals with profound hearing loss. In this section we review the hardware and software components of a cochlear implant, present patient selection criteria for an implant, and discuss speech perception results in postlingually deafened adults with multichannel cochlear implants. The same cochlear implants are used for management of profound deafness in children deafened prelingually (before age 2) and postlingually. The indications and results for children are discussed in Chapter 7.

Cochlear Implant Devices

Cochlear implants attempt to replace the transducer function of damaged inner ear hair cells. Most causes of sensorineural deafness result in injury to the hair cells rather than to auditory nerve fibers. Prolonged deafness eventually affects the auditory nerve, as its neurons rely on neurotrophic factors (proteins produced by hair cells) for their survival. It has been shown that electrical stimulation provided by cochlear implants can prevent neural degeneration (Leake, Hradek, and Snyder, 1999). The devices are continually undergoing modification and upgrading; however, the basic components of the systems have not changed.

The early pioneers of cochlear implants include William House (1976), Blair Simmons (1965, 1966), and Robin Michelson (1971). These individuals were the first to describe the clinical benefits of electrically stimulating the inner ear. House and Michelson described the placement of single electrodes within the scala tympani of the inner ear, while Simmons introduced multiple electrodes directly into the auditory nerve. Their reports in the 1960s were strongly criticized by the scientific community.

The first commercially available implants were produced in 1972 as the House-3M single channel implant. This device was an aid to speechreading and provided an awareness of environmental sounds to several thousand postlingually deafened adults and a few hundred children. Graeme Clark (Clark et al., 1977) and his research team in Australia focused on multichannel stimulation. A commercially available (Cochlear Corporation) multichannel implant with 22 separate channels began clinical trials in 1983. The University of California at San Francisco implant team also began clinical trials in 1985 with a multichannel implant. A variant of this device is now manufactured by Advanced Bionics (the Clarion cochlear implant). Major advances in microcircuitry and speech coding algorithms have been developed over the past 20 years.

In 2003, there were three companies that made commercially available cochlear implants for use in the United States—Cochlear Corporation, Advanced Bionics, and Med El. Each has a slightly different electrode array that is inserted into the inner ear and a different way of encoding speech information into an electrical signal. There is substantial variability in results with all devices and subject populations, and the results have improved as more is learned about the way the human brain processes speech signals. It is important to recognize that results with implants will likely continue to improve as device technology advances and indications for implantation expand. The results reported here are most likely to be out of date in two to three years.

The basic components of a cochlear implant (shown in Figure 5-1) include:

- a microphone to pick up auditory information from the environment,
- a speech processor that changes the mechanical acoustic sound energy into electrical signals,
- a headpiece with transmitter coil to send the information via radio frequency through the skin,
- an implanted receiver/stimulator that interprets the electrical signal sent by the speech processor, and
- an intracochlear electrode array that distributes the electrically processed speech information to the auditory nerves.

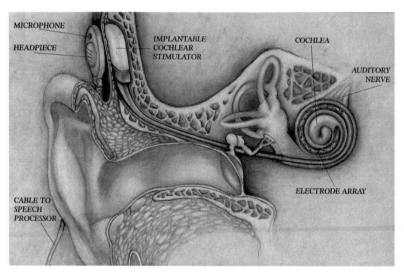

FIGURE 5-1 The components of a cochlear implant.
NOTE: In some models, the speech processor is incorporated with microphone and batteries in "behind-the-ear" unit.
SOURCE: Advanced Bionics Company, reprinted with permission.

Multichannel cochlear implants that deliver different temporal information to different parts of the cochlea (place or spectral information) have been the most successful in generating speech perception in postlingually deafened adults with profound hearing loss and in postlingually and prelingually deafened children (Cohen, Waltzman, and Fisher, 1993; Gantz, McCabe, and Tyler, 1988). Innovative methods of processing speech have been developed by many independent research programs and cochlear implant manufacturers.

Most cochlear implants today employ a band-pass filter system to separate the acoustic signal into discrete frequency bands that can be delivered to the appropriate frequency regions of the cochlea, providing spectral information about the speech signal. Temporal and intensity cues are delivered by varying the rate of stimulation and the amount of stimulating current. Multichannel implant systems use between 8 and 24 channels, depending on the implant manufacturer.

Current cochlear implant systems are designed to take advantage of the tonotopic organization of the cochlea. Thus, place coding is used to transfer spectral information in the speech signal as well as to encode durational and intensity cues (American Speech-Language-Hearing Association, 2004). The number of channels may not be as important as the speech processing algorithm. Most implant systems use a nonsimultaneous stimulation paradigm, which prevents stimulation of more than one channel at a time and eliminates electrical field interaction across electrodes; however, newer speech coding algorithms employing simultaneous stimulation are now in development. Electrical field interaction can induce excessive current loads causing increased loudness and distortion from overlapping signals.

One type of speech processing that has been shown to improve speech perception scores has been labeled continuous interleaved sampling (CIS) (Wilson, Lawson, Finley, and Wolford, 1991). CIS speech processing employs a rapid pulse rate (up to 25 microseconds/phase) to deliver envelope cues similar to an analog signal. The CIS processing is available in the Advanced Bionics Clarion, the Nucleus CI24M, and the MedEl implants.

The Nucleus implant has additional proprietary Spectral Peak (SPEAK) and Advanced Combination Encoders (ACE) speech coding algorithms. The ACE strategy claims to combine advantages of the SPEAK and the CIS strategies (Cochlear Corporation, 2004). The Clarion implant can be programmed in a pulsatile, compressed analog, or combination pulsatile/analog format. It is capable of stimulating at a rate of 82000 Hz, allowing presentation of more fine temporal information in their proprietary coding strategy, "Hi Res." A new implant by the Cochlear Corporation (RP-8), now in feasibility trials by the Food and Drug Administration

(FDA), also incorporates a faster stimulating chip set. Adding more fine temporal information may allow improved word understanding in background noise as well as appreciation of quality changes in voice and music. Changes in speech processing strategies surely will continue as the technology advances, and new implant systems are being designed to enable adaptation to a broad array of speech processing software changes without requiring surgical hardware reimplantation.

A recent addition to cochlear implant systems is the on-board telemetry capability to measure the electronic functioning of the implanted electrode package. Each implant manufacturer has developed its own proprietary system. For all devices, impedance measures of individual channels can be obtained as well as measures of the electronic signal being transmitted by each channel. Auditory whole nerve action potential measures developed by Brown and Abbas (Brown, Abbas, and Gantz, 1990) have been incorporated into the Nucleus (neural response telemetry, NRT) and Clarion (neural response imaging, NRI) implant systems, but not into the Med El systems at this time. The telemetry systems can measure the activity of the residual auditory nerve. The whole nerve action potential measures have a moderate correlation with speech perception skills with an implant. Presumably these measures are based on the integrity and number of residual auditory nerve fibers, so it may be possible to use this capability to identify different areas in an individual cochlea that have better surviving neural populations. It is expected that this information will be useful in developing unique speech coding algorithms for individual subjects, thereby improving their speech perception. Ongoing studies of residual auditory nerve function may be an important method of enhancing performance in individual patients.

Audiological Criteria for Implantation in Adults

The selection criteria for adults continue to evolve as cochlear implant hardware and software are able to reliably provide improved speech understanding. Successful restoration of speech perception with cochlear implants in adults has been limited to postlingually deafened individuals (adults who have learned spoken language and speech prior to losing their hearing). Prelingually deafened adults who use primarily spoken language obtain some important speech cues from the device. Prelingually deafened adults who use sign language have not been able to obtain much benefit from the devices. Cochlear implantation is also limited to individuals with bilateral moderate to profound sensorineural hearing loss in the low frequencies and profound loss in the high frequencies. The present FDA guidelines for adult cochlear implant candidacy include the following or similar criteria that may differ by implant manufacturer and model (Advanced Bionics, 2004; Cochlear Corporation, 2004; Food and Drug Administration, 2001): If the subject can detect speech at 70 dB sound pressure level (SPL), a series of speech perception tests are performed, bilaterally aided in a sound field at 70 dB SPL. Candidates unable to detect speech in a sound field with the assistance of appropriately fitted hearing aids are considered audiological candidates for an implant. Individuals who can understand some speech in the test condition are considered to be candidates for an implant if they understand 50 percent correct or less on a recorded sentence test (many centers use the HINT hearing in noise sentence test for cochlear implant evaluation) in the ear to be implanted and 60 percent or less in the best binaural aided condition. The above indications are in transition as speech coding algorithms and devices continue to provide improved speech understanding results. Continued research and careful documentation of these findings are necessary to expand the clinical selection criteria for electrical speech processing.

Adults with prelingual, long-term deafness demonstrate a poor prognosis for developing speech understanding following cochlear implantation (Busby, Roberts, Tong, and Clark, 1991; Dawson et al., 1992; Zwolan, 2000). A number of these individuals can learn to recognize environmental or warning sounds and may demonstrate limited speech-reading enhancement with their cochlear implants. Other individuals have reported some improvement in their own speech production following implantation (Zwolan, Kileny, and Telian, 1996). Prelingually deafened adults with previous auditory or oral training or experience (those who communicate primarily with speech rather than sign language) have a better prognosis for accepting and using their devices. It is suspected that central neural processing of auditory information is not possible using current cochlear implant technology if the central auditory pathways have not been stimulated either through normal hearing mechanisms or electrical stimulation with a cochlear implant prior to puberty.

Medical Considerations for Implantation

There are very few medical conditions that limit the use of a cochlear implant in an adult or child. The ability to undergo a general anesthetic must be assessed. Certain personal characteristics, such as onset of profound deafness, educational environment, and history of chronic ear disease and surgery should be ascertained. The medical history is important because it can identify potential problems that might result in less than optimal outcome with a cochlear implant. This information should be considered when counseling the candidate and planning rehabilitation.

Rarely is a candidate eliminated from consideration for an implant based on medical history.

Almost all diseases and disorders that induce profound deafness primarily affect the cochlear hair cells, which are responsible for transducing acoustical signals into electrical responses. This has enabled candidates with almost all causes of profound deafness to be candidates for cochlear implantation. Exceptions to this are those who have had tumors removed from their hearing and balance nerves and those with severe trauma severing the auditory nerve. Studies have failed to identify any etiology except meningitis with severe labyrinthine ossification with obliteration of the cochlea as a disadvantage for cochlear implantation (Gantz, Woodworth, Abbas, Knutson, and Tyler, 1993).

Radiographic imaging of the cochlea is essential to determine the presence of a congenital inner ear deformity. Absence of the cochlea (Michele deformity) or a small internal auditory canal (similar to the fallopian canal) are contraindications for implantation on that side. Congenital malformations, such as Mondini deformities, are not contraindications for implantation, but they should alert the implant team that complications may be encountered during implantation and the candidate must be carefully counseled as to possible limited hearing outcome (Jackler, Luxford, and House, 1987; Miyamoto, Robbins, Myres, and Pope, 1986).

Recurrent acute or chronic ear disease must be controlled prior to placing a cochlear implant. If acute otitis media occurs following implantation, it should be treated with appropriate antibiotics.

In the recent past it has been recognized that there may be an increased risk of meningitis associated with cochlear implantation. Because of this, the Centers for Disease Control and Prevention (2003), the FDA (2003), and the American Academy of Pediatrics (2004) have recommended that all young children who receive a cochlear implant, as well as adults at high risk of invasive pneumococcal disease, be vaccinated against meningitis. It is recommended that vaccination take place prior to implantation in children and the elderly.

Finally, a history of a congenitally deafened ear should be noted. The congenitally deafened ear in a postlingual deaf adult should not be implanted. Case reports indicate that these ears perform similarly to implants in prelingually deafened adults, in that a sensation of sound may not be perceived in a prelingually deafened ear.

Other Considerations

The characteristics of an individual cochlear implant user play a large role in the communication outcomes he or she achieves (Wilson, Lawson, Finley, and Wolford, 1993). Two important factors are age at implantation and duration of deafness (Battmer, Gupta, Allum-Mecklenburg, and Lenarz, 1995; Gantz et al., 1993; Geir, Barker, Fisher, and Opie, 1999; Shipp, Nedzelski, Chen, and Hanusaik, 1997). Individuals implanted at a younger age with a corresponding shorter period of auditory deprivation are more likely to achieve good outcomes. In addition, cochlear implant outcome improves with increasing device use for many recipients (Rubinstein and Miller, 1999; Rubinstein, Parkinson, Tyler, and Gantz, 1999). Other factors that may influence adult outcomes include speech-reading ability and degree of preimplant residual hearing (Cohen et al., 1993; Gantz et al., 1993; Rubinstein et al., 1999).

Cochlear Implant Results

Evaluation of cochlear implant performance has required the development of new test materials for both children and adults, because existing test materials were too difficult or they were used so frequently that subjects could learn the test material. As with routine auditory testing, speech perception material should be presented from audiotape or videotape standardized material (see Chapters 3 and 4). A battery of tests of varying difficulty is needed, assessing temporal or intonation patterns of speech, sound + vision tests to evaluate speech reading enhancement, closed-set and open-set sound-only sentence tests or single word tests. The most difficult are open-set monosyllabic word tests, such as the CID W-22 word lists, NU-6, or CNC monosyllabic word tests (see Chapters 3 and 7 for test descriptions).

Postlingual Adult Performance

Multichannel implant strategies have been shown to provide postlingually deafened adults more auditory information than single channel implants in comparative studies (Gantz et. al., 1988a) and in the prospective randomized Veterans Administration clinical trial (Cohen et. al., 1993). Open-set sentence test and monosyllabic word test score results from subjects using multichannel implants have improved as speech coding strategy advances have been incorporated in clinical trials. It should also be kept in mind that during this same period the selection criteria for implantation have been liberalized. Subjects receiving implants in 2003 have much more residual auditory function than the individuals with no response to audiometric testing implanted in the early 1980s.

Initial prospective randomized clinical trials using the four-channel Ineraid cochlear implant and the Nucleus CI-22 (feature extraction, F0F1F2 coding) implant demonstrated an average open-set sentence score of 30-

38 percent correct after 9 months of device experience (Gantz et al., 1993). Monosyllabic NU-6 word score averages ranged between 9 and 12 percent at 9 months.

It is of interest that the Iowa trial (Gantz et. al., 1988b) could not demonstrate any performance differences between the 22-channel Nucleus device using a feature extraction speech coding algorithm and the Ineraid 4 channel vocoder compressed analog speech processing paradigm. Speech scores improved with the development of the CIS-like speech coding used in the Clarion implant and the SPEAK band-pass filter strategy of the Nucleus 22. Average sentence scores for the Clarion CIS implant are in the range of 65 percent; NU-6 word scores are 30-38 percent (Tyler, Fryauf-Bertchy, Gantz, Kelsay, and Woodworth, 1997). Similar results have been obtained with the Nucleus CI-22 implant using SPEAK speech coding (Hollow et al., 1995). Multiple speech coding strategies are available in most cochlear implants. A recent comparison of five different speech coding strategies in the Clarion device, including CIS, simultaneous analog stimulation (SAS), paired pulsatile sampler (PPS), quadruple pulsatile sampler (QPS), and hybrid strategies (HYB), showed no statistically significant difference between CIS and SAS strategies on vowel and sentence recognition tasks (Loizou, Stickney, Mishra, and Assman, 2003). About one-third of the group benefited from PPS and QPS strategies. There were individual preferences for each strategy. A similar study with the Nucleus implant compared SPEAK, ACE, and CIS speech coding strategies (Skinner et al., 2002). The outcomes in postlingually deafened adults indicated individual preferences for each strategy; however, group means demonstrated similar performance for all three coding strategies.

It is recommended that clinicians fit each coding strategy for an individual in order for the user to obtain maximum benefit from the implant. A period of trial (4-6 weeks) for each is recommended, as the initial preferred strategy may not be the final best speech coding strategy.

In all published trials of cochlear implant performance, a wide range of scores is seen among individual subjects. Ranges have widened as speech coding has improved. Average scores for monosyllabic word understanding for different devices are 40-50 percent correct in the sound-only condition. Average sentence understanding scores range between 60 and 70 percent. Duration of profound deafness has been shown to be the most significant patient variable that contributes to intersubject score differences (Gantz et al., 1993; Rubinstein et al., 1999).

Cognitive abilities, residual hearing, and speech-reading skills have also had a small influence on performance with an implant. Implanting individuals with more residual hearing has shown that preoperative sentence recognition scores and duration of deafness can account for 80 percent of the variance in single word recognition scores (Rubinstein et al., 1999).

The etiology of deafness, except for meningitis with labyrinthine ossification, has not contributed to performance differences. It is suspected that residual auditory nerve function has some influence on performance, but until auditory nerve integrity tests are available on large populations, this remains speculative. Over the past 15 years, speech perception scores have demonstrated steady improvement. Much of the improvement is attributed to advancing technology and speech processing; however, it must be kept in mind, as mentioned above, that the subject population being implanted today has more residual hearing than the people implanted several years ago. The cochlear implant has also been able to elevate the functional health status of older adults (Francis, Chee, Yeagle, Cheng, and Niparko, 2002). A team at the Johns Hopkins University evaluated the quality of life of individuals between ages 50 and 80 who were using cochlear implants. There was a strong correlation between increases in emotional utility scores and improvements in speech understanding scores; 65 percent of this group could conduct interactive conversations on the telephone. These studies also demonstrated that cochlear implantation was cost-effective in this patient population, similar to findings for young adults and children. The cost utility analysis of $9,480 per quality-adjusted life year (QALY) in this age group was well below the threshold of $20-25,000 per QALY for procedures that are considered to be acceptable value for the money. Costs for children ranged between $5,197 and $9,029/QALY (Cheng et al., 2000).

Bilateral Implantation

The increasing clinical success of cochlear implants has prompted the exploration of bilateral implantation (Gantz et al., 2002; van Hoesel and Tyler, 2003). Preliminary results suggest that the greatest benefit from bilateral implantation is sound localization. The head shadow effect in a noisy environment was also a benefit to most individuals. A small percentage of the subjects improved speech recognition in quiet with two implants compared with one device. Much more research in larger groups of individuals must be undertaken to determine whether bilateral implantation should become standard clinical care.

Hybrid (Combined Acoustic and Electrical) Stimulation

The improved speech perception scores achieved by an increasing number of individuals implanted with multichannel cochlear implants, along with the implants' record of safety, has enabled the gradual expansion of implant selection criteria to those with more residual hearing. Individuals with severe hearing loss who use hearing aids complain of poor word understanding that is not improved with conventional hearing aids. Amplifying the sound does not improve their word perception scores. Most adults with severe to profound age-related deafness and noise exposure have substantial low-frequency hearing but cannot hear the high-frequency consonants that are essential for word understanding. While the speech communication performance of postlingually deafened patients with cochlear implants is quite good, acoustic hearing (if the damage to the ear is not too severe) still offers considerable advantages for appreciation of the aesthetic qualities of sound (such as music and voice quality), as well as for understanding speech in background noise (Fu, Shannon, and Wang, 1998). Many users of cochlear implants complain that the sound is very mechanical and background noise reduces the ability to perceive speech. The loss of the aesthetic quality of sound is most likely to be related to the inability to discriminate the pitches of sound (Gfeller et al., 2002). The loss of pitch perception is a consequence of the limited spectral resolution of current speech coding strategies (Fishman, Shannon, and Slattery, 1998). Hearing in background noise requires even finer spectral resolution (Fu et al., 1998).

Residual low-frequency hearing (125-750 Hz) has the potential to provide more low-frequency spectral resolution than the current generation of speech coding algorithms. However, placement of the standard intracochlear electrode usually results in loss of residual hearing. To circumvent this loss, a novel "short" 10 mm multichannel cochlear implant was developed for use in severely impaired individuals with residual low-frequency acoustic hearing (Gantz and Turner, 2003). Recipients of this device have preserved low-frequency acoustic hearing and have been able to combine acoustic and electrical speech processing to substantially improve speech perception in quiet and in multitalker noise (Gantz and Turner, 2003). These early experiences suggest that residual low-frequency hearing is important and should be preserved as individuals with more hearing are considered for cochlear implantation.

The cochlear implant has been shown to be safe and effective in providing significant improvements in speech perception skills for postlingually deaf adults. The results with cochlear implants are encouraging and have continued to improve as indications for implantation expand and software and hardware advances become clinically available. Newer implant designs are in development, and the combination of acoustic and electrical stimulation strategies may greatly expand the application of this technology to more individuals with hearing loss in the future.

AUDITORY BRAINSTEM IMPLANTS

Neurofibromatosis Type II (NF-2) is a disease in which patients develop multiple tumors of the central nervous system, including bilateral acoustic neuromas (vestibular schwannomas). Profound deafness is the usual outcome following removal of the acoustic neuromas in these individuals. Researchers have developed auditory brainstem implants that can deliver stimulation to the cochlear nucleus, bypassing the damaged nerve, in patients undergoing such surgery (House and Hitselberger, 2001).

The present auditory brainstem implant (ABI) is approved by the FDA for use in patients with NF-2. The device has a Silastic pad with 22 electrode contacts that are placed adjacent to the dorsal cochlear nucleus in the brainstem following tumor removal. Some patients who receive an ABI do not receive any auditory benefit from the device, and the patients must fully understand this, as well as the risks and potential side effects of surgery, prior to implantation. The most recent results with the ABI can be found in an article by Otto et al. reporting on the 55 subjects that were included in the FDA clinical trial with this device (Otto, Brackmann, Hitselberger, Shannon, and Kuchta, 2002).

OTHER ASSISTIVE LISTENING DEVICES

In addition to conventional hearing aids and cochlear implants, there is a category of technologies called ALDs. These devices are typically used part-time either instead of, or in addition to, hearing aids or implants. They are usually targeted toward improving communication functionality in specific limited situations, such as talking on the telephone, communicating over a distance, attending the theater, or detecting a doorbell ring. A recent review of ALD types and technologies is found in Compton (2000).

Varieties of ALDs may be partitioned into two categories: acoustic and alerting. Acoustic ALDs facilitate the reception of acoustic signals by reducing the corruption of desired sounds that occurs in many everyday listening situations, for example, background noise (including speech babble), reverberation effects in auditoria, large distance between talker and listener, and limited visual cues resulting from poor lighting or a talker who cannot be seen.

Amplified telephones are probably the most widely used and effective acoustic ALDs (Kochkin, 2002). Another effective type of device employs a wireless system composed of a transmitter and receiver pair. The transmitter is driven by a microphone that is held by or near the talker. The signal is broadcast to the receiver using FM radio, induction loop, or infrared transmission. The receiver routes the signal to the hearing aid (or other amplifier), from which it is delivered to the listener. A related category of ALDs converts the acoustic speech signal into a visual representation. Examples of these are real-time captioning and speech recognition technology such as that used by CapTel. There are also other visually based technologies such as TTY (a keyboard and display device connected to the phone system), e-mail, and instant messaging.

Alerting ALDs are designed to improve detection of warning and alerting signals by substituting visual or vibratory signals for auditory signals. Examples of this category include vibrating alarm clocks, light-up telephone signalers, and doorbells and fire alarms that activate flashing lights.

ALDs are often considered appropriate in addition to a conventional hearing aid or in cases in which a hearing aid is not effective or desired. Despite enthusiastic support from some professionals (e.g., Loovis, Schall, and Teter, 1997) and considerable popularity in some other countries, ALDs are not used very much in the United States (with the exception of amplified telephones). It is not clear whether this results from a culturally based reluctance to embrace devices that are more obvious, or whether it results more from lack of their promotion by hearing care professionals.

Although both alerting and acoustic ALDs seem to be used quite effectively in some home situations, their penetration into work settings and other settings outside the home is reported to be limited (Bowe, 2002; Kochkin, 2002; Wheeler-Scruggs, 2002). The reasons for this are not clearly established. Reluctance of workers to request accommodations may be a contributing factor; lack of knowledge about available and appropriate devices is another.

In addition, there is evidence that persons with hearing loss are often reluctant to utilize ALDs that they know to be helpful because they are conspicuous and potentially stigmatizing. For example, with a personal FM system, the talker must be close to the microphone (typically holding it or wearing it) before the device will be helpful to the listener with the hearing loss. It is difficult to achieve this in an inconspicuous, flexible manner that does not inconvenience communication partners in the work setting.

This presumption has been supported in two studies that have compared hearing aids and ALDs in fairly large groups of persons with hearing loss. Jerger et al. (1996) noted that although many subjects preferred the sound quality of an ALD (a personal FM system), 97 percent of them still preferred to use a conventional hearing aid in daily life. Yueh et al. (2001) reported that use of conventional hearing aids produced substantial reported improvements in hearing-related quality of life, whereas the quality of life improvement reported to result from use of an ALD was very small.

RECOMMENDATIONS FOR RESEARCH

The committee recommends that SSA support research efforts that are directed toward increasing the knowledge base in the area of amplification effectiveness. Despite the long history of study of amplification, fitting strategies, and outcomes, there is a lack of empirically based information about the use and benefit of modern sensory aids and prostheses that are used by persons with severe/profound hearing loss. Such data potentially would be of interest to SSA in judging the likely employability of individuals with hearing loss.

Research Recommendation 5-1. There is very limited information about the efficacy and effectiveness[1] of modern high-technology wearable hearing aids in adults with severe or profound hearing loss. Reports in the literature tend to be on small samples that are rather loosely defined. Results are probably of limited generalizability to the population of adults with work potential. It would be valuable to have information from large groups of adults with severe and profound hearing loss about the effectiveness of conventional amplification. Data describing both laboratory measures of speech understanding and self-reports of real-world performance should be obtained. Basic linguistic abilities would be an important variable in such studies. Individuals with adult-acquired hearing loss should be investigated separately from those whose hearing losses originated in early life.

Research Recommendation 5-2. Research should be undertaken to determine: (1) performance for hearing aid wearers with severe/profound losses on the tests recommended in Chapter 4 of this report (monosyllabic words in quiet and in noise); and (2) the ability of the same hearing aid wearers to function in real work environments.

Research Recommendation 5-3. After work environments are meaningfully categorized using dimensions such as typical background noise level, noise modulation, and need for oral communication (as recommended elsewhere in this report), data describing: (1) performance on tests for SSA disability determination, and (2) performance with hearing aids in different work environments should be combined in attempts to develop reasonably accurate models to predict likely abilities of given individuals to function auditorily in given jobs.

---

[1]"Efficacy" refers to whether controlled trials show a treatment effect. "Effectiveness" refers to whether the treatment transfers well to real-world populations.

Research Recommendation 5-4. Overall, it seems likely that ALDs have the potential to be quite efficacious in the workplace, but they are underutilized at this time. Because many of them are less costly to purchase, adjust, and maintain and less individually specialized than either hearing aids or cochlear implants, they could provide a cost-effective approach to facilitating integration of some persons with hearing loss into the workforce. The committee recommends that SSA support research directed toward determining the benefits and cost-effectiveness of ALDs in the workplace. It may be valuable to develop a program that facilitates the purchase, maintenance, and promotion of ALDs by employers who have, or could have, workers with hearing loss.

6

Impact of Hearing Loss on Daily Life and the Workplace

As people move through the activities of daily living at home, at work, and in social or business situations, basic auditory abilities take on functional significance. Audition makes it possible to detect and recognize meaningful environmental sounds, to identify the source and location of a sound, and, most importantly, to perceive and understand spoken language.

The ability of an individual to carry out auditory tasks in the real world is influenced not only by his or her hearing abilities, but also by a multitude of situational factors, such as background noise, competing signals, room acoustics, and familiarity with the situation. Such factors are important regardless of whether one has a hearing loss, but the effects are magnified when hearing is impaired. For example, when an individual with normal hearing engages in conversation in a quiet, well-lit setting, visual information from the speaker's face, along with situational cues and linguistic context, can make communication quite effortless. In contrast, in a noisy environment, with poor lighting and limited visual cues, it may be much more difficult to carry on a conversation or to give and receive information. A person with hearing loss may be able to function very well in the former situation but may not be able to communicate at all in the latter.

In this chapter we examine what is known about the impact of hearing loss on adults as they function in daily life; the impact of hearing loss in the workplace; the effectiveness of sensory aids, prosthetic devices, and assistive devices; and the implications and challenges for disability determination.

HEARING IN DAILY LIFE

Impact of Hearing Loss for Adults

Early Versus Late Onset

It is important at the outset to distinguish between adults who have experienced an early onset of severe or profound hearing loss and adults whose hearing loss was acquired later in life. When hearing loss occurs at an early age (i.e., prelingually, defined in this report as before age 2 years), there is an impact on the development of spoken language, on reading ability and educational attainment, and, ultimately, on employability (discussed further in Chapter 7). These persons are usually considered deaf, and a good number may use American Sign Language or a similar sign system as their preferred mode of communication. When hearing loss occurs after the development of spoken language, and particularly when it occurs slowly, as it does in aging or as the result of prolonged noise exposure, there is a loss of functional hearing ability, but other cognitive skills and competencies are not greatly affected. The terms "hard-of-hearing" and "late deafened" are often used to describe these individuals. In the sections that follow, we examine the impact of hearing loss in adults, with only occasional reference to etiology or time of onset. Nevertheless, each issue or research finding has greater relevance for one of these groups than for the other.

Education and Employment

Communication Access. Communication access for people with hearing loss can be described as "the right of deaf and hard of hearing people to receive and understand information and signals presented directly . . . and . . . the lack of barriers to, and the concomitant presence of access to, visual or auditory communication" (Barnartt, Seelman, and Gracer, 1990, p. 50). Individuals with hearing loss can perform as well as their counterparts without hearing loss when equitable educational and employment opportunities are provided (Schroedel and Geyer, 2000). These equitable opportunities are dependent on the individual student or worker having access to the information necessary for learning or for getting the job done. The nature of this communication access depends on individual needs and the auxiliary aids available to address these needs. For example, a deaf person who is unable to use the telephone can use a TTY or computer system and can communicate with hearing peers through telephone or Internet relay systems. These systems provide operators who type or, via video, sign the hearing person's spoken words for the deaf caller and voice the deaf person's typed words or signed phrases for the hearing caller.

In the educational setting, an individual with a hearing loss is most likely to have trouble hearing what is said. In these situations, communication access is enhanced with the use of FM systems and other assistive listening devices (see Chapter 5), computer-assisted note-taking systems, and other accommodations. However, for various reasons, including background noise in the classroom, communication is often less than clear, thereby affecting access to the English language and educational achievement. Chapter 7 discusses hearing loss in an educational setting in greater detail.

Those with education are less likely to be in need of Social Security Disability Insurance and Supplemental Security Income (SSI) than those without education (Clarcq and Walter, 1997-1998). Most worrisome, however, is the 44 percent high school dropout rate among deaf students (Blanchfield, Feldman, Dunbar, and Gardner, 2001), compared with a general population rate of 19 percent. With high-stakes testing now being instituted by the states, the potential for this dropout rate to increase is high.

Buchanan (1999) notes that in addition to employer resistance to hiring deaf individuals, the automation of many work functions has disadvantaged the unskilled deaf worker. The implication here is that education is a critical factor that facilitates occupational entry and mobility for the deaf worker. The generally lower educational achievement of deaf persons continues to contribute to vocational difficulties. Those who lose their hearing later in life, and whose jobs depend on effective communication, run the risk of eventually losing their jobs if satisfactory accommodations, including the provision of auxiliary aids that meet their communication needs, are not instituted.

Americans with Disabilities Act. Title V of the Rehabilitation Act of 1973 was landmark legislation enacted to address job discrimination in federally supported programs that affected qualified people with disabilities (National Association of the Deaf, 2000). Under the Americans with Disabilities Act of 1990 (ADA), which was enacted in part because of pervasive ongoing discrimination in the mainstream of American public life, the removal of communication barriers (which deny information access for individuals with hearing loss equivalent to what hearing persons might have) became a legal right for deaf and hard-of-hearing people (National Association of the Deaf, 2000). The legal protection of both acts covers individuals who can demonstrate that, even with corrective devices such as hearing aids or cochlear implants, they have a substantial impairment to a major life activity—for example, the inability to distinguish words due to background noise on the job. Public venues must provide auxiliary aids or services when necessary. A comprehensive list of auxiliary aids and services required by the ADA is included in the corresponding regulations, with the understanding that evolving technology will create new devices.

Psychosocial Impact of Hearing Loss

Perspectives of the Deaf Community

The deaf community is defined as an entity that shares the common goals of its members and works toward these goals (Padden, 1980). These goals include, for example, telecommunications and entertainment access, captioning, sign language and oral interpreting, and accommodations in the work setting. For the most part, the deaf community comprises individuals who have been deaf from birth or early in life (Lane, Hoffmeister, and Bahan, 1996). Some of these individuals prefer oral communication but see themselves as part of the deaf community. Most are deaf individuals who rely on some form of signed communication or American Sign Language and identify with Deaf Culture. These individuals value American Sign Language as their language, and they tend to devalue speech when they interact with each other. Socialization with other deaf persons is strongly emphasized, particularly through local, state, and national associations, sports leagues, deaf clubs, religious settings, and Deaf festivals (Lane et al., 1996; Padden and Humphries, 1988).

Within the deaf community, hearing loss is not a detriment to socialization; rather, it brings people with common issues together into a vibrant entity (Andrews, Leigh, and Weiner, 2004). As Lane, Hoffmeister, and Bahan (1996) indicate, hearing loss as measured in decibels is not a significant issue for those who identify with Deaf Culture as defined above. Rather, what is significant is how deaf community members relate to each other and how they communicate with each other. The use of vision rather than audition to communicate, most often using sign language, is integral to their daily living (Andrews et al., 2004). Many wear hearing aids to alert them to environmental noises at the very least, but audition is still not primary in their lives. While some value their previous speech and auditory therapy to maximize spoken English abilities, others may experience such exposure as stressful and potentially inadequate in providing them with functional expressive and receptive spoken English skills (Bain, Scott, and Steinberg, 2004). It must be kept in mind that most individuals whose hearing loss goes back to the early years of life do have the ability to speak with varying degrees of clarity ranging from speech indistinguishable from hearing peers to speech that is incomprehensible, depending not necessarily on level of hearing loss, but rather on background training, ability to benefit from hearing devices, and the use of speech (Blamey, 2003).

Generally, those identifying with Deaf Culture see sign language as providing them with critical access to language, communication, and positive social experiences. Because they have a language acquired through vision and a means to education, they do not see themselves as disabled per se, although many will acknowledge having a disability regarding the lack of hearing that entitles them to coverage under the ADA and its provisions for more equal opportunities. Hearing disability per se is not as much an issue for them as is the disability engendered by society's reluctance to accommodate to their needs by providing interpreter services, captioning, and other means of access to communication (Lane et al., 1996). This reluctance of society is what they see as profoundly disabling.

Psychosocial Adjustment and Hearing Loss

The majority of those with hearing loss acquire it later in life at a time following the acquisition of spoken language. The prevalence is particularly high among those who are over 65 years of age and among those who have been exposed to noise. Because hearing loss tends to disrupt interpersonal communication and to interfere with perception of meaningful environmental sounds, some individuals experience significant levels of distress as a result of their hearing problems. For example, some express embarrassment and self-criticism when they have difficulty understanding others or when they make perceptual errors. Others have difficulty accepting their hearing loss and are unwilling to admit their hearing problems to others. Anger and frustration can occur when communication problems arise, and many individuals experience discouragement, guilt, and stress related to their hearing loss. These negative reactions are also associated with reports of negative attitudes and uncooperative behaviors of others (Demorest and Erdman, 1989).

Interestingly, the association between degree of hearing loss and psychosocial adjustment to hearing loss per se is not strong (Erdman and Demorest, 1998). Individuals with virtually identical audiograms and clinical test results may differ greatly in their self-reported adjustment problems. This finding is not unique to the impact of hearing loss on psychosocial adjustment; low (negative) correlations between severity of impairment and degree of psychosocial adjustment have been found repeatedly in the disability literature for a wide variety of health-related problems (Shontz, 1971).

Given the high variability in how individuals adjust to their hearing problems, it is not surprising that hearing loss does not seem to affect basic personality structure (Thomas, 1984). Although many adults are resilient, acquired hearing difficulties are nevertheless responsible for a high level of general psychological distress for a significant number of people due in part to isolation, loneliness, and withdrawal (Meadow-Orlans, 1985). This distress, which may be manifested in heightened anxiety, depression, sleep disturbance, and the like, is observed not only among those who seek audiological evaluation, but also among those reluctant to acknowledge a hearing problem (Hallberg and Barrenas, 1995; Hetu, Riverin, Getty, Lalande, and St-Cyr, 1990; Hetu, Riverin, Lalande, Getty, and St-Cyr, 1988) and among those who have already acquired hearing aids (Thomas, 1984, 1988). This psychological distress can significantly impact the family or significant others as well as the individual (Schein, Bottum, Lawler, Madory, and Wantuch, 2001).

Similarly to what has been found for psychosocial adjustment, studies to date have consistently demonstrated that there is no overall association between hearing loss and psychopathology. Rosen (1979) has confirmed this for individuals with acquired hearing loss, and Pollard (1994) has confirmed it from an analysis of public mental health records on deaf and hard-of-hearing individuals in the Rochester, New York, vicinity. Despite this lack of association, it is important to acknowledge that psychological distress can be a factor in adjustment difficulties.

Knutson et al. (1998) have investigated whether the use of cochlear implants can affect the social adjustment of those with acquired hearing loss. In a study of psychological change over 54 months of cochlear implant use by 37 postlingually deafened adults, the researchers used standard psychological measures of affect, social function, and personality prior to implantation, and then at regularly scheduled intervals after implantation, to assess the impact of audiological benefit. There was evidence of significant improvement on measures of loneliness, social anxiety, paranoia, social introversion, and distress. To a lesser extent, improvement was also noted for depression. Improvement of marital distress and assertiveness took comparatively longer to emerge. One caveat is that because of the complexities of individual life issues and personality attributes, it is not possible to attribute the improvement in psychological measures solely to the influence of audiological benefits. How well the improvement noted on self-report measures translates into actual social and job situations has not been determined.

Hearing in the Workplace

Prevalence of Hearing Loss in the Workplace

Although there have been numerous surveys used to estimate the prevalence of hearing loss in the general population, there is no comparable survey of prevalence in the workplace. Prevalence rates in the general population, broken down with respect to age and gender, can be used, with appropriate weights, to derive such estimates. For example, according to a survey of 80,000 households in the National Family Opinion (NFO) panel conducted in November 2000, 275 per 1,000 households reported having a person with a hearing difficulty, in one or both ears, without the use of hearing aid (Kochkin, 2001). The NFO panel is balanced to reflect U.S. census information, and the survey results translate to an estimated 28.6 million households reporting hearing loss.[1] Although the age distribution reported by Kochkin leads to an estimate of 17.4 million adults of working age (18-64) in the United States, it is very difficult to estimate the numbers actually in the workplace. The disabling outcomes of hearing loss are likely to reduce this number, but as discussed by Mital (1994), the median age of the population is increasing and many older workers are delaying retirement for financial reasons, thereby increasing the numbers of older adults in the workplace.[2]

Despite our inability to derive an estimate of the number of individuals with hearing loss in the workplace, it is clear that many such individuals function, and function quite well, despite their impairment. As noted in Chapter 1, a great many factors influence employability and performance, and these must be taken into account when accurate prediction of disability for an individual is needed.

Employment Status of Adults with Hearing Loss

Educational level is a key factor in understanding the employment status of adults with hearing loss. For those individuals with early onset of hearing loss, the challenges for acquisition of spoken language, devel-

---

[1]Although the sampling unit for this estimate is the household, the estimate is often reported and interpreted as the number of individuals with hearing loss. Because a given household can have more than one individual with hearing loss, 28.6 million is probably an underestimate of the prevalence of hearing loss in the population that was sampled. Current estimates (see Chapter 1) are closer to 34 million individuals.

[2]A recent report (National Research Council, 2004) from the National Academies, *Health and Safety Needs of Older Workers*, may be of interest to readers concerned with the aging workforce and its special needs.

opment of reading skills, and educational achievement result in limited job opportunities. These problems, combined with needs for better career guidance, job training, and job placement, result in poor preparation for entering the workforce on a competitive basis (Phillippe and Auvenshine, 1985).

Positive career outcomes are statistically related to educational level, although this relationship does not imply a causal linkage. Clarcq and Walter (1997-1998) compared graduates of high schools for the deaf ages 28-32 with individuals who had attended or graduated from the postsecondary National Technical Institute for the Deaf (NTID). They found that 33 percent of the high school graduates were receiving SSI benefits compared with 12 percent of those with some college education and 0 percent of those who had graduated from NTID. Schroedel and Geyer (2000) examined the long-term career attainments of deaf and hard-of-hearing college graduates and found that most were successfully employed and satisfied with life. Many had completed graduate degrees and were employed in white-collar positions.[3] Similarly, Welsh (1993) examined factors affecting the career mobility of deaf adults and recommended that they pursue the highest degree of education possible and that they target careers in which the demand for workers is greatest.

When hearing loss occurs during adulthood, after the completion of formal education and after establishment of a work history or career, it poses challenges for job performance and future job mobility. Because these adults have already acquired the knowledge and skills needed to perform their jobs, the difficulties they face are related to communication barriers, such as working conditions and employer attitudes, as discussed in the following sections.

Communication Barriers

For an individual with hearing impairment, the most obvious communication problem in the workplace is the presence of background noise. Noise is highly prevalent in industrial settings and, among workers with noise-induced hearing loss, noise is mentioned most frequently as an obstacle and a source of annoyance in the workplace (Hetu, 1994; Laroche,

---

[3]It is clear that many variables, such as intelligence, motivation, family support, and academic preparation, influence which young people attend and graduate from college, among youth with normal hearing as well as those who are deaf and hard-of-hearing. These comparative studies did not control for such factors, but they provide evidence that, like their hearing peers, those deaf and hard-of-hearing youth who are able to attain a college education fare better in the world of work.

Garcia, and Barrette, 2000). Other surveys and focus groups of workers with hearing loss have highlighted physical aspects of the work environment, the need to use telephones or videoconferencing, the difficulty of group communication situations, and difficulties presented by various speaker characteristics (Laroche et al., 2000; Scherich and Mowry, 1997).

Employer attitudes are another barrier. According to the National Association of the Deaf, "employer attitudes create the largest single barrier to employment opportunities" (National Association of the Deaf, 2000, p. 123). Schroedel and Geyer (2000) cite studies indicating that communication stress, social isolation, and unsupportive supervisors are among the difficulties encountered by many deaf and hard-of-hearing workers. Of concerns expressed by employers of adults with hearing loss, 62 percent were communication-related and 24 percent were safety-related (Dowler and Walls, 1996). When these concerns are addressed, employer satisfaction tends to increase (Dowler and Walls, 1996).

Effectiveness of Sensory Aids, Prostheses, and Assistive Devices

As described in Chapter 5, there are a great many devices available today that can restore some of the function that is lost as a result of hearing impairment. However, most studies of the potential effectiveness of these devices are based on laboratory or clinical research, not on assessment of actual functioning in the workplace.

For persons with severe or profound hearing loss, the literature on cochlear implants provides data showing significant restoration of function for many implant recipients. Studies have confirmed, however, that individuals with lifelong profound deafness who undergo cochlear implantation do not do as well with speech recognition as individuals with late-onset hearing loss (e.g., Dorman, 1998), primarily because of limited exposure to auditory experiences and limited understanding of what auditory stimuli mean. Nonetheless, an increasing number of these adults with strong ties to the deaf community are considering cochlear implants in order to gain access to the world of sound (Christiansen and Leigh, 2002). For the most part, these individuals desire to maintain contact with the deaf community and do not necessarily reject the values of Deaf Culture. The level of hearing loss is important only insofar as it qualifies them to become candidates for the surgery, if they are so inclined. After implantation, rarely do they pick up skills such as using telephones effectively or understanding speakers in groups and in other listening situations.

ADA and Accommodation

Although the ADA has mandated accommodations in the workplace, and there are devices and other methods of accommodation that can reduce or eliminate disability for those with hearing loss, there is evidence that such accommodations are underutilized. According to results of a series of focus groups with over 100 members of Self Help for Hard of Hearing People (SHHH) (Stika, 1997), several factors account for this. Lack of knowledge on the part of both employees and employers concerning what is available and what is required by the ADA is one factor. Perhaps more pervasive, however, are apprehension, concern, and anxiety about the consequences of making one's hearing loss known to others (Glass and Elliott, 1993; Stika, 1997). Workers with hearing loss report high levels of psychological stress associated with fears of appearing (or being) incompetent, feelings of self-consciousness, overcompensation, and lowered self-esteem. Indeed, Hétu and his colleagues (Hetu, Getty, and Waridel, 1994) found that fears of stigmatization due to hearing loss are not without foundation. Mark Ross (1994, p. xii) states that "the greatest challenge we face regarding communication access is neither technological nor legislative, but societal attitudes toward hearing loss—attitudes that seem to be shared fully by many people with hearing losses." These findings point to the need for education and intervention both with the individual with hearing loss and with his or her coworkers and supervisors.

DISABILITY DETERMINATION

Different Perspectives

As discussed in Chapter 1, the term "disability" has been defined in different ways over time, and this is quite apparent in the differing approaches to disability found today. The earlier conceptualization, based on a medical model, viewed disability as a direct consequence of impairment and therefore measurement of impairment could be used, with suitable medical criteria, for disability determination. This approach is embodied in the medical listings used by the Social Security Administration (SSA) to determine that an individual is unable to work.

In contrast, the approach taken by the World Health Organization, and embodied in the ADA, is based on a social model of disability. This approach is a more positive one, in which the emphasis is on what an individual with an impairment *can* do, and the capabilities the person *does* have. The new emphasis is on accommodation and restructuring of the environment so as to maximize each individual's functioning in daily life.

These differing perspectives on disability create challenges and apparent inconsistencies in disability determination. For example, is it reasonable for deaf adults to claim on one hand that they *are* disabled and hence entitled to accommodations at work, while at the same time arguing forcefully that hearing loss is *not* a disability and that the only thing a deaf person cannot do is to hear? In the sections that follow, disability assessment is discussed from a measurement perspective, and elements of both of these approaches are apparent. In agreement with the social model, however, we note that disability is usually not absolute, and that as conditions change and accommodations are made available (and accessed), disability may be reversed.

Direct Assessment

In previous chapters the nature of hearing loss and its impact on auditory function was described in terms of clinical tests that have proven diagnostic value or that are assumed to assess auditory skills that are important in daily life. Conspicuously lacking, however, are empirical studies establishing the link between the clinical measures and performance in natural settings. In their review of the literature on sound localization, Middlebrooks and Green (1991) note that laboratory studies are designed to isolate the effects of one particular variable, with the effects of other factors controlled and held constant. In daily life, these factors are free to vary and to interact, and hence generalization from the laboratory to the real world cannot readily be made. As they state: "there is often no evidence to indicate the importance of that cue in a more realistic setting" (p. 136).

As discussed in Chapter 1, the social model of disability implies that disability, as an outcome, is a function not only of the individual's hearing loss, but also of other factors internal and external to the individual. This highlights the dilemma posed by trying to predict the consequences of hearing loss that occur in daily life: the farther one moves from testing the ear per se, the more meaningful the measure may be, but the less it is a function of hearing ability alone. This implies that impairment in a specific auditory ability may not be strongly correlated with disability, and indeed this has been shown to be true for the relation between degree of hearing loss measured audiometrically and self-reported communication function in daily life. Correlations are high enough to support the assumption of a causal link between impairment and disability (as well as the validity of the self-reports), but low enough to preclude accurate prediction of disability for individuals from the auditory measures alone.

In principle, it is possible to develop clinical tests with acceptable predictive validity, but in practice it will likely require testing conditions that are more representative of how the person functions in the real world. Some of the issues that would need to be considered are binaural versus monaural hearing, free field testing versus testing using headphones, testing with more complex stimulus materials (such as real-world sounds and sentences, connected discourse, or competing noise), and the role of visual information and auditory-visual integration, to name just a few.

The challenge of validating clinical tests in terms of performance in daily life is magnified by the complexity of real-world auditory environments and by the fact that clinical tests differ from those that are needed for functional assessment. A model for the functional approach (Laroche et al., 2003) illustrates the complexity of identifying hearing requirements and noise environments in specific jobs. Laroche et al. used the Hearing in Noise Test (Nilsson, Soli, and Sullivan, 1994) to screen for functional hearing. First, hearing-critical tasks and locations in the workplace (the Canadian Coast Guard and the conservation and protection departments of Fisheries and Oceans Canada) were identified, and performance parameters for those tasks (e.g., accuracy level, distance) were determined. Noise recordings were made in those environments, simulated in the laboratory, and used with normal-hearing listeners to develop a screening test. Statistical modeling was used to derive performance tables, and the listening tests were then validated on listeners with hearing loss. In the final stage, minimal acceptable performance criteria were established and screening scores were determined. This comprehensive and systematic approach, integrating theoretical and statistical models, psychometric instrument evaluation, and empirical determination of workplace characteristics, clearly illustrates the challenges involved in direct assessment of functional hearing abilities.

Indirect Assessment

Many forms of assessment can be considered indirect; that is, they do not involve direct observation of target behaviors. One way, discussed in previous chapters, is the use of a measurement on one variable (such as a clinical test of pure-tone thresholds) to predict or estimate performance on a different target variable (such as speech communication at work). A strong relation between the predictor and the target validates the use of the predictor in place of direct measurement of the target.

Another type of indirect assessment occurs when a self-report or self-assessment is used in lieu of direct behavioral observation. This method has been used extensively in audiology to obtain information about communication problems and communication strategies that could, in principle, be measured by direct observation. Interestingly, such instruments have also been used to obtain direct measures of the respondent's attitudes, beliefs, feelings, and reactions to experiences in everyday life. These cognitive and affective variables are not directly observable and, as a result, they are usually measured using self-reports.

A third type of indirect assessment may be termed *doubly indirect*. This occurs when a self-report on one variable, or a difference between two such reports, is used as a measure of another variable. For example, self-reported communication with a hearing aid (an indirect measure of aided communication) might be interpreted as measure of "health-related quality of life" (another variable), or a change in self-reported communication problems after receiving a cochlear implant (a difference between two indirect measures of communication) might be used as a measure of "benefit from the implant" (another variable). These measures are quite different from asking the individual to report on quality of life per se or using behavioral measures of performance to evaluate benefit from the cochlear implant. Doubly indirect assessment compounds the difficulties in arriving at valid conclusions because of the many additional assumptions that must be made about the relation between the target variable and the one actually assessed. In the sections that follow, examples of all three types of indirect assessment can be found.

Assessment of Hearing Disability, Handicap, and Benefit from Interventions

Efforts to assess hearing handicap and disability through self-report questionnaires have been ongoing since publication of the Hearing Handicap Scale by High, Fairbanks, and Glorig (1964) and the Hearing Measurement Scale (Noble and Atherley, 1970). The essential role of self-report in assessment of disability and handicap and the unique perspective of the affected individual are widely acknowledged and now generally accepted (Baldwin, 2000; Dobie and Sakai, 2001).

The earliest scales focused on self-reported abilities and difficulties experienced by the hearing-impaired individual in daily life. The use of terminology has been inconsistent, however, and the targeted constructs suggested by an instrument's name have not always been consistent with the content of its questions or items. The Hearing Handicap Scale, for example, contains items dealing primarily with detection of sounds and understanding of speech—functions that today are considered aspects of hearing disability. Similarly, early surveys of hearing aid users did not adequately distinguish among hearing aid use, hearing aid benefit, and satisfaction with a hearing aid. Attention to psychometric principles in the development, evaluation, and application of self-assessment tools has been strongly advocated (e.g., Demorest and Walden, 1984; Hyde, 2000), and surveys and recent critical reviews of self-assessment instruments (e.g., Bentler and Kramer, 2000; Demorest and DeHaven, 1993; Noble, 1998) have generally been positive.

As sophistication in instrument design has increased, so has the conceptualization of the constructs to be measured. The most dramatic changes have occurred in the assessment of hearing aid outcomes, as documented by a collection of eight articles devoted to that topic in two issues of the 1999 volume of the *Journal of the American Academy of Audiology* (Cox, 1999a, 1999b). Distinctions between objective and subjective outcomes, and conceptual distinctions among hearing aid benefit, satisfaction, and use, along with statistical analysis of their interrelationships, have led to the conclusion that hearing aid outcomes are truly multidimensional (Humes, 1999). Another important development has been the recognition that standardized assessments, in which the same questions are asked of all respondents, can fail to assess areas of function that are important to the individual. Examples of personalized assessments are the Client Oriented Scale of Improvement (COSI) (Dillon, Birtles, and Lovegrove, 1999) and the Glasgow Hearing Aid Benefit Profile (GHABP) (Gatehouse, 1999).

Quality of Life. Among the most popular approaches to outcomes assessment has been the attempt to measure a global outcome called "quality of life." Quality of life is a concept that encompasses physical, social, psychological, and environmental aspects of an individual's life. In the social and medical sciences, the concept has defied precise and distinct conceptualization (Rogerson, 1995), and operational definitions range from health economists' quality-adjusted life years (QALY) to scores on disease-specific self-report questionnaires. In Rogerson's conceptualization, environmental and health-related quality of life are each viewed as a sense of satisfaction and well-being that is multiply determined: by external factors and their characteristics and by the characteristics of the individuals themselves. Palmore and Luikart (1972), Flanagan (1978), and Bowling (1995) have taken an empirical approach to determining what is most important to adults in the general population. Their studies revealed similar factors, with health (both one's own and that of significant others) high on the list and physical welfare/finances/standard of living also in the top five. Bowling reported that "relationships with family and relatives" was the most frequently mentioned and most frequently first-ranked item.

Health-Related Quality of Life. Given the impact of hearing loss on communication and interpersonal functioning and the importance of interpersonal relationships in determining quality of life, it is not surprising that there has been significant interest in incorporating health-related quality-of-life measures into the diagnosis of rehabilitative needs of persons with hearing loss and the evaluation of rehabilitative interventions. In a causal chain that begins with hearing loss and its effects on disability and handicap (World Health Organization, 1980), quality of life is an ultimate state or outcome that is a function of all three (Ebrahim, 1995). As might be expected, issues of conceptualization and operational definition have been no less difficult in audiology than in other behavioral domains.

Global measures of health-related quality of life (HRQL) serve several purposes, both at a population level and at an individual level. Clinically, they may be useful in diagnosis of disease, assessment of prognosis, treatment outcome evaluation, and determination of etiology (Ebrahim, 1995). Examples of global HRQL instruments include the Self Evaluation of Life Function (SELF) scale (Linn and Linn, 1984), the Sickness Impact Profile (Bregner, Bobbitt, Carter, and Gilson, 1981), the EuroQOL (The EuroQol Group, 1990), the Medical Outcomes Study Short Form 36 (SF-36) (Ware and Sherbourne, 1992), the World Health Organization's WHOQOL (1993), and the Dartmouth COOP Functional Health Assessment (Nelson, Wasson, Johnson, and Hays, 1996).

There is evidence of an association between some global quality-of-life scales and degree of hearing loss. Bess, Lichtenstein, Logan, Burger, and Nelson (1989) found a systematic relation between degree of hearing impairment and scores on the physical, psychosocial, and overall scales of the Sickness Impact Profile. Similarly, Dalton et al. (2003) have reported that hearing loss, self-reported hearing handicap, and communication difficulties were associated with small but significant differences in quality of life, as measured by the SF-36.

Despite the attractiveness of having such global measures, their usefulness has been questioned on conceptual and psychometric grounds (Ebrahim, 1995), and they have not been found to be sufficiently sensitive to detect clinically meaningful changes in adults with hearing loss. Bess (2000) reviewed studies that used the Sickness Impact Profile, the SELF, the SF-36, and the Dartmouth COOP Functional Health Assessment to evaluate the outcomes of hearing-aid fitting, often in conjunction with more communication-specific assessments. The benefits of amplification were typically found on the latter measures but not on the more general quality-of-life measures. This lack of sensitivity is understandable, given the myriad factors that influence outcomes far removed from the causal agents one wishes to evaluate. Perhaps for this reason, Ebrahim concludes that measures of impairment, disability, and handicap have advantages over global health-related quality-of-life measures for clinical purposes. Disease-specific instruments that are grounded in an understanding of predictable disease consequences and precise treatment outcome goals afford greater potential, ipso facto, of being sensitive to treatment effects.

Appropriate Uses of Self-Assessment Instruments

Self-assessment scales have been used widely in research and in clinical settings. Scales focusing on disability and handicap have been used successfully to evaluate the need for audiological rehabilitation and to measure the outcomes of treatment interventions, such as hearing aids, cochlear implants, and specific rehabilitation programs. Such uses are appropriate when there is psychometric evidence of the tests' validity for these purposes. However, despite the considerable progress that has been made in the conceptualization and assessment of hearing disability and handicap (as defined by the World Health Organization), these measurements have little to offer in disability determination as defined by SSA. When a client seeks treatment for a hearing loss, it is usually assumed that symptoms are reported conscientiously. In contrast, when assessment is conducted for purposes of determining compensation, there is an inherent conflict of interest, and self-reports cannot be used with confidence (Dobie, 1996).

What, then, is the role of self-assessed disability or handicap in a compensation context? Dobie and Sakai (2001) argue that direct measurement of disability and handicap through self-report constitutes a gold standard, but that surrogate measures must be used in contexts in which compensation is involved. Despite the fact that audiometric measures of pure-tone threshold and speech recognition are imperfectly correlated with disability/handicap, they argue that these (more objective) measures can serve as surrogates in a compensation context. Moreover, based on the available data, they find insufficient evidence to support a change from the 1979 AAO-HNS/AMA (American Medical Association, 2001) method of estimating hearing handicap. Research is needed to more fully understand the relations and interactions among objective measures of hearing abilities, demographic and psychological factors, and self-reported communication outcomes and to evaluate the unique contribution of hearing loss among these other influences.

RECOMMENDATIONS

Disability Determination

The committee examined the use of self-reports and concludes that self-reports should *not* be used as criteria for disability determination. In clinical settings, there is little motivation for exaggeration of problems, but in the context of disability determination, conflict of interest poses a serious threat to the validity of self-reports.

The committee examined the potential usefulness of quality of life as an outcome variable. First, because quality of life is assessed through self-report, the conflict of interest that arises with all self-reports in disability determination applies equally to measures of quality of life. In addition, the committee concludes that definitions of quality of life, including health-related quality of life, are not sufficiently precise for such assessments to provide useful outcome measures. Finally, the labeling of hearing-related self-assessments as measures of quality of life is to be discouraged, as it is a doubly indirect form of assessment.

Self-reports can provide valuable, albeit indirect, information about an individual's functioning in daily life. For this reason, they can and should be used as outcome measures in predictive validation studies that do not involve claimants.

Tests that purport to measure or predict functional hearing ability in daily life must be validated against real-world criteria measured in natural settings. Validation in a simulated test environment is appropriate if a strong relation between the simulated and naturalistic settings can be demonstrated or assumed.

Research Recommendation

Research Recommendation 6-1. Research is needed on the prevalence of hearing loss in the workplace and on its effects on worker performance. In conjunction with this, the effectiveness of workplace accommodations, including devices and other types of accommodation, needs to be established.

7

Hearing Loss in Children

Spoken communication is uniquely human. If the sense of hearing is damaged or absent, individuals with the loss are denied the opportunity to sample an important feature of their environment, the sounds emitted by nature and by humans themselves. People who are deaf or hard-of-hearing will have diminished enjoyment for music or the sound of a babbling brook. We recognize that some deaf and hard-of-hearing children are born to deaf parents who communicate through American Sign Language. Without hearing, these children have full access to the language of their home environment and that of the deaf community. However, the majority of deaf and hard-of-hearing children are born to hearing parents. For these families, having a child with hearing loss may be a devastating situation. The loss or reduction of the sense of hearing impairs children's ability to hear speech and consequently to learn the intricacies of the spoken language of their environment. Hearing loss impairs their ability to produce and monitor their own speech and to learn the rules that govern the use of speech sounds (phonemes) in their native spoken language if they are born to hearing parents. Consequently, if appropriate early intervention does not occur within the first 6-12 months, hearing loss or deafness, even if mild, can be devastating to the development of spoken communication with hearing family and peers, to the development of sophisticated language use, and to many aspects of educational development, if environmental compensation does not occur.

Hearing loss can affect the development of children's ability to engage in age-appropriate activities, their functional speech communication skills, and their language skills. Before we consider the effects of hearing loss on this development, we will review briefly the extensive literature on the development of speech and language in children with normal hearing. Although the ages at which certain development milestones occur may vary, the sequence in which they occur is usually constant (Menyuk, 1972).

This chapter discusses the nature of the emergence of communication skills in normally hearing children as well as the unique effects of early hearing loss and deafness on this process for infants and children. We give details of the special nature of assessments and rehabilitation strategies appropriate for infants and children with hearing loss and finally discuss how considerations for disability determination need to be tailored to the special needs of this population.

DEVELOPMENT OF PERCEPTION, SPEECH PRODUCTION, AND LANGUAGE

Children with Normal Hearing

Speech Skills

Infants begin to differentiate among various sound intensities almost immediately after birth and, by 1 week of age, can make gross distinctions between tones. By 6 weeks of age, infants pay more attention to speech than to other sounds, discriminate between voiced and unvoiced speech sounds, and prefer female to male voices (Nober and Nober, 1977).

Infants begin to vocalize at birth, and those with normal hearing proceed through the stages of pleasure sounds, vocal play, and babbling until the first meaningful words begin to occur at or soon after 1 year of age (Bangs, 1968; Menyuk, 1972; Quigley and Paul, 1984; Stark, 1983). Speech-like stress patterns begin to emerge during the babbling stages (Stark, 1983), along with pitch and intonational contours (Bangs, 1968; Quigley and Paul, 1984; Stark, 1983).

According to Templin (1957), most children (75 percent) can produce all the vowel sounds and diphthongs by 3 years of age; by 7 years of age, 75 percent of children are able to produce all the phonemes, with the exception of "r." Consonant blends are usually mastered by 8 years of age, and overall speech production ability is generally adult-like by that time (Menyuk, 1972; Quigley and Paul, 1984).

Language Skills

Language studies have described vocabulary and grammatical development of children with normal hearing. Studies of grammatical development have focused on both word structure (e.g., prefixes and suffixes), termed "morphology," and the rules for arranging words into sentences, termed "syntax." Vocabulary development up to young adulthood is estimated at roughly 1,000 word families per year, with vocabulary size estimated at approximately 4,000-5,000 word families for 5-year-olds and 20,000 word families for 20-year-olds (see Schmitt, 2000, for discussion). A word family is defined as a word plus its derived and inflectional forms. Most morphological and syntactic skills are fully developed by the age of 5 years, and grammatical skills are fully developed by age 8 (Nober and Nober, 1977). By age 10 to 12, most children with normal hearing have reached linguistic maturity (Quigley and Paul, 1984). In summary, by age $4^{1}/_{2}$ years, children with normal hearing are producing complex sentences. Although a majority of the speech sounds in English are mastered by age 4, and most of the grammatical categories by age 5, it is not until age 8 that a normally hearing child has fully mastered grammar and phonology and has an extensive vocabulary (Nober and Nober, 1977).

Children with Hearing Loss

A review of speech and language development in children with hearing loss is complicated by the heterogeneity of childhood hearing loss, such as differences in age at onset and in degree of loss; we review these complicating factors separately following a more general overview. Mental and physical incapacities (mental retardation, cerebral palsy, etc.) may also coexist with hearing loss. Approximately 25-33 percent of children with hearing loss have multiple potentially disabling conditions (Holden-Pitt and Diaz, 1998; McCracken, 1994; Moeller, Coufal, and Hixson, 1990). In addition, independent learning disabilities and language disabilities due to cognitive or linguistic disorders not directly associated with hearing loss may coexist (Mauk and Mauk, 1992; Sikora and Plapinger, 1994; Wolgemuth, Kamhi, and Lee, 1998). For example, Holden-Pitt and Diaz (1998) reported the following incidences of additional impairments in a group of children with some degree of hearing loss:

1. blind/uncorrected vision problem (4 percent),
2. emotional/behavioral problem (4 percent),
3. mental retardation (8 percent), and
4. learning disability (9 percent).

The coexistence of other disabilities with hearing impairment may impact the way in which sensory aids are fitted or the benefit that children receive from them (Tharpe, Fino-Szumski, and Bess, 2001). A recent technical report from the American Speech-Language-Hearing Association stated that pediatric cochlear implant recipients with multiple impairments often demonstrate delayed or reduced communication gains compared with their peers with hearing loss alone (American Speech-Language-Hearing Association, 2004).

In this chapter, we focus on speech and language development in children with prelingual onset of hearing loss (before 2 years of age) without comorbidity. However, it should be kept in mind that the presence of multiple handicapping conditions may place a child at greater risk for the development of communication or emotional disorders (Cantwell, as summarized by Prizant et al., 1990). In addition, these children may require adaptations to standard testing routines to accommodate their individual capacities.

Natural acquisition of speech and spoken language is not often seen in individuals with profound hearing loss unless appropriate intervention is initiated early. One of the primary goals in fitting deaf or hard-of-hearing children with auditory prostheses (hearing aid or cochlear implant) is to improve the ease and the extent to which they can access and acquire speech and spoken language. It should be kept in mind that the children under discussion typically are not born to deaf parents; those children may acquire American Sign Language as their native language.

Speech Skills

Speech and voice characteristics of persons who are deaf or hard-of-hearing are generally acknowledged to differ significantly from those of individuals with normal hearing (Abberton and Fourcin, 1975; Hood and Dixon, 1969; Monsen, 1974, 1978, 1983b; Monsen and Engebretson, 1977; Monsen, Engebretson, and Vemula, 1978, 1979; Nickerson, 1975; Nober and Nober, 1977; Stark, 1983; Wirz, Subtelny, and Whitehead, 1981). A congenital or prelingually acquired hearing loss reduces the intelligibility of talkers who are deaf or hard-of-hearing and impairs the production and tonal aspects of their speech (John and Howarth, 1965; Markides, 1970; McGarr and Osberger, 1978; Monsen, 1979; Osberger and Levitt, 1979; Smith, 1975).

Difficulties with speech sound production include problems with the articulation of vowels and consonants, such as substitutions, distortions, and omissions (Hudgins and Numbers, 1942; Zimmerman and Rettaliata, 1981); excessive use of a neutral vowel, such as schwa (/ə/), the unstressed vowel sound in the second syllable of the word "kitten" (Markides, 1970); lack of adequate differentiation between various vowels (Angelocci, Kopp, and Holbrook, 1964; Levitt and Stromberg, 1983); and failure to differentiate between voiced and voiceless consonant sounds, for example "b" and "p" (Calvert, 1962; Monsen, 1976; Whitehead, 1983). These problems are accompanied by a significantly slowed rate of general speech sound awareness (phonological development) in children with hearing loss (Subtelny, 1983). Although many talkers who are deaf or hard-of-hearing can correctly produce phonemes in isolation, they may still be unable to smoothly combine the phonemes in connected speech. Thus, reduced speech intelligibility can result.

Language Skills

Vocabulary knowledge in children with hearing loss may be age appropriate or reduced, with results showing large variability (Gilbertson and Kamhi, 1995; Seyfried and Kricos, 1996; Yoshinaga-Itano, 1994). In general, however, the rate of vocabulary growth is slowed, and may plateau prematurely (Briscoe, Bishop, and Norbury, 2001; Carney and Moeller, 1998; Davis, 1974; Davis, Elfenbein, Schum, and Bentler, 1986; Moeller, Osberger, and Eccarius, 1986). Word entries may have less breadth or flexibility of meaning (Moeller et al., 1986; Yoshinaga-Itano, 1994). In particular, nonliteral or abstract word usage may be impoverished. The dynamic time course of accessing the meanings of words may also be slowed (slowed lexical retrieval) in children with hearing loss, although again, large unpredictable variability among individuals occurs (Jerger, Lai, and Marchman, 2002). In concert with vocabulary development, grammatical knowledge is also reduced in children with hearing loss.

For example, in a sentence construction task, 14-year-old children who were deaf or hard-of-hearing performed similarly to 6- to 8-year-old children with normal hearing (Templin, 1966). In spoken language samples, the sentences of children who were deaf or hard-of-hearing were of shorter lengths with simpler sentence constructions and syntax (Brannon and Murray, 1966; Seyfried and Kricos, 1996). Sentences in the passive voice were not successfully comprehended or produced by about half of 17- to 18-year-old children who were deaf or hard-of-hearing (Power and Quigley, 1973). In studies of the morphological rules for different types of suffixes (e.g., -s as in sings and -er as in singer), children who are deaf or hard-of-hearing generally show inferior performance (Bunch and Clarke, 1978; Cooper, 1967; Elfenbein, Hardin-Jones, and Davis, 1994). The extent to which specific language skills are delayed versus deviant in the presence of childhood hearing loss continues to be pursued. It should also be noted that language proficiency is a strong predictor of reading achievement (Carney and Moeller, 1998). Thus, age-appropriate literacy skills typically are not observed in children with hearing loss and language problems.

Complicating Factors

One factor that influences the extent to which speech and language development is affected by hearing loss is the child's age when the loss occurs. Auditory deprivation early in life has serious consequences for subsequent development (Davis, 1965). In general, children with early, prelingual hearing losses more frequently display deficits in the respiratory, articulatory, and phonatory aspects of speech (Binnie, Daniloff, and Buckingham, 1982; de Quiros, 1980; Itoh, Horii, Daniloff, and Binnie, 1982; Nober and Nober, 1977). Three important periods for onset of hearing loss have been described by de Quiros (1980). Children whose hearing loss occurs during the first 2 years of life are considered prelingually deafened. If profound deafness occurs prior to 2 years of age and intervention is delayed, speech can be severely disturbed. Hearing losses that occur between ages 2 and 5 will result in the loss of speech skills unless appropriate sensory aids and aural rehabilitation are provided. Finally, de Quiros suggests that deafness occurring after age 5 can result in appropriate articulation; however, good articulation skills may deteriorate if sensory input is not reestablished with amplification. Again, these detrimental outcomes may be ameliorated if the child is provided with a sensory aid that can provide auditory access to the acoustic properties of speech.

Age at onset of hearing loss is not the only important prognostic indicator for speech and language development in children who are deaf or hard-of-hearing. A second critical factor is the degree of hearing loss. In a classic study, Hudgins and Numbers (1942) described an inverse relationship between articulatory errors and audiometric scores. Other authors have suggested that speech intelligibility decreases as the degree of hearing loss increases (Jensema, Karchmer, and Trybus, 1978; McGarr and Osberger, 1978; Monsen, 1983a). Similarly, Quigley and Paul (1984) reported that deficits in language comprehension and usage increase with degree of hearing loss. In spite of this overall trend, however, a general finding is that degree of hearing loss cannot perfectly predict speech and language abilities in individual children (Davis et al., 1986; Gilbertson and Kamhi, 1995; Mayne, Yoshinaga-Itano, and Sedey, 1998; Seyfried and Kricos, 1996).

Unilateral Hearing Loss

A study published in 1998 estimated that the prevalence of unilateral hearing loss in school-age children ranged from 6.4 to 12.3 per 1,000 and at that time there were 391,000 school-age children with unilateral hearing loss (Lee, Gomez-Marin, and Lee, 1998). There is a pervasive misunderstanding that unilateral hearing loss is of no consequence and that this problem can be disregarded. Consequently, children with unilateral hearing loss often receive no direct intervention, such as amplification or therapeutic services. However, research now has shown that children with unilateral hearing loss are disadvantaged. In particular, children with unilateral hearing loss have difficulty in understanding speech in noisy environments and are deficient relative to their peers in localization of a sound source (Bess, Tharpe, and Gibler, 1986). Another study found that 32 percent of children in a cohort with unilateral hearing loss failed a grade in school and were significantly delayed in language compared with a matched group of children with normal hearing (Klee and Davis-Dansky, 1986).

Age at Intervention

Because speech and language develop rapidly during the early years in children's lives (up to age 5), the importance of early intervention, including suitable amplification or cochlear implantation, can be seen. It is generally agreed that such intervention procedures are most effective when initiated as early as possible after the identification of the hearing loss (Silverman, 1983). According to Ling (1979), the motor skills required for speech can be learned at any time, but they are most likely to be transferred to the spontaneous level if children have not developed firmly established error patterns. Intervention techniques should be initiated at an early stage and should mirror the pattern of development in children with normal hearing (Ling, 1979).

EFFECTS OF HEARING LOSS ON LITERACY AND EDUCATION

Recent data from the Gallaudet Research Institute's annual survey indicate that approximately 51.2 percent of children and youth with hearing loss are white, 15.4 percent black, 24.5 percent Hispanic, 4.3 percent Asian-Pacific Islander, and 0.8 percent American Indian, with the rest falling under the "other" or multiethnic categories (Gallaudet Research Institute, 2002). About 54 percent are male and 46 percent are female. This survey represents a database of roughly 60 percent of children in the United States who are deaf and hard-of-hearing and is based on reports from educational programs in which these children are enrolled (Karchmer and Mitchell, 2003). Current racial/ethnic proportions now mirror those found in the United States (Holden-Pitt and Diaz, 1998).

The following is a condensation of information presented by Karchmer and Mitchell (2003). In terms of educational placement, 31.7 percent are in regular education settings, 12.6 percent are in resource rooms in these settings, 27.5 percent are in self-contained classrooms in regular education settings, 24.7 percent are in specialized schools, and the rest of the children (3.5 percent) are in other types of settings. In essence, two-thirds of all such children are now receiving at least some academic instruction in a regular classroom. Slightly more than 90 percent come from homes where only one spoken or written language (primarily English or Spanish) is used regularly. Self-contained educational settings have a larger percentage (almost 25 percent) of students from Spanish-speaking homes, almost twice the percentage found in the other three settings taken in aggregate. Special schools tend to enroll children with profound hearing impairments while self-contained classrooms serve students across the hearing spectrum, and regular school settings serve mostly those with less than severe degrees of hearing loss. The primary communication mode in educational settings is strongly related to degree of hearing loss. Specifically, those with profound losses are typically educated in programs that use signing or signing with speech, while students with milder hearing losses are most typically in speech-based programs. Students in regular education settings are least likely to have additional disabilities.

With regard to academic achievement, children who lose their hearing after learning English generally achieve higher scores on standardized tests, including reading, than those with hearing loss at younger ages. The exception is deaf children of deaf parents, who tend to have higher English-language achievement scores than those with limited access to linguistic interaction both inside and outside the home. It is important to keep in mind, however, that the range of results is considerable. Mathematics performance, while higher than for language-based achievement, is not equivalent to that for hearing peers.

In addition, students with hearing loss tend to demonstrate the same relative academic performance differences as their hearing peers across racial and ethnic groups. Karchmer and Mitchell (2003) emphasize the confound between race/ethnicity and lower socioeconomic status (SES), which makes it difficult to identify the impact of SES for students who are deaf and hard-of-hearing. Sex differences are minimal.

In the recent past, it has been reported that the vast majority of persons educated in deaf schools (95 percent) reach a reading age of only 9 years (Stern, 2001; Traxler, 2000). Reading achievement scores are reduced even for students with minimal sensorineural hearing loss (Bess, Dodd-Murphy, and Parker, 1998). Reading deficits are exacerbated by reduced vocabulary, as previously discussed. More important, however, are deaf children's deficits in phonological awareness. This is a crucial skill in the development of sound-symbol associations and consequently in reading ability. Paul (2003) emphasizes that deaf readers who use phonological codes for processing print do better than those who use nonphonological codes. Consequently, access to phonological information is critical. Reading and generalized linguistic difficulties can also be manifested in deficits in other areas of academics, including mathematics (Hyde, Zevenbergen, and Power, 2003) and science (McIntosh, Sulzen, Reeder, and Kidd, 1994).

Although children are not in the workforce, they do spend considerable time in school. It is known that poor classroom acoustics (Acoustical Society of America, 2000) exacerbate difficulties in development of speech perception and eventually contribute to language and cognitive problems (Nelson, Soli, and Seltz, 2002). Perceptual difficulties in children due to poor classroom acoustics are especially challenging for children with even mild to moderate hearing loss (Bess et al., 1998), especially if English is not their primary language (Nelson et al., 2002). Poor classroom acoustics can result from too much noise intruding into the classroom from outside, leading to a poor signal-to-noise ratio for speech communication (Soli and Sullivan, 1997). Many classrooms also are poorly designed in terms of controlling for reverberation time (Knecht, Nelson, Whitelaw, and Feth, 2002). As explained earlier, reverberation time is a measure of the amount of time that a sound remains in the room after the original sound source has ceased, due to the reflections within the room (Acoustical Society of America, 2000). Long reverberation times mean that sounds already produced can interfere with newly produced sounds, leading to low speech intelligibility. It is known that normally hearing children's auditory processing capabilities are adversely affected by long reverberation times (Johnson, 2000; Litovsky, 1997). Children with hearing loss are at risk in their ability to understand spoken communication in many schools. This difficulty can lead to reduced language and cognitive development.

A clinical entity known as central auditory processing disorder (CAPD) is a dysfunction in perceiving auditory signals that is not attributed to peripheral hearing loss (McFarland and Cacace, 1995). CAPD is believed to subsume specific language and reading disabilities in school-age children. The area of CAPD assessment and remediation is not considered in this report, because this disability by definition is not attributed to hearing impairment. Children suspected of this disorder would be evaluated more appropriately in the domain of developmental disabilities.

In summary, even mild hearing loss places children at risk for speech, language, and educational problems. A view expressed in the literature, however, is that strong familial support and early enrollment in high-quality intervention programs can increase the chances of successful speech and language outcomes in the presence of childhood hearing loss (Moeller, 2000; Yoshinaga-Itano and Apuzzo, 1998a, 1998b; Yoshinaga-Itano, Sedey, Coulter, and Mehl, 1998). Appropriate early intervention, for example, educational intervention, hearing aids, or cochlear implantation, can help to improve the performance of deaf children in areas of language and academic performance (Boothroyd and Boothroyd-Turner, 2002; Tomblin, Spencer, and Gantz, 2000). Next we turn to diagnosing and quantifying hearing loss in infants and children.

INFANT HEARING SCREENING

Hearing loss in infants is not obvious, and without specific measures to test for the condition it will go undetected for a significant period of time. As recently as 1996, the average age of identification of hearing loss in the United States was 30 months (Harrison and Roush, 1996). The means to evaluate infants for hearing loss with clinical tools, such as auditory brainstem response (ABR) and otoacoustic emissions (OAEs) have emerged in the past 20 years. However, until recently newborn hearing loss screening programs have existed in only a few hospitals for high-risk infants. In 1993, the National Institute on Deafness and Other Communication Disorders (NIDCD) of the National Institutes of Health issued a consensus statement (National Institutes of Health, 1993) calling for screening of all infants for hearing loss by 3 months of age. By 2000, the American Academy of Pediatrics (1999, 2000) endorsed universal newborn hearing screening for all infants prior to hospital release. Currently all 50 states have legislation either passed or pending to mandate universal newborn hearing screening, or they are conducting screening for most newborns without legislation.

Neonatal hearing screening programs have proven effective as the first step in early identification of infants with congenital hearing loss. These programs identify infants at risk for a mild or more serious hearing loss. It is important to note that screening identifies only which infants are in need of a more complete assessment to determine if hearing loss exists. Infants failing this screening require a diagnostic audiological assessment by a qualified audiologist to confirm the presence of hearing loss and determine the exact type and degree of hearing loss in each ear. Results of the diagnostic evaluation are used to determine the degree of disability, to determine eligibility for rehabilitation programs and financial assistance, and to form the basis for fitting of amplification and placement in appropriate educational settings.

Although the screening process for newborn hearing loss is excellent, it is not perfect. Children with mild hearing loss or hearing loss in restricted frequency regions may pass the screening. Some children develop significant permanent hearing loss after the newborn period, which is not detected by the screening. Infants with neural hearing loss, such as auditory neuropathy, will pass a screening if an OAE test alone is used for screening (Sininger, 2002). Infants with late-onset hearing loss will be missed in the newborn screening; and constant surveillance is needed by the medical community to find these infants and begin remediation as soon as possible (Joint Committee on Infant Hearing, 2000).

The screening and diagnostic testing process is designed to expedite intervention for children with hearing loss and maximize the opportunity to provide audition during critical learning periods (Sininger, Doyle, and Moore, 1999; Yoshinaga-Itano et al., 1998). The goal of early hearing detection and intervention programs is to identify hearing loss and begin intervention including fitting of hearing aids at or before 6 months of age.

Assessment of hearing loss in infants requires age-appropriate procedures. Infants under 6 months of age cannot give an accurate response to sounds at threshold levels, regardless of their ability to detect them. These infants require an audiological test battery based on objective physiological tests that reveal threshold-level responses, as well as information regarding the functioning of the peripheral auditory system.

AUDIOMETRIC DIAGNOSTIC EVALUATION

General agreement exists in the United States regarding the essential elements of an appropriate protocol for diagnostic audiological assessments of infants and young children. An audiologist with appropriate state licensure or equivalent credentials must perform such assessments. The complete battery includes a history and parent interview, evaluation of middle ear function, OAE testing, and an age-appropriate assessment of auditory behaviors. The core of the diagnostic evaluation protocol is an estimate of audiometric thresholds using auditory brainstem response or other proven electrophysiological assessment with frequency-specific stimuli. According to the American Academy of Pediatrics (2000, p. 804):

> Audiologists providing the initial test battery to confirm the existence of a hearing loss in infants must include physiological measures and developmentally appropriate behavioral techniques. . . . For infants birth to six months of age, the test battery . . . must contain an electrophysiological measure of threshold such as ABR or other appropriate electrophysiological test using frequency-specific stimuli.

Threshold Audiometry

Unlike vision, human auditory sensitivity is adult-like within a few days of birth (Adelman, Levi, Linder, and Sohmer, 1990; Klein, 1984; Sininger, Abdala, and Cone-Wesson, 1997). Consequently, hearing loss degree and configuration are judged by the same standards for newborns as for adults.

The basic hearing evaluation for persons of any age is the pure-tone audiogram. Thresholds are also measured using speech stimuli. Establishing thresholds for tonal and speech stimuli by air and bone conduction using standard adult procedures is possible with children who have a developmental age of 4-5 years. Prior to that age, procedures must be modified to meet developmental demands. For all pediatric assessments, multiple-procedure test batteries are recommended to ensure the consistency of results.

Pure-tone or frequency-specific threshold tests in infants and children are classified either as physiological tests, in which a response is determined by some objectively measured change in physiological status, or behavioral tests, in which an overt response is elicited from children in response to sound and their responses are judged by an audiologist. Physiological tests do not actually measure perception of sound but can generally predict hearing thresholds or the range of hearing with a great deal of precision. The most valuable of these tests for threshold prediction for infants less than 6 months old is the ABR. A promising but as yet less proven technique for threshold prediction in these very young children is the auditory steady-state response (ASSR). Other physiological measures that correlate with hearing levels and support the test battery include tympanometry, acoustic middle ear muscle reflex, and OAEs.

Behavioral threshold tests for children under 5 are classified in Table 7-1. It is generally assumed that reliable behavioral responses to sound in infants under the developmental age of 6 months will be suprathreshold. By 6 months of age, normally developing children can be trained to respond to threshold-level stimuli using an operant conditioning paradigm known as visual reinforcement audiometry (VRA). Consequently, before

TABLE 7-1 Behavioral Tests of Hearing Threshold

Developmental Age	Test	Description	Accuracy
0-6 months	Behavioral observation audiometry	Systematic observation of behaviors in response to sound	Response is suprathreshold
6 months-2 years	Visual reinforcement audiometry	Conditioned response to head-turn reinforced by visual stimulus	Thresholds obtained
2-5 years	Play audiometry; tangible reinforcement audiometry	Test involves a game or tangible reinforcement for correct response	Thresholds obtained

6 months of age, audiometric thresholds must be inferred from physiological tests such as ABR.

However, during the 0- to 6-month age period, it is possible to obtain unconditioned responses to sound, such as a change in sucking behavior, startle reflex, or eye widening. This test paradigm is known as behavioral observation audiometry (BOA). These responses will be suprathreshold and cannot rule out mild or moderate hearing loss. BOA is nonetheless a valuable part of the test battery for infants under age 6 months to substantiate overall impressions.

Children with normal vision at the developmental level of typical 6-month-olds naturally turn their heads to find the source of an interesting sound. VRA takes advantage of that fact by reinforcing head turns with a pleasant visual stimulus, usually an animated toy that is lit to become visible for a short time following a head turn that is time-locked to the presentation of an auditory stimulus. Tones and speech can be used. The test must be administered quickly after appropriate conditioning to maintain the child's interest. A variety of visual reinforcers can be used to elicit head turns in response to near-threshold level stimuli. VRA can be administered using insert earphones for an ear-specific response or with a bone-conduction vibrator. If a child will not tolerate earphones, the stimuli can be presented through a speaker into the sound field of a sound-treated chamber. This procedure limits the conclusions of the tests to hearing in the better ear and cannot determine a unilateral hearing loss. Generally, normally hearing 6-month-old infants will respond to stimuli of 20 dB HL or better (Widen and O'Grady, 2002).

VRA may no longer hold the interest of children who have reached the developmental status of a 2-year-old. In that case, the children's interest can usually be maintained by involving them in a play activity. Play audiometry involves making a game of hearing sounds. Children respond to the sound presentation, for example, by dropping a block into a bucket or stacking a ring on a peg. Devices are available that dispense a tangible reward, such as a piece of candy or a token, when an appropriate response to sound is given. This is known as tangible reinforcement audiometry (TROCA). As long as the interest of the child can be maintained, these techniques will yield accurate audiometric threshold evaluations.

Otoacoustic Emissions

OAE tests are described in detail in Chapter 3. The objective nature of these measures and the ease with which they generally can be obtained make OAEs ideal for assessment of cochlear function in infants, toddlers, and all cooperative children. These measures are used in newborn hearing screening because the presence of a response can be interpreted as indicating normal cochlear function sufficient to indicate hearing levels generally better than 30 to 40 dB. These levels correspond to no more than mild hearing loss and are in line with screening levels for newborns.

As emphasized in Chapter 3, OAEs used to assess children must be used in a test battery to avoid common pitfalls. The presence of an OAE alone does not indicate normal hearing and the absence of a response can be due to factors other than cochlear dysfunction, such as middle ear dysfunction.

Auditory Brainstem Response

The ABR as described in Chapter 3 is an important part of any audiometric evaluation of infants and children. The ABR is present in infants as young as 28 weeks gestation (Starr, Amlie, Martin, and Sanders, 1977). ABR is stable in infants and is unaffected by sleep or sedation. Frequency-specific ABR is the test universally recommended to determine thresholds in infants who do not pass newborn hearing screening (Joint Committee on Infant Hearing, 2000). The accuracy of predicting the actual hearing threshold using ABR is quite good, generally within 10 dB (Sininger et al., 1997; Stapells, Picton, Durieux-Smith, Edwards, and Moran, 1990).

ABRs generated in infants for threshold prediction may require specific recording parameters that differ from those that are standard for use with adults. Infant ABRs are slower and later than those of adults and generally require a long analysis window of 20-30 ms and a lowered band-pass filter (30 to 1000 Hz). Infants' recordings, especially those made during natural sleep, may be noisy, requiring longer averaging time to achieve adequate signal-to-noise ratio for reliable response detection.

The ABR can sometimes be absent or severely abnormal, even when the inner ear is functioning well, due to auditory neuropathy. Children with this disorder will have an abnormal or absent ABR but usually will also show a present OAE. When this condition exists, neither the ABR nor the OAE can be used to predict hearing levels. The hearing loss in patients with auditory neuropathy can be of any degree, and their speech perception ability is severely disordered. Therefore, it is very important to include the measurement of OAEs in any assessment of hearing using ABR. If the ABR and OAE are disparate in the prediction of threshold, then auditory neuropathy must be suspected, and neither will be a good indicator of hearing level.

Auditory Steady-State Response

The ASSR, previously known as the steady-state evoked potential (SSEP), is another way of objectively assessing frequency-specific responses, and it is described fully in Chapter 3. For infants and children, the appropriate modulation frequency range is about 80-100 Hz. Long segments of these stimuli are presented and ongoing electroencephalographic activity is sampled and analyzed in the frequency domain. When the neural activity shows a preference for the modulation frequency over other frequencies in the analysis, it is assumed that the auditory system is responding to the carrier frequency.

One reservation about the use of ASSR for measurement of hearing in infants and children is the lack of good data on them (Stapells, 2002). Rickards has found that normally hearing infants may not have a reliable response below about 40 dB (Rickards et al., 1994). This would make it impossible to distinguish between mild hearing loss and normal hearing, which is critically important for determination of amplification needs. Data from Perez-Abalo and colleagues (Perez-Abalo et al., 2001) showed that although they were able to determine hearing loss in the severe and profound range, in general, there was only fair agreement between ASSR thresholds and hearing levels in children with hearing loss. Her data also showed that ASSR was unable to determine thresholds below 40 to 50 dB nHL (stimuli calibrated relative to thresholds in normally hearing individuals) in the children at any frequency. At this time it would be not be prudent to recommend the use of ASSR to determine hearing loss in infants and young children, especially those with mild and moderate hearing loss.

Immittance Audiometry

Immittance audiometry, as described in Chapter 3, is used to determine the physical status of the middle ear by assessing the mobility of the tympanic membrane. From these measures one can infer whether the membrane is intact or perforated, the pressure of the middle ear, and the functional status of the Eustachian tube. When middle ear function is impaired, for example due to reduced tympanic membrane mobility from otitis media with effusion, hearing sensitivity is reduced and generally the audiogram will show an air-bone gap.

Immittance audiometry is an objective measure requiring no overt response from patients, although cooperation for fitting of a pressure-tight ear canal probe and a few minutes of sitting still are required. Consequently, immittance is an important part of any pediatric audiometric assessment, because of the possibility of limited cooperation for standard bone conduction measures. Also, the incidence of otitis media with effusion is quite high in infants and toddlers.

When tympanic membrane mobility is normal, the acoustic stapedial reflex can be used as an assessment of brainstem auditory system function. Children with moderate hearing loss or greater will show elevated reflex thresholds or no reflex. Auditory neuropathy will also eliminate the acoustic stapedial reflex.

Immittance measures in children are essentially the same as those used for adults with one exception. Based on the physical properties of the ear canal, the probe frequency recommended for neonates and young infants is 1000 Hz (Rhodes, Margolis, Hirsch, and Napp, 1999).

COMMUNICATION ASSESSMENT

The ability to hear and understand speech can have a profound impact on all aspects of children's communication development and daily functioning. Clinicians must have available a wide array of age-appropriate outcome measures that allow them to target different aspects of communication skills (Kirk, 1999, 2000; Kirk, Pisoni, and Osberger, 1995). A battery of communication tests should be employed that includes measures of spoken word recognition, speech production, and receptive and expressive language abilities. The tests and administration procedures for each communication area are considered independently below. It may be necessary to select other tests or adapt the procedures for children who have other impairments in addition to hearing loss. For example, closed-set picture tests may be needed for children who cannot produce verbal or signed responses. Similarly, questionnaires completed by parents or caregivers may be used for children who cannot participate in structured testing situations.

Spoken Word Recognition

Tests utilizing speech stimuli can help to determine the extent to which a hearing loss affects the ability to perceive, recognize, and discriminate speech sounds. This information can be useful in diagnosing the type and severity of the hearing disorder, in assessing candidacy for sensory aid use (hearing aid versus cochlear implant), in informing aural rehabilitation strategies, and in estimating a child's listening abilities in real-world listening situations.

There are a number of factors that must be considered when selecting tests of spoken word recognition and interpreting their results. Characteristics that can impact performance on such measures include the child's chronological age, vocabulary and language level, speech production abilities, and cognitive abilities. Children with congenital or prelingually acquired hearing loss often are delayed in the development of speech and language skills and have restricted vocabularies. Thus, test measures with unfamiliar vocabulary may underestimate their auditory skills. Similarly, the task must be appropriate for the child's language and developmental abilities. If children do not have the cognitive ability to understand and perform a task, the testing will be invalid.

Methodological variables that impact performance outcomes include presentation level (Gravel and Hood, 1999), the method of stimulus presentation, the response format of the tests, the use of competing stimuli, and the sensory modality in which the speech signal is presented.

Recorded Versus Live Voice Stimulus Presentation

There are merits and drawbacks to the use of both live voice and recorded test administration. Live voice testing is problematic because the results depend, in part, on the characteristics of the person administering the test. Thus, results obtained with live voice stimulus presentation are not comparable across clinics or research centers unless talker equivalence can be demonstrated. Several clinicians and researchers have argued that consistency in presentation between listeners or over time can be maintained only through the use of recorded test stimuli (Carhart, 1965; Mendel and Danhauer, 1997). However, this is true only when a standard recording of a particular test is used. The use of different versions of a recorded test (i.e., those recorded by different talkers) can introduce as much variability in the acoustic signal as when two different talkers administer live voice tests. The advantages of live voice test administration are that it allows the examiner greater flexibility and often takes less time than using recorded materials. The use of live voice tests may be desirable for young children because the rate of stimulus presentation can be varied to ensure that children are attending to the task. In general, the use of recorded tests is preferred for assessing performance in older children, so that results can be compared across centers or testing intervals. There are no absolute age guidelines for converting from live voice to recorded test administration. It depends, in part, on the child's previous auditory experience and developmental level. It seems reasonable to attempt recorded testing by the time children are 5 years old. In fact, this age guideline for recorded test administration has been adopted in recent clinical trials of cochlear implant use in children.

Open-Set Versus Closed-Set Test Formats

Open-set tests are those in which listeners theoretically have an unlimited number of response possibilities. That is, no alternatives are provided from which to select a response. Closed-set tests restrict the listener to one of a fixed number of possible responses (e.g., as in a multiple-choice test). Closed-set tests reduce vocabulary and cognitive demands inherent in the speech perception task; they often are used to assess speech recognition in listeners with reduced language skills or limited speaking and writing abilities. However, closed-set tests may not adequately evaluate the perceptual processes that support word recognition in daily life.

In contrast, open-set tests are thought to better reflect the types of communication demands encountered in natural listening situations. For example, performance on open-set tests of spoken word recognition is influenced by cognitive (top-down) processing, just as is speech comprehension in the real world. Cognitive processing is facilitated by an individual's general knowledge (including vocabulary and linguistic knowledge), as well as by expectations based on the situational or linguistic context of the speech event.

Sometimes clinicians or researchers wish to evaluate an individual's sensory capabilities without the influence of cognitive or linguistic factors (see Tyler, 1993) in order to obtain information about the speech cues that are well conveyed by the individual's sensory aid. This information may be helpful in planning therapeutic intervention. Closed-set tests of word or nonsense syllable recognition can be used to assess perception of speech features in the absence of cognitive influences; these tests typically use foils that are acoustically or phonetically similar to the target item. Such closed-set tests of speech-feature perception also can be used to assess the performance of children who have limited auditory-only speech understanding.

Sources of Variability in the Speech Signal

In daily listening, children must cope with a great deal of variability in the speech signal introduced by different talkers, different speaking rates, different dialects, and competing noise, to name a few factors. Although clinical tests of spoken words in quiet yield estimates of children's speech understanding in optimal listening situations, they may not accurately estimate performance in daily living in which there are many sources of competing noise. Whenever possible, it is best to evaluate word recognition using tests containing multiple talkers or competing stimuli.

Multimodal Spoken Word Recognition

Information in the speech signal is conveyed through both the auditory and the visual modalities in face-to-face conversation. Children with similar degrees of hearing loss can differ greatly in their ability to understand speech through listening alone, and also in their ability to integrate auditory and visual speech information (Lachs, Pisoni, and Kirk, 2001). Assessing perceptual performance in the auditory-only, visual-only, and auditory + visual modalities provides information about how well speech is understood through listening alone, and also about the enhancement in speech perception obtained when auditory and visual cues are combined. Furthermore, assessing performance in the auditory + visual modality may better estimate real-world performance.

Measures for Preschool-Age Children

For the very youngest children, subjective communication scales, such as the Infant-Toddler Meaningful Auditory Integration Scale (IT-MAIS) (Zimmerman-Phillips, Robbins, and Osberger, 2000) have been used to assess auditory development. This scale assesses a variety of meaningful auditory behaviors used in everyday life. There are 10 questions. Parents are asked to respond on a scale from 0 to 4 indicating how often their child demonstrates a particular behavior. A 0 indicates that the child never demonstrates a given listening behavior, and a 4 indicates that the child always demonstrates a listening behavior. Thus the total score on the scale can range from 0 to 40.

By the time children reach the age of 3 years, they may be able to participate in formal spoken word recognition testing. Many measures of spoken word recognition have been developed over the years. We briefly present information on some of the more commonly used assessment tools that currently are available. (Interested readers may wish to review the work of Jerger, 1983, for a more thorough description and a comparison of the psychophysical characteristics of pediatric speech tests.) All of the tests described below require the administration of a standard number of test items across children. Other tests, such as the Early Speech Perception Test—Low Verbal Version (ESP-Low Verbal) (Moog and Geers, 1990) and the Early Speech Perception Test (Moog and Geers, 1990) follow a hierarchical approach, in which children move on to successive test items only after they achieve a minimum score on a previous level of the test. Although such tests can be useful in informing aural habilitation programs, the committee's view is that a more consistent test administration procedure is preferable for the purposes of determining disability in children.

The Northwestern University-Children's Perception of Speech Test (NU-CHIPS) (Elliott and Katz, 1980) is a closed-set test of speech discrimination. The test consists of 50 monosyllabic words that can be depicted in simple pictures and fall within the vocabulary of very young children. This is a closed-set picture-pointing task with four pictures per page. The test is intended for children who demonstrate a vocabulary recognition age of at least 2.5 years as measured by the Peabody Picture Vocabulary Test (Dunn and Dunn, 1997).

The Pediatric Speech Intelligibility Test (PSI) (Jerger and Jerger, 1984; Jerger, Lewis, Hawkins, and Jerger, 1980) was developed for children as young as 3 years of age for evaluating a range of auditory disorders. Both monosyllabic words and sentence materials were generated from words produced by children with normal hearing between 3 and 7 years of age. The test consists of 20 words depicted on four picture plates with five items per plate, and 10 sentences depicted on two five-picture plates. The child responds by pointing to the word or sentence that is presented. Jerger, Jerger, and Abrams (1983) found that test-retest reliability of the PSI word test was high for both children with normal hearing and children with hearing loss (r = .92). No significant differences were noted among the four lists of monosyllabic words. The reliability of performance on the PSI sentences also was high (r > .82) for children with normal hearing and those with hearing loss.

The Multisyllabic Lexical Neighborhood Test (MLNT) is an open-set word recognition test whose theoretical underpinnings are the Neighborhood Activation Model (NAM) of spoken word recognition (Luce and Pisoni, 1998). The NAM proposes that words are organized into "similarity neighborhoods" based on their frequency of occurrence (i.e., how often words occur in the language) and the density (i.e., acoustic-phonetic similarity) of words within the lexical neighborhood. The MLNT consists of two lists of 24 two- and three-syllable words containing vocabulary that is suitable for children age 3 years and older. On each list, half of the words are lexically "easy"; that is, they occur often in the language of young children and have few acoustically phonetically similar words with which they can be confused. The remaining "hard" words on the test have the opposite lexical characteristics.

The MLNT can be administered either via live voice or in recorded form. Children respond by repeating the word they perceive. Their responses are scored as the percentage of lexically easy and hard words that are correctly identified. One also can derive a total composite percentage-correct score. It is typical to observe better performance on the easy than the hard words. This suggests that children are sensitive to the acoustic-phonetic similarity among words and that they use this information to encode, store, and retrieve words from their mental lexicon. Use of the MLNT can provide diagnostic information regarding spoken language processing. For example, if children show very large differences in the ability to recognize easy and hard words, it would suggest that they are unable to make fine acoustic-phonetic distinctions among words. Test-retest reliability and interlist equivalency are high (Kirk, Eisenberg, Martinez, and Hay-McCutcheon, 1999).

Measures of Spoken Word Recognition for School-Age Children

The Word Intelligibility by Picture Identification (WIPI) test (Ross and Lerman, 1970) was developed to assess spoken word recognition in children with limited vocabularies who could not read. The test consists of six-picture plates that can be used to evaluate recognition of four different lists of 25 monosyllabic words. Children must make relatively fine acoustic-phonetic distinctions to correctly identify the target word from among the five foils on each plate. The WIPI is recommended for children with mild to moderate hearing loss ages 5-6 and children with severe hearing loss ages 6-7. Ross and Lerman (1970) found good interlist equivalency and test-retest reliability for this measure.

The Lexical Neighborhood Test (LNT) (Kirk et al., 1995) is an open-set monosyllabic word recognition test. Test motivation, administration, and scoring are identical to the MLNT. The LNT consists of two lists of 50 monosyllabic words. Half of the items on each list are lexically hard and half are lexically easy. As for the MLNT, interlist equivalency and test-retest reliability are high.

The Phonetically Balanced Kindergarten Word Lists (PB-K) test (Haskins, 1949) was developed to assess open-set monosyllabic word recognition. The test consists of four lists of 50 monosyllabic words that are phonetically balanced (that is, the sounds in the test items occur in the same proportion in which they occur in spoken English). This test has been the most widely used measure of isolated word recognition in clinics and research centers throughout the United States for more than 50 years. Because the requirement of phonetic balancing within lists constrains test item selection, some words on the PB-K may not be familiar to young children with limited vocabularies (Kirk, Sehgal, and Hay-McCutcheon, 2000). The test can be administered via live voice or recordings. Children respond by repeating the item heard. Responses are scored as the percentage of words or phonemes correctly identified.

The Hearing in Noise Test for Children (HINT-C) was developed by Nilsson, Soli, and Gelnett (1996), based on the work of Bench, Bamford, and colleagues (Bench and Bamford, 1979; Bench, Bamford, Wilson, and Clift, 1979). This test consists of a number of lists of 12 sentences each. Vocabulary was selected to be familiar to children age 6 and older. A recorded version of the test is used to test children in quiet or in the presence of speech-spectrum-shaped noise. The test has been administered in two ways. In one method, the reception threshold for sentences is determined adaptively with the speech and speech-spectrum noise presented from 0° azimuth (directly in front of the patient) and with the noise at 90° (left of the patient) and 270° (right of the patient) relative to the speech signal (0°). In another method, the percentage of words correctly identified in quiet and in noise are determined.

The Common Phrases Test (Robbins, Renshaw, and Osberger, 1995b) was developed to assess the understanding of familiar phrases used in everyday situations. This test was motivated by the idea that children would better be able to recognize familiar phrases than monosyllabic words in an open-set format. Furthermore, such a test has greater face validity than an isolated word test. The test consists of 6 lists of 10 sentences; separate lists can be administered in the auditory-only, visual-only, and auditory + visual modality. Children may respond by correctly repeating all of the words in the sentence or by responding appropriately to a question. Performance is scored as the percentage of sentences correctly identified.

Speech Production Outcome Measures

A battery of tests also is needed for assessing speech production skills in children who are deaf or hard-of-hearing. One common approach is to evaluate vowel and consonant production in a variety of tasks ranging from imitation of nonsense syllables through elicited and spontaneous productions in words and sentences (Tobey, Geers, and Brenner, 1994). Speech tasks that use imitation require children to reproduce an examiner's utterance accurately. Speech tasks that elicit productions (such as picture naming or object description) require children to produce target sounds in the absence of a model from the examiner, in this case, yielding information about the children's speech and expressive language abilities. Finally, spontaneous samples provide a representative sample of the child's usual speech and expressive language skills. When assessing speech production skills, it is common for the examiner to score children's responses on-line, or to record the responses for later transcription by another clinician. This type of scoring may be influenced by the examiner's familiarity with the children or with the speech of other talkers who are deaf or hard-of-hearing.

Language Tests

Researchers have applied several different strategies to examine the same types of behaviors in children with hearing loss. One school of investigators (Geers and Moog, 1994) has developed and applied measures specifically for children with hearing loss, such as the Grammatical Analysis of Elicited Language. Other schools (e.g., Robbins, Osberger, Miyamoto, and Kessler, 1995a) have applied tests developed for children with normal hearing, such as the Reynell Scales of Language Development, using caution in the interpretation of results. Still others (Moeller, 1988) have argued for integrating formal and informal measures, prudently incorporating standardized tests with informal measures, such as following directions, narrative (re)production, spontaneous language samples, etc. Many tests of language development are available. The committee does not recommend any particular test for use in SSA disability determination.

USE OF AUDITORY PROSTHESES

When children are born with a hearing loss, prosthetic devices can be used to amplify the environmental sounds to levels that make them audible (see Chapter 5). If the hearing loss is quite severe, acoustic amplification, such as that provided by hearing aids, may not have enough power to provide audibility, especially for soft speech sounds. In those cases, surgically administered cochlear implants can be used to sample environmental sounds, transduce sounds into a series of electrical impulses, and present these representations of the sound to the auditory nerve directly through the inner ear. Fitting of prosthetic devices to children is a complex process. When care is taken to fit appropriately and follow with educational intervention to train them in the use of the altered signal and to augment development of communication, the communication ability and auditory development of children can be dramatically improved.

Hearing Aids

When hearing loss is identified in infants or toddlers, hearing aids can and should be fitted as soon the degree and type of hearing loss is known in each ear. Hearing aids can be adjusted or programmed to provide a frequency response that is appropriate for the hearing loss of the individual and to provide the appropriate amount of amplification based on the degree of loss for sounds of specific frequency. The amount of amplification and maximum power can also be adjusted in most aids to be appropriate for the hearing loss and the acoustic environment. The characteristics of the hearing aids are selected or programmed to match the severity and frequency response of the child's hearing loss. Consequently, any hearing aid fitting begins with the diagnostic audiological assessment discussed earlier.

Styles of Hearing Aids

Infants and young children are generally fitted with a behind-the-ear (BTE) model of hearing aid. These devices hang behind the pinna, and amplified sound is routed to the ear canal via tubing ending in a custom earmold. Infants' and toddlers' pinnas grow very rapidly, requiring new earmolds on a regular basis to ensure proper acoustic coupling between the device and the child.

Exceptions to the use of BTE aids in children do occur. In rare instances, a young child may need a "body style" hearing aid. These aids are housed in a body-worn case, which is attached to the custom fit earmold via a cord and external receiver. These devices are used only in special cases, such as when a bone-conduction device is needed for a child with no external pinnas on which to attach a BTE or when an ear-worn device is not practical for a bedridden child. Older children and adolescents may be able to use in-the-ear (ITE) or in-the-canal (ITC) hearing aids, depending on the degree of hearing loss.

Special Features and Assistive Devices

Children in learning situations both at home and in classrooms need as clear and quiet a signal as possible. Assistive listening devices such as frequency modulation (FM) or induction coil systems (described in Chapter 5) are often quite beneficial to children and are usually recommended to be used alone or in conjunction with personal amplification devices. Hearing aids equipped with direct audio input connectors can be adapted for this application. Infants and children may not have the sophistication to participate in loudness discomfort measures or to manipulate a volume control to avoid loud sounds. Their amplification systems will require flexibility to set loudness growth and limiting and to allow for manipulation of such parameters as the child learns to respond. Wide dynamic range compression (WDRC) may be a particularly important feature of amplification for an infant or child on whom loudness discomfort levels are not obvious. Amplification devices fitted to children should have flexibility to adjust the gain and frequency response to accommodate changes in the external ear and ear canal due to growth and to respond to any possible changes in hearing sensitivity over time. Because of their flexibility, digitally programmable aids may be advantageous for use by infants and children.

Hearing Aid Candidacy

Infants and children who are in the process of developing language and speech have a critical need to hear. Children with permanent, bilateral average hearing loss of 20-25 dB (or greater) should be evaluated for the use of amplification. Children with unilateral hearing loss should be considered for fitting with amplification whenever possible. Those with a profound unilateral loss that is not helped by conventional aids may receive benefit from an FM system or contralateral routing of signal (CROS) hearing aid, in which a microphone is placed at the nonfunctioning ear and the signal is routed to the contralateral, normally functioning ear.

Fitting and Verification of Amplification

Proper fitting of amplification begins with determination of audiometric thresholds. As in all audiometric procedures, modifications must be made to adult procedures to accommodate the capacity of infants to provide feedback. Prescriptive formulae, such as the NAL-NL1 or DSL (see Chapter 5), should be used to determine the appropriate hearing aid characteristics based on the children's audiometric thresholds, and they should be modified based on the individual acoustic characteristics of each child's ear. Procedures to determine the appropriateness of the fitting compare the prescribed performance to the actual acoustic output. These comparisons can be measured from the child's ear (real ear measures) or in a hearing aid coupler with appropriate corrections made based on actual measurements from that child's ear, called real ear to coupler difference (RECD) (Moodie, Seewald, and Sinclair, 1994). These corrections to coupler measures are especially important when fitting infants and small children to avoid overamplification because of increased sound levels in tiny ear canals.

Outcomes of Hearing Aid Use

For linguistically sophisticated adults, the goal of amplification use is the enhanced perception of speech in a variety of listening environments. For infants or young children, for whom speech has not yet acquired meaning, the audibility of sounds in a wide frequency range is the initial primary goal. Consistent exposure to sounds in environmental context is the basis for development of auditory neural networks that will ultimately be responsible for the organization of auditory information and learning about complex patterns of sounds including speech. If the infant or toddler with hearing loss can be provided with consistently audible speech through amplification, he or she should be able to learn to recognize speech, distinguish voices, and develop spoken vocabulary. Children with significant hearing loss will not be able to monitor their own voice and speech sounds unless these are audible to them. Other more rudimentary skills also are developed through auditory experience, such as awareness and recognition of environmental sounds and development of the ability to find sound-emitting objects in space (sound localization). As children develop, speech perception ability is monitored as a metric of aided performance.

Stelmachowicz (1999, p. 16) describes the most common outcome measures used in children who use amplification as "auditory awareness, audibility of speech, speech intelligibility, accuracy of speech production, rate of language acquisition, loudness discomfort and social development." Normal developmental time-courses exist for many of these skills in all children, as discussed earlier in this chapter. Such skills can be assessed only after they are expected to be present, regardless of the hearing status. For example, there are few measures of speech recognition for children under 3 years of age. For older children, it is important to distinguish the effects of amplification on outcome measures from normal developmental patterns and from the effects of the therapy and early intervention that necessarily accompany the fitting of amplification.

Surveys and Inventories for Pediatric Hearing Outcome Measures. Hearing loss is now often identified in very young infants due to the advent of newborn hearing screening. Few outcome measures can be used directly with these children. Consequently, it is increasingly common for professionals to use questionnaires or surveys of parents, caregivers, or teachers to gain insights into the early development of auditory behaviors. As children age, more direct objective measures can be taken if allowances for normal developmental patterns of ability are taken into account. However, questionnaires and inventories can be very useful for pre- and postintervention assessment over time, for example in assessing the use of amplification or devices such as FM systems.

Among parent-teacher survey tests is the Screening Instrument for Targeting Educational Risk (SIFTER) (Anderson, 1989), used by educators for school-age children. A preschool version is also available (Anderson and Matkin, 1996). The Meaningful Auditory Integration Scale (Robbins, Renshaw, and Gerry, 1991) and the IT-MAIS infant-toddler version (Zimmerman-Phillips et al., 2000) are parent inventories used generally with children who demonstrate severe to profound hearing loss. These scales probe for hearing aid use, acceptance, and basic auditory development.

The Listening Inventories for Education (LIFE) (Smaldino and Anderson, 1997) is a classroom inventory that includes student and teacher appraisals of listening difficulty and a teacher opinion and observation list.

Kopun and Stelmachowicz (1998) have used an adapted version of the Abbreviated Profile of Hearing Aid Benefit (APHAB) (Cox and Alexander, 1995) successfully with children ages 10-15 with hearing loss as well as with their parents. Discrepancies were found between the children's assessments and those of their parents, which points out the need for development and validation of tools that can be used with children.

Many other functional assessments based on report of behaviors are being developed for assessing outcomes in children with hearing loss. For example, the Functional Auditory Performance Indicators (FAPI), from Stredler-Brown and Johnson (2001), address many functional areas, including localization, discrimination, and short-term auditory memory. It can be used over time to map a given child's progress. Each of these inventories has strengths in evaluating certain aspects of auditory development and may best be suited to a particular environment or degree of hearing loss.

Direct Measures for Toddlers and Young Children. To be appropriate for infants and toddlers, measures of speech perception ability that can be used to evaluate adequacy of amplification must be modified to be age appropriate for both the task and the perceptual skills of the children. If speech stimuli are used, the influence of the children's linguistic capacity on speech perception must be considered carefully. For example, it is easier to perceive words in one's vocabulary or to perceive a sentence when one has the grammatical capacity to construct such a sentence. Eisenberg and Dirks (1995) looked at children's ability to judge speech clarity using paired comparison and category rating tasks. They found that by 5 years of age, children could make reliable clarity judgments of distorted speech, especially with the paired comparison method. Dawson, Nott, Clark, and Cowan (1998) evaluated a test procedure using a play paradigm for assessing the ability of young children to discriminate between pairs of speech sounds. They found that 82 percent of 3- and 4-year-old children and 50 percent of 2-year-old children could perform this task and would reliably indicate when two stimuli were discriminated. Boothroyd and colleagues have developed an imitative speech perception test that allows for evaluation of speech feature perception in toddlers and has the added attraction of allowing a comparison of visual, auditory, and auditory + visual perception ability (Kosky and Boothroyd, 2003). This simple task (IMSPAC) can be used with toddlers as young as 3 years of age. To date, we know of no studies that have used these measures to evaluate the outcome of amplification in children.

Age at Amplification. Both Yoshinaga-Itano et al. (1998) and Moeller (2000) have found that language outcomes in children with hearing loss are significantly related to age at intervention. Specifically, both studies found that if infants are enrolled in an early-intervention program for deaf and hard-of-hearing children before 1 year of age (Yoshinaga-Itano found 6 months to be critical and Moeller found 11 months), there is a significant positive effect on the child's later language ability. Conversely, delayed intervention leads to poorer language outcomes in children. However, in neither study was the intervention necessarily tied to amplification fitting. Consequently, although conventional wisdom based on consistent widespread clinical observations supports the value of fitting amplification as soon as a hearing loss is diagnosed (Joint Committee on Infant Hearing, 2000; Pediatric Working Group, 1996), published data on communication outcomes (language, speech perception, speech production) that confirm the utility of early amplification are not currently available.

Device Efficacy and Features in Children—Audibility. The outcomes of children using amplification can be measured in many ways. At the most basic are tests that evaluate the audibility of sounds when using a device. The most important factor is the audibility of sounds within the frequency range that comprises speech signals. In addition, Stelmachowicz, Pittman, Hoover, and Lewis (2002) emphasize that infants and children may have specific additional needs for adequate audibility of frequencies considered to be high in the speech spectrum (above 3000 Hz). She points out that children who are learning language need to be able to hear and perceive these very high frequency sounds that include "s" because of its importance in denoting possession, plurality, and verb tense. Also, infants and children are often listening to female speech, which is higher in frequency content than male speech.

Assessing the audibility of sounds has become a routine procedure in the process of fitting and evaluating amplification for infants and children (Pediatric Working Group, 1996; American Academy of Audiology, 2003). Procedures such as the desired sensation level input/output (DSL i/o) (Cornelisse, Seewald, and Jamison, 1995) or NAL NL1 (Dillon, Birtles, and Lovegrove, 1999) allow comparison of amplified signals to target prescription levels. Appropriate signals, such as speech or speech-shaped noise, are directed to the hearing aid, and the amplified output is measured in the ear canal of the infants or children under optimal conditions, or in a standard hearing aid coupler with corrections appropriate for estimating sound levels that would occur in infants' or toddlers' ears. Applied stimulus type and level can be manipulated to simulate real listening conditions, and the characteristics of the amplification can be adjusted to maximize the response in a particular infant's ear and to document the audibility of the signal, based on the hearing loss of each child. Scollie et al. (2000) have provided support for the 4.1 version of the DSL by demonstrating that the DSL target levels for amplified speech are very similar to the preferred listening levels of children with hearing loss.

Aided audibility can be also be quantified by the articulation index (American National Standards Institute, 1969). The articulation index is a number from 0 to 1 which approximates the percentage of the speech spectrum that is audible. Stelmachowicz and colleagues have developed a system to provide a visual display of the audibility of speech at various input levels and to take into account the amplification and output-limiting characteristics of the hearing aid. This system is known as the situational hearing aid response profile (SHARP) (Stelmachowicz, Lewis, Kalberer, and Cruetz, 1994). Presently, the above measures of audibility in an aided situation are used clinically as initial indicators of aided performance in infants and children, or a sort of early outcome measure.

Measuring Outcomes of Hearing Aids and Features. Standard measures of hearing aid fitting often include determining speech recognition scores for words or sentences with the speech presented in the context of background noise. Often the level of the noise that can be tolerated relative to the level of the speech is the metric of performance. These measures can be used only with older children (over about age 7). Pettersson (1987) demonstrated that children with hearing loss ages 8 to 20 performed better on speech perception when using their own amplification devices than when evaluated with amplified speech presented through an audiometer. She attributes much of this finding to the fact that the children had accommodated to their amplification and were familiar with the amplification characteristics.

School-age children with all degrees of hearing loss have been shown to have an advantage in listening through hearing aids while using a directional microphone (Gravel and Hood, 1999; Hawkins, 1984; Kuk, Kollofski, Brown, Melum, and Rosenthal, 1999). Gravel et al. (1999) noted that the directional advantage is greatest for older children with more advanced language skills.

FM Systems. Several studies have shown that a significant advantage is afforded to children with hearing loss for perceiving speech in real-life situations when an FM transmission system is used. These advantages have been demonstrated in the classroom (Boothroyd and Iglehart, 1998; Hawkins, 1984; Pittman, Lewis, Hoover, and Stemachowicz, 1999) and to a lesser degree in the home (Moeller, Donaghy, Beauchaine, Lewis, and Stelmachowicz, 1996). Most studies point out that while speech perceived from a distance may be enhanced using FM systems, the need for local microphones must be addressed in order to allow children to monitor their own voices and speech as well as to interact with classmates.

Outcomes with Minimal and Unilateral Hearing Loss. There is clear evidence that children with even unilateral or mild hearing loss are at a significant disadvantage when listening in noisy situations, such as classrooms

(Crandell, 1993). However, there are few outcome data on the use of amplification with these children. Kenworthy, Klee, and Tharpe (1990) compared the use of a CROS hearing aid and personal FM devices on children with unilateral hearing loss in a variety of listening conditions. They found an advantage to the CROS aid but only in limited conditions, whereas the personal FM provided uniform advantage for speech perception in these children. However, device fitting for children with unilateral hearing loss is not universally accepted as a clinical procedure. English and Church (1999) reported that only 27 percent of children with unilateral hearing loss are using amplification in the classroom.

COCHLEAR IMPLANTS IN CHILDREN

Determining Candidacy for Cochlear Implants

Cochlear implants are approved by the FDA for use in children as young as 12 months of age. For very young children, measures of unaided and aided speech detection are the primary determinants of cochlear implant candidacy. In addition, the IT-MAIS (Zimmerman-Phillips et al., 2000) has been used to assess auditory development in relation to cochlear implant candidacy. That is, candidacy is determined by a lack of development of auditory skills over a 3-6 month time span. For older children, spoken word recognition tests are an important part of candidacy determination and post-implant assessment of benefit. Recent clinical trials have employed open-set measures of word recognition, such as the LNT (Kirk et al., 1995) and measures of sentence recognition, such as HINT-C (Nilsson et al., 1996) to determine candidacy in school-age children. For preschool-age children, the open-set MLNT (Kirk et al., 1995) and less difficult closed-set tests, such as the ESP Test (Moog and Geers, 1990), have been utilized to determine candidacy and monitor long-term communication skill development.

Cochlear Implant Communication Outcomes in Children

Spoken Word Recognition

In early investigations, children who used previous generations of cochlear implant systems demonstrated significant improvement in closed-set word identification but very limited open-set word recognition (Miyamoto et al., 1989; Staller, Beiter, Brimacombe, Meckelenburg, and Arndt, 1991). The introduction of newer processing strategies yielded greater speech perception benefits in children, just as in adults. Like adults (see Chapter 5), children with cochlear implants demonstrate a wide range of postimplant communication abilities (Gantz, Tyler, Woodworth, Tye-Murray, and Fryauf-Bertschy, 1994; Miyamoto et al., 1991; Staller et al., 1991; Waltzman, Cohen, and Shapiro, 1995). The majority of children with current cochlear implant devices achieve at least moderate levels of open-set word recognition.

For example, Cohen, Waltzman, Roland, Staller, and Hoffman (1999) reported word recognition scores for a group of 19 children that ranged from 4 to 76 percent words correct with a mean of 44 percent words correct. Osberger, Barker, Zimmerman-Phillips, and Geier (1999) reported average scores of approximately 30 percent correct on a more difficult measure of isolated word recognition in children with the Clarion cochlear implant. More recently Geers, Brenner, and Davidson (2003a) reported average word recognition scores of 50 percent correct when the stimuli were presented auditorily only, and scores of 80 percent when the children had access to both auditory and speech-reading cues.

The rate of development of auditory skills following surgery for a cochlear implant seems to be increasing as cochlear implant technology improves and as children are implanted at younger ages (Cohen et al., 1999; Osberger et al., 1999; Young, Carrasco, Grohne, and Brown, 1999). In contrast to adults with postlingual deafness, children's postimplant speech perception skills continue to develop over a relatively long time course. Continued improvements with increasing device use have been noted in children who have used their devices for as long as 5 to 8 years (Tyler, Fryauf-Bertchy, Gantz, Kelsay, and Woodworth, 1997).

Further evidence of the success of cochlear implants in children with congenital or early-acquired deafness was demonstrated by Tyler, Rubenstein, Teagle, Kelsay, and Gantz (2000). They used sentence materials to compare the performance of such children with that of adults with a later onset of deafness. Tyler et al. found that 60 percent of the adults and 70 percent of the children tested correctly identified at least half of the words presented in sentences. These data suggest that the auditory system of children with congenital or prelingually acquired hearing loss will develop spoken language processing abilities similar to those of adults who had the benefit of learning language through a normal auditory channel.

Several investigators have compared the performance of children with cochlear implants to that of their peers who use conventional amplification. The speech perception abilities of pediatric cochlear implant recipients met or exceeded those of their peers with unaided pure-tone average thresholds ≥ 90 dB HL who use hearing aids (Meyer, Svirsky, Kirk, and Miyamoto, 1998; Svirsky and Meyer, 1999).

Demographic Factors

A number of demographic factors have been shown to influence speech perception and spoken word recognition in children with cochlear implants. Early results suggested better speech perception performance in children deafened at an older age with a corresponding shorter period of deafness (Fryauf-Bertschy, Tyler, Kelsay, and Gantz, 1992; Osberger, Todd, Berry, Robbins, and Miyamoto, 1991; Staller et al., 1991). Those children who lost their hearing after acquiring spoken language (usually becoming profoundly deaf after age 2 years) are categorized as postlingually deafened. This group of children is able to use multichannel cochlear implants in a manner similar to adults with postlingual deafness. In most instances, the speech perception skills of children with postlingual deafness improved over a few months and were at the upper end of adult performance curves for sentence and monosyllabic word understanding (Gantz et al., 1994). It is most likely that the short duration of deafness as well as a young and adaptive central nervous system was responsible for the outstanding results in this group of cochlear implant recipients.

When only children with prelingual deafness are considered, age at onset of hearing loss does not appear to significantly impact speech perception and spoken word recognition outcomes (Miyamoto, Osberger, Robbins, Myers, and Kessler, 1993). It is clearly evident that earlier implantation yields superior cochlear implant performance in children (Fryauf-Bertschy, Tyler, Kelsay, Gantz, and Woodworth, 1997; Illg et al., 1999; Lenarz et al., 1999; Nikolopoulos, O'Donoghue, and Archbold, 1998; O'Donoghue, Nikolopoulos, Archbold, and Tait, 1999). Although the critical period for implantation of congenitally or prelingually deafened children has not been determined (Brackett and Zara, 1998), preliminary evidence suggests that implantation prior to age 3 years may yield improved results (Waltzman and Cohen, 1998; Waltzman et al., 1995, 1997). Finally, the variables of communication mode and unaided residual hearing also influence speech perception performance (Cowan et al., 1997; Hodges, Ash, Balkany, Scholffman, and Butts, 1999; Osberger and Fisher, 1998; Zwolan et al., 1997). Oral children and those who have more residual hearing prior to implantation typically demonstrate superior speech understanding.

Speech Intelligibility and Language

Improvements in speech perception are the most direct benefit of cochlear implantation. However, if children with cochlear implants are to be fully integrated into the hearing world, they must also acquire the language of their surrounding community and be able to produce it intelligibly. The speech intelligibility and language abilities of children with cochlear implants improve significantly over time (Allen, Nikolopoulos, and O'Donoghue, 1998; Moog and Geers, 1999; Svirsky, Robbins, Kirk, Pisoni, and Miyamoto, 2000; Waltzman et al., 1995) and, on average, exceed those of their age- and hearing-matched peers with hearing aids (Tomblin, Spencer, Flock, Tyler, and Gantz, 1999; Svirsky, 2000; Svirsky et al., 2000). Tobey and her colleagues reported average speech intelligibility scores of greater than 65 percent for a large group of children with cochlear implants (Tobey, Geers, Brenner, Altuna, and Gabbert, 2003). That is, more than half of what they said could be understood by listeners who were not familiar with the speech of deaf talkers. This is far greater than previous reports for children with profound deafness who used hearing aids (Smith, 1975). Speech intelligibility and spoken language acquisition are significantly correlated with the development of auditory skills (Moog and Geers, 1999; Tomblin et al., 1999). Although a great deal of variability exists, the best pediatric cochlear implant users demonstrate highly intelligible speech and age-appropriate language skills. These superior performers are usually implanted at a young age and are educated in an oral/aural modality (Moog and Geers, 1999).

The relationship between language development and literacy (reading and writing skills) in children with prelingual deafness who use a cochlear implant was investigated by Spencer, Barker, and Tomblin (2003). Children with cochlear implants scored within one standard deviation of their age-matched peers on measures of language comprehension, reading comprehension, and writing accuracy. The researchers reported that the children with cochlear implants differed from children with normal hearing in their ability to utilize correct grammatical structures and verb forms. This information should be useful in designing appropriate educational models for children with cochlear implants.

A comprehensive investigation of the factors that influence cochlear implant outcomes recently was completed by Geers and her colleagues (Geers, 2003; Geers and Brenner, 2003; Geers et al., 2003a; Geers, Nicholas, and Sedey, 2003b; Tobey et al., 2003). The primary goal of this study was to identify the impact of educational factors on cochlear implant outcomes. Because the characteristics of the family and the cochlear implant recipient also contribute to postimplant outcomes, these characteristics were carefully documented and controlled in the data analyses. The study evaluated postimplant outcomes in 181 children who were 8-9 years of age and who were implanted by the time they were 5 years of age. Performance outcomes included measures of speech perception, speech production, language, and reading skills development. The predictors of performance were very similar for the development of speech perception and speech production abilities. These included a higher nonverbal intelligence quotient (IQ), longer use of the newest generation of speech processing strategies, a fully active electrode array and higher electrical dynamic range, and a greater growth of loudness on the electrodes. When these characteristics were controlled, educational placement did have a significant impact on cochlear implant outcomes (Geers et al., 2003a; Tobey et al., 2003). That is, children who were educated in settings that emphasized the development and use of speaking and listening skills had the best prognosis for spoken language processing. Predictors of good language skills included a higher nonverbal IQ, smaller family size, higher SES, and being female (Geers et al., 2003b). These factors similarly impacted language development for children who used oral communication and those who used total communication. Finally, predictors of reading success included a higher nonverbal IQ, higher SES, being female, and later onset of deafness within the period from birth to 36 months (Geers, 2003). When the variance due to these factors was controlled, the development of good reading skills was associated with mainstream educational placement, use of a current generation of speech processor strategy with a wide dynamic range, a longer memory span, and the use of phonological coding strategies. Geers (2003) reported that reading competence was best predicted by language competence and speech production abilities.

In summary, cochlear implant technology and candidacy criteria have evolved greatly over the past 20 years. Today, patients with severe to profound deafness as young as 12 months old may be implanted. With earlier implantation and improved cochlear implant systems come continued increases in the benefits of cochlear implantation. Although wide variability in outcomes is noted, cochlear implant use by children with severe to profound hearing loss promotes the development of speaking and listening skills and the development of a spoken language system beyond what previously could be achieved with hearing aids. Children who are implanted at a young age and use oral communication have the best prognosis for developing intelligible speech and age-appropriate language abilities. However, it is also helpful to note that data from a Gallaudet Research Institute survey returned by 439 parents of children with cochlear implants indicate that roughly 50 percent continue to use sign language with their children as a supplement to spoken language (Christiansen and Leigh, 2002).

The potential for optimal speech and language development in young children is greatly influenced by parent intervention. This requires considerable time commitment on the part of motivated parents, directed toward ongoing activities that reinforce spoken language, as well as extensive speech and auditory therapy (Christiansen and Leigh, 2002). Generally, parents believe that their children's communication skills improve following implant (Christiansen and Leigh, 2002; Kluwin and Stewart,

2000). While this improvement does result in improved socialization with hearing peers, obstacles related to speech intelligibility and receptive understanding of what is communicated as well as attitudes of hearing peers continue to be ongoing factors (Bat-Chava and Deignan, 2001; Boyd, Knutson, and Dahlstrom, 2000). Psychological difficulties following implant, as reported by parents, are generally associated with getting the implant closer to adolescence and not being happy with it (Christiansen and Leigh, 2002).

RECOMMENDATIONS

Disability Determination Tests and Criteria

Action Recommendation 7-1. The recommended criteria for determination of disability in children who are deaf or hard-of-hearing are presented in tabular format in Table 7-2. To be considered disabled, children under 3 years of age must meet the criterion for hearing level only. Children older than 3 years must meet the pure-tone average criterion *and either* the criterion for deficit in speech perception *or* the criterion for delay in language. Children with marked mental retardation who cannot be evaluated for speech perception or language should be considered disabled if the hearing level criterion alone is met.

Action Recommendation 7-2. Speech perception tests are administered in quiet using recorded test materials at 70 dB SPL (based on peak levels or the equivalent in dB HL if available). Presentation of the speech perception test is via sound field using personal amplification or cochlear implant if such is used by the child. A preliminary check of the functioning and appropriateness of the cochlear implant or amplification should precede the aided testing (see Chapter 5). If no device is used by the child, testing is performed unaided.

Action Recommendation 7-3. In general, average hearing levels will be determined from thresholds at 500, 1000, 2000, and 4000 Hz (PTA 5124). This differs from the PTA of 500, 1000, and 2000 Hz (PTA 512) used for adults. When thresholds are obtained with ABR, a minimum of two frequencies, one low (500 to 1000 Hz) and one high (2000 to 4000 Hz), can be used to determine average hearing level. It should be noted that when conditions indicate that auditory neuropathy may be present (absent ABR and normal OAE), it will not be possible to determine hearing thresholds by ABR. In those cases, disability should be presumed unless or until proven otherwise by age-appropriate behavioral testing (see Table 7-1). Behavioral threshold testing by VRA should be possible once the infant is older than 6 months of developmental age.

Action Recommendation 7-4. The committee carefully considered

TABLE 7-2 Summary of Recommended Disability Determination for Children Who Are Deaf or Hard-of-Hearing

Age in Years: Months	Hearing Levels: Pure-tone average (.5, 1, 2, 4), better ear, air conduction	Speech Perception Test	Criterion	Language Test	Criterion
0 to 2:11	$> = 35$ dB HL	Not Applicable		Not Applicable	
3 to 5:11	$> = 35$ dB HL	Age-appropriate, standardized test with normative data by age.	Scores that are significantly ($P <= 0.05$) below expected normal (see Table 7-3).	Age-appropriate, standardized test with published normative data by age.	$> = 1.64$ standard score below norm for age.
6-14:11	$> = 50$ dB HL	Age-appropriate, standardized test with normative data by age.	Scores that are significantly ($P <= 0.05$) below expected normal (see Table 7-3).	Age-appropriate, standardized test with published normative data by age.	$> = 1.64$ standard score below norm for age.
15-18 years	$> = 70$ dB HL	NU-6	Scores that are significantly ($P <= 0.05$) below expected normal (see Table 7-3).	PPVT-III	$> = 1.64$ standard score below norm for age.

these guidelines in the preparation of recommendations. In contrast to the suggested adult standards for PTA hearing level, we are suggesting that the degree of hearing loss that is considered disabling in infants and children is 35 dB HL or greater before the age of 6 years, 50 dB from 6 to 12 years, and 70 dB from 12 to 18 years of age. We have selected these criteria for the reasons stated below.

As emphasized in the text of this chapter, a loss of hearing sensitivity can have a more detrimental effect on infants and children who are in critical learning periods for speech, language, and general communication ability than on their adult counterparts. School-age children depend on communication skills for all means of learning. Development of communication skills may be the most important task for an infant because it provides the basis for almost all subsequent learning.

The committee chose 35 dB HL as the minimum hearing loss criterion on the basis of studies that have documented significant delays in speech production, language, verbal intelligence, and associated areas of learning (Briscoe et al., 2001; Davis et al., 1986) in children with hearing loss, including those with mild loss. The strongest evidence that even mild bilateral hearing loss is debilitating to young children comes from the endorsement of groups like the National Institutes of Health (1993), the American Academy of Pediatrics Task Force on Newborn and Infant Hearing (1999), and the American Academy of Pediatrics (2000), that endorse programs for early detection of mild hearing loss of 30 to 40 dB because of evidence that this degree of loss will cause significant communication and educational delays.

The needs for intervention for children with hearing loss are particularly acute in the infant and preschool period, when peak gains are attained in language and speech. Particularly if language skills are developing well, the elementary-school-age child should be able to tolerate slightly more hearing loss and the criterion level for disability is adjusted to moderate (50 dB) rather than mild. It should be noted that at this age and older, assessments of speech perception and language skills are also recommended as part of the disability determination evaluation. Although the hearing level criterion for disability is less stringent at this age for a child than for an adult, it should be noted that a child with a moderate hearing loss whose speech perception skills and language ability are normal for his or her age may not be considered disabled. As these communication skills emerge, more emphasis is placed on them and the criterion for hearing level is raised.

Finally, we recommend a 70 dB HL criterion for high school students, which is less strict than the 90 dB recommended for adults. The child of high school age with a hearing loss is significantly challenged by the hostile acoustic environment in which he or she must function and learn and by the increased social-emotional pressure that accompanies this period of development. Therefore, we do not recommend the adult standard of 90 dB HL average hearing loss until the child has reached 18 years of age. We recommend that speech perception be evaluated in the auditory mode that is optimal for individual children. In most instances, the optimal mode will be binaural, well-fitted amplification or a cochlear implant. We recognize, however, that some children may not use amplification devices for a variety of reasons. The determination of disability in these children should be without amplification. A guiding principle is that disability determination should reflect the real-world situation of the child.

It is clear that the degree of hearing loss alone is not a perfect predictor of functional communication competencies. Therefore, the determination of disability requires assessment of a variety of communication skills. We chose the domains of speech perception and language processing because they are directly affected by childhood hearing loss and provide an important foundation for spoken language communication, reading, and multiple facets of educational achievement.

Given the SSA criterion, it would be ideal to select and administer standardized measures that yield normative scores allowing comparable cutoff criteria for both types of tests. At present, this may be possible for language testing but not for speech perception testing.

Standardized language measures provide normative data for children as a function of their age at time of testing. That is, within a given age range, normally developing, hearing children exhibit a normally distributed range of performance scores. By using normative data, we can determine where on the normal distribution an individual child's performance lies. Standard language assessment scores are normalized to a mean of zero and a standard deviation of 1. Because abnormally poor performance occurs in only one tail of the distribution, we use a standard score of > = 1.64 units below the age norm to indicate performance below the 5th percentile.

In contrast, spoken word recognition instruments containing age-appropriate vocabulary and response tasks should yield a skewed distribution with expected scores of 90-100 percent in normally developing, hearing children. This homogeneity of performance on speech perception tasks makes it impossible to derive a standard score for performance. Thus, we have taken a different approach in recommending guidelines for determining marked or extreme impairment in the areas of speech perception performance. We specified as the criterion for abnormality, scores that are significantly different from 90 percent correct ($P <= 0.05$). The percentage

TABLE 7-3 Cutoff Scores Determined to Be Significantly < 90 Percent at p <= 0.05

	Number of Test Items				
	15	20	25	40	50
Items correct	< 10	< 15	< 19	< 32	< 40
Percentage correct	66%	75%	76%	80%	80%

NOTE: 90 percent correct is low end of normal performance range.

score deemed abnormal will vary based on the number of items in the test as indicated in Table 7-3. Table 7-4 summarizes the characteristics of the spoken word recognition measures described in this chapter.

The committee has not recommended assessment of speech perception in noise for children, although to do so in our view would increase the sensitivity of the testing for disability. Such testing was not recom-

TABLE 7-4 Description of Speech Recognition Tests for Children

Test	Recommended Age Range	Test Format	Presentation Format
NU-Chips	> 3 years	Closed set	Auditory only
PSI	3-10 years	Closed set	Auditory only
WIPI	> 5 years for children with mild loss; > 7 years with severe loss	Closed set	Auditory only
MLNT	> 3 years	Open set	Auditory only
LNT	> 5 years	Open set	Auditory only
Common phrases	> 5 years	Open set	Auditory only; visual only; auditory + visual
HINT-C	> 6 years	Open set	Auditory only

[a]This criterion applies only for whole word scoring of tests of isolated word recognition. It cannot be applied to phoneme scores or to words tested in a sentence context.

mended because of the lack of appropriately standardized tests across the age groups of interest. When tests exist, they may not be readily available to audiologists. With young children, test time and cooperation often are limited, and these test scores are not often available for scrutiny. However, checks for functional disability in Step 3 testing should detect the child's significant difficulty hearing in noise. As standardized testing protocols to assess this function become more available, this information should be incorporated into a complete assessment of ability of children with hearing loss.

Action Recommendation 7-5. In addition to the administration of standard audiometric and language tests, the evaluation for determination of disability for children who are deaf or hard-of-hearing should include a checklist to be completed by the audiologist. The checklist presented in Box 7-1 will ensure that information needed for test interpretation is available to SSA. For each checklist item, a response in the shaded box indicates that the response is invalid or needs explanation, as discussed below.

Stimuli	Test Items per List / # of Lists	Response	Score significantly < 90 percent correct[a]
Monosyllabic words	50 / 4	Picture pointing	< 40 words correct
Monosyllabic words	20 / 1	Picture pointing	< 15 words correct
Sentences	10 / 1		Not applicable
Monosyllabic words	25 /4	Picture pointing	< 19 words correct
2-3 syllable words	24 /2	Imitation	< 18 words correct
Monosyllabic words	50 / 2	Imitation	< 40 words correct
Sentences	10 / 6	Imitation	Not applicable
Sentences	10 / 13	Imitation	Not applicable

BOX 7-1
Pediatric Checklist for Audiological Evaluation
for Disability Determination

Question   Response

1. Are hearing thresholds indicated for individual ears?   [Yes] [No]
2. Are hearing thresholds obtained for at least two frequencies
in each ear?   [Yes] [No]
3. Is the test validity/reliability indicated on the audiogram?   [Yes] [No]
4. Was the child cooperative during the testing?   [Yes] [No]
5. Was speech testing performed with age- and language-
appropriate materials?   [Yes] [No]
6. Were tympanograms normal at the time of the threshold
testing?   [Yes] [No]
7. Does the child use personal amplification or a cochlear
implant?   [Yes] [No]
8. If yes to question 7, was the device functioning as expected
on the day of testing?   [Yes] [No]
9. If yes to question 7, was the child tested with the device?   [Yes] [No]

Comments from audiologist:

_____

_____

_____

_____

Interpretation of the checklist above is as follows.

Item 1. For a variety of reasons including lack of patient cooperation, some pediatric evaluations are performed without earphones; rather the stimuli are presented through speakers or in the "sound field." In this instance, thresholds will be

Recommendations for Further Research

This chapter reveals many unresolved issues with respect to determination of disability status for infants and children with hearing loss. Persons involved in the care and management of these children rely on published laboratory and clinical science for direction. Many of the questions raised could be answered with appropriate scientific investigation.

indicated with the symbol "S" rather than O or X. These scores indicate the hearing thresholds of the better-hearing ear. These scores may serve to indicate the overall hearing loss level until ear-specific scores can be obtained.

Item 2. When ABR is used to predict thresholds, occasionally only a click stimulus is used for the evaluation. For purposes of disability determination, we recommend that a minimum of two frequency-specific stimuli should be tested to determine average hearing level in each ear. A click threshold alone may not give an accurate estimate of the degree of hearing loss and could underestimate the average loss. In special circumstances, if a click threshold alone is available as an indication of hearing level, it can be used as evidence of disability until a more complete evaluation is available.

Item 3. It is important to obtain cooperation when testing a young child. There are a variety of reasons why the test results might not be considered valid or reliable on any given test date. If results are not valid and reliable, additional testing should be considered.

Item 4. Augments item three. If the child was not cooperative during testing, the results should be deemed unreliable and additional testing should be considered.

Item 5. Examples of measures for speech perception that are appropriate for various ages of children are listed in Table 7-4. If the test is not age appropriate or the language level is beyond the skills of the child, the test will not be valid.

Item 6. The tympanogram is a measure of the mobility of the eardrum. If the tympanogram is not normal, the child may have had a transient middle ear condition, such as fluid behind the eardrum, on the day of the test. This condition can exacerbate the degree of loss. When "no" is indicated on item 6, a treatment plan from a physician, preferably an otolaryngologist, should indicate if the hearing loss is stable or if treatment may improve the hearing levels. The status of the hearing may need to be reevaluated after treatment to determine accurate hearing levels. During treatment, the average bone conduction threshold, if available, can give an indication of the degree of permanent hearing loss.

Item 7. Speech testing should be performed with the child using the hearing aid or cochlear implant if it is regularly used.

Item 8. The audiologist should perform basic checks of the status of devices before testing. This information should be in the report. If not, it is possible that the maximum ability of the child was not assessed.

Item 9. If the device was not worn for testing, it is possible that the maximum ability of the child was not assessed.

We recommend that the SSA partner with other research funding agencies for whom these questions are also relevant, such as the U.S. Department of Education and the National Institutes of Health, particularly the NIDCD and the National Institute of Child Health and Human Development. Issues that are particularly relevant to SSA are emphasized below. The top three listed here are considered highest priority research aims for SSA purposes; the others listed are not in order of priority.

Research Recommendation 7-1. There is a distinct need for standardized speech perception measures for infants and children that take into account developmental age and degree of hearing loss. Such tests should be developed in English as well as in other languages spoken in homes across the United States. When possible, such tests should incorporate evaluation of perception both in quiet and with relevant competing messages to simulate real-life situations, such as classrooms.

Research Recommendation 7-2. Often children with similar audiograms have very different higher-level auditory abilities, such as spoken word recognition. There are even less-direct relationships between severity of hearing loss and such long-term outcomes as educational achievement, vocational status, and overall psychosocial development. It is important to identify other factors that contribute to these outcomes in persons who have been deaf or hard-of-hearing since early childhood. Specifically, it is important to determine how the following factors influence long-term outcomes for children who are deaf or hard-of-hearing:

- complexities of linguistic environment in the home and in the educational setting, such as multilingual environments, signed or spoken instruction.
- the complexities of educational intervention, including the types of intervention, age at inception and duration, educational setting (mainstream, self-contained, home), and training of intervention specialists.

Research Recommendation 7-3. Many studies have documented the expected outcomes for children using cochlear implants, yet documenting benefits and outcomes of amplification use in children is a more complex task, and few controlled studies exist. More prospective studies of children using amplification are needed to determine related outcomes for communication, socialization, and educational achievement. For example, better studies are needed to determine how factors specific to the amplification fitting process and specific to the child influence such outcomes as language development, speech production, perception development, and social development. Examples of factors surrounding amplification fitting include type of aid fitted, features used such as directional microphones, feedback suppression, type of compression, or specific fitting formula selected. Factors specific to the child that could influence outcomes include the child's age at fitting, degree of hearing loss, and other disabling conditions.

The following research aims may do less to refine disability criteria for SSA but are extremely important in terms of understanding auditory issues relevant to communication development in infants and children who are deaf and hard-of-hearing.

Research Recommendation 7-4. Little is known about the interaction between vision and audition in the development of communication skills. Children with hearing loss often rely heavily on visual perception of speech (speech reading or speech feature cueing) to supplement their auditory capacity. Large individual differences may occur in the reliance on visual information when auditory information is incomplete. Currently, there are no standards for measuring visual, auditory, or combined perception of speech. There is a great need for the development of standard clinical measures that incorporate auditory and visual assessments.

Research Recommendation 7-5. There is a need to understand the effects of slight and unilateral hearing loss on the development of communication skills, educational performance, and social adjustment. Studies are needed to reveal the true nature of the dysfunction these children experience, especially in educational settings, and the possibilities for intervention that may help to mitigate such disturbances.

References

CHAPTER 1

Alberti, P.W. (1993). Occupational hearing loss in Canada. In R.T. Sataloff, and J. Sataloff (Eds.), *Occupational hearing loss* (2nd ed.). New York: Marcel Dekker.

American Medical Association. (1955). Principles for evaluating hearing loss. *Journal of the American Medical Association, 157*(16), 1408-1409.

American Medical Association. (2001). *Guides to the evaluation of permanent impairment* (5th ed.). Chicago, IL: American Medical Association.

American National Standards Institute. (1996). ANSI S3.6-1996. *Specification for audiometers.* New York: American National Standards Institute.

American National Standards Institute. (1997). ANSI S3.21-1978 (R1997). *Method for manual pure-tone threshold audiometry.* New York: American National Standards Institute.

American National Standards Institute. (2002a). ANSI S3.13-1987 (R2002). *Mechanical coupler for measurement of bone vibrators.* New York: American National Standards Institute.

American National Standards Institute. (2002b). ANSI S3.5-1997. *Method for the calculation of the Speech Intelligibility Index.* New York: American National Standards Institute.

American National Standards Institute. (2003). ANSI S3.1-1999 (R2003). *Maximum permissible ambient noise levels for audiometric test rooms.* New York: American National Standards Institute.

American Speech-Language-Hearing Association. (1981). On the definition of hearing handicap. *ASHA, 23*, 293-297.

Bilger, R.C. (1977). Psychoacoustic evaluation of present prostheses. *Annals of Otology, Rhinology and Laryngology, 86*(Suppl 38), 92-140.

Blanchfield, B.B., Feldman, J.J., Dunbar, J.L., and Gardner, E.N. (2001). The severely to profoundly hearing-impaired population in the United States: Prevalence estimates and demographics. *Journal of the American Academy of Audiology, 12*(4), 183-189.

Corthals, P., Vinck, B., De Vel, E., and Van Cauwenberge, P. (1997). Audiovisual speech reception in noise and self-perceived hearing disability in sensorineural hearing loss. *Audiology, 36*(1), 46-56.

Cruickshanks, K.J., Wiley, T.L., Tweed, T.S., Klein, B.E., Mares-Perlman, J.A., and Nondahl, D.M. (1998). Prevalence of hearing loss in older adults in Beaver Dam, Wisconsin. *American Journal of Epidemiology, 148*, 879-886.

Davis, H. (1948). The articulation area and the social adequacy index for hearing. *Laryngoscope, 58*, 761-778.

Davis, H. (1960). Audiometry. In H. Davis and S.R. Silverman (Eds.), *Hearing and deafness* (revised ed.). New York: Holt Rinehart and Winston.

Demorest, M.E., and Walden, B.E. (1984). Psychometric principles in the selection, interpretation, and evaluation of communication self-assessment inventories. *Journal of Speech and Hearing Disorders, 49*(3), 226-240.

Dempsey, J.J. (1994). Hearing aid fitting and evaluation. In J. Katz (Ed.), *Handbook of clinical audiology* (4th ed., pp. 723-735). Baltimore, MD: Williams and Wilkins.

Dobie, R.A., and Sakai, C.S. (2001). Estimation of hearing loss severity from the audiogram. In D. Henderson, D. Prasher, R. Kopke, R. Salvi, and R. Hamernik (Eds.), *Noise induced hearing loss basic mechanisms, prevention and control* (pp. 351-363). London, England: Noise Research Network Publications.

Dubno, J.R., Lee, F.S., Klein, A.J., Matthews, L.J., and Lam, C.F. (1995). Confidence limits for maximum word-recognition scores. *Journal of Speech and Hearing Research, 38*(2), 490-502.

Flynn, M.C., Dowell, R.C., and Clark, G.M. (1998). Aided speech recognition abilities of adults with a severe or severe-to-profound hearing loss. *Journal of Speech Language and Hearing Research, 41*(2), 285-299.

Fowler, E.P. (1941). Hearing standards for acceptance, disability rating, and discharge in the military services and in industry. *Laryngoscope, 51*, 937-956.

Gallaudet Research Institute. (2002). *Regional and national summary report of data from the 2000-2001 annual survey of deaf and hard of hearing children and youth.* Washington, DC: GRI, Gallaudet University.

Gatehouse, S. (1990). Determinants of self-reported disability in older subjects. *Ear and Hearing, 11*(5 Suppl), 57S-65S.

Gatehouse, S. (1998). Speech tests as measures of outcome. *Scandinavian Audiology Supplemental, 49*, 54-60.

Gordon-Salant, S., and Fitzgibbons, P.J. (1997). Selected cognitive factors and speech recognition performance among young and elderly listeners. *Journal of Speech Language and Hearing Research, 40*(2), 423-431.

Grant, K.W., and Seitz, P.F. (2000). Measures of auditory-visual integration in nonsense syllables and sentences. *Journal of the Acoustical Society of America, 104*, 2438-2450.

Hardick, E.J., Melnick, W., Hawes, N.A., et al. (1980). *Compensation for hearing loss for employees under jurisdiction of the U.S. Department of Labor: Benefit formula and assessment procedures.* Columbus, OH: Ohio State University.

Heinemann, A., Mallinson, H., Chen, C., Findley, P., Fisher, B., Amir, H., Raju, N., and Schiro-Geist, C. (2002). *Social Security job demands project: Methodology to identify and validate critical job factors (Deliverable 9).* Unpublished technical report submitted by Disability Research Institute: The University of Illinois at Champaign-Urbana, Northwestern University, Rehabilitation Institute of Chicago. Available: http://www.dri.uiuc.edu/research/p02-06c/final_report_p02-06c.doc.

Hone, S.W., Norman, G., Keogh, I., and Kelly, V. (2003). The use of cortical evoked response audiometry in the assessment of noise-induced hearing loss. *Otolaryngology, Head and Neck Surgery, 128*, 257-262.

Houtenville, A.J. (2002). Employment and economic consequences of visual impairment. In Committee on Disability Determination for Individuals with Visual Impairments, P. Lennie, and S.B. Van Hemel (Eds.), *Visual impairments: Determining eligibility for Social Security benefits* (pp. 275-321). Washington, DC: National Academy Press.

International Organization for Standardization (ISO). (2003). ISO 7731:2003 Ergonomics— Danger signals for public and work areas—Auditory danger signals. International Organization for Standardization.

King, P.F., Coles, R.R.A., Lutman, M.E., and Robinson, D.W. (1992). *Assessment of hearing disability: Guidelines for medicolegal practice.* London, England: Whurr.

Mueller, H.G. (2001). Speech audiometry and hearing aid fittings: Going steady or casual acquaintances? *Hearing Journal, 54,* 19-29.

National Center for Health Statistics. (1996). *Vital and health statistics series 10, No. 200.* Washington, DC: National Center for Health Statistics.

National Center for Health Statistics. (2002). *Trends and differential use of assistive technology devices: United States, 1994.* Washington, DC: National Center for Health Statistics.

National Institute for Deafness and other Communication Disorders (NIDCD). (2004). *Who gets Cochlear Implants.* Available: http://www.nidcd.nih.gov/health/hearing/coch.asp#c. [Accessed March 2004.]

National Research Council. (2002). *Visual impairments: Determining eligibility for Social Security benefits. Committee on Disability Determination for Visual Impairments.* Washington, DC: National Academy Press.

Niskar, A.S., Kieszak, S.M., Holmes, A.E., Esteban, E., Rubin, C., and Brody, D.J. (2001). Estimated prevalence of noise-induced hearing threshold shifts among children 6 to 19 years of age: The Third National Health and Nutrition Examination Survey, 1988-1994, United States. *Pediatrics, 108*(1), 40-43.

Pleis, J.R., and Coles, R. (2002). Summary health statistics for U. S. adults: National Health Interview Survey, 1998. *Vital Health Statistics Vol. 10*(209). Washington, DC: National Center for Health Statistics.

Pledger, C. (2003). Discourse on disability and rehabilitation issues: Opportunities for psychology. *American Psychologist, 58*(4), 279-284.

Popelka, M.M., Cruickshanks, K.J., Wiley, T.L., Tweed, T.S., Klein, B.E., and Klein, R. (1998). Low prevalence of hearing aid use among older adults with hearing loss: The Epidemiology of Hearing Loss Study. *Journal of the American Geriatrics Society, 46*(9), 1075-1078.

Rickards, F.W., DeVidi, S., and McMahon, D.S. (1996). Audiological indicators of exaggerated hearing loss in noise-induced hearing loss claims. *Australian Journal of Audiology, 18,* 89-97.

Rizer F.M., Arkis, P.N., Lippy, W.H., and Schuring A.G. (1988). A postoperative audiometric evaluation of cochlear implant patients. *Otolaryngology—Head and Neck Surgery, 98,* 203-209.

Social Security Administration. (2003a). *Disablitity evaluation under Social Security.* (Blue Book) SSA Pub. No. 64-039. Available: http://www.ssa.gov/disability/professionals/bluebook/2003-version.pdf. [Accessed August 2004.]

Social Security Administration. (2003b). *Program Operations Manual System: DI 24535.010– Evaluation of Hearing Impairments–10/02/2003.* Washington, DC: Social Security Administration.

Social Security Administration. (2004) *20CFR Parts 404 and 416.* Available: http://www.gpoaccess.gov/cfr/index.html. [Accessed March 2004.]

Social Security Advisory Board. (2001). *Agenda for social security: Challenges for the new congress and the new administration.* Washington, DC: Social Security Advisory Board.

Social Security Advisory Board. (2003). *The Social Security definition of disability.* Washington, DC: Social Security Advisory Board.

Thornton, A.R., and Raffin, M.J. (1978). Speech-discrimination scores modeled as a binomial variable. *Journal of Speech and Hearing Research, 21*(3), 507-518.

U.S. Department of Health and Human Services. (1991). *Healthy people 2000: National health promotion and disease prevention objectives.* (DHHS Publication No. 91-50121). Washington, DC: Government Printing Office.

U.S. Public Health Service. (1990). *Healthy people 2000.* Washington, DC: Government Printing Office.

World Health Organization. (1980). *International classification of impairments, disabilities and handicaps: A manual of classification relating to the consequences of disease.* Geneva: World Health Organization.

World Health Organization. (2001). *The international classification of functioning, disability and health: ICF.* Geneva: World Health Organization.

CHAPTER 2

American Medical Association. (2001). *Guides to the evaluation of permanent impairment* (5th ed.). Chicago, IL: American Medical Association.

American National Standards Institute. (2002). ANSI S3.5-1997. *Method for the calculation of the Speech Intelligibility Index.* New York: American National Standards Institute.

American National Standards Institute. (2003). ANSI S3.4-1980 (R2003). *Procedure for the computation of loudness of noise.* New York: American National Standards Institute.

Baskill, J.L., and Coles, R.R.A. (1999). Relations between tinnitus loudness and severity. In *Proceedings of the sixth international tinnitus seminar* (pp. 424-428). London, England: British Society of Audiology.

Bregman, A.S. (1990). *Auditory scene analysis: the perceptual organization of sound.* Cambridge, MA: MIT Press.

Brookhouser, P.E. (1993). Sensorineural hearing loss in children. In C.W. Cummings and L.A. Harker (Eds.), *Otolaryngology—Head and Neck Surgery* (2nd ed., pp. 3080-3102.). St. Louis, MO: Mosby.

Cherry, C. (1953). Some experiments on the recognition of speech with one and two ears. *Journal of the Acoustical Society of America, 25,* 975-983.

Ching, T.Y., Dillon, H., and Byrne, D. (1998). Speech recognition of hearing-impaired listeners; predictions from audibility and the limited role of high-frequency amplification. *Journal of the Acoustical Society of America, 103*(2), 1128-1140.

Dahl, H.H., Saunders, K., Kelly, T.M., Osborn, A.H., Wilcox, S., Cone-Wesson, B., Wunderlich, J.L., Du Sart, D., Kamarinos, M., Gardner, R.J., Dennehy, S., Williamson, R., Vallance, N., and Mutton, P. (2001). Prevalence and nature of connexin 26 mutations in children with non-syndromic deafness. *Medical Journal of Australia, 175*(4), 182-183.

Dobie, R.A. (1999). A review of randomized clinical trials in tinnitus. *Laryngoscope, 109*(8), 1202-1211.

Dorland, W.A.N. (1974). *Dorland's illustrated medical dictionary, 25th edition.* Philadelphia: W.B. Saunders.

Erbe, C.B., Harris, K.C., Runge-Samuelson, C.L., Flanary, V.A., and Wackym, P.A. (2004). Connexin 26 and connexin 30 mutations in children with nonsyndromic hearing loss. *Laryngoscope, 114*(4), 607-611.

Gurtler, N., Kim, Y., Mhatre, A., Muller, R., Probst, R., and Lalwani, A.K. (2003). GJB2 mutations in the Swiss hearing impaired. *Ear and Hearing, 24*(5), 440-447.

Hallpike, C.S., Harriman, D.G.F., and Wells, C.E.C. (1980). A case of afferent neuropathy and deafness. *Journal of Laryngology and Otology, 94,* 945-964.

Hazell, J.W.P., and Sheldrake, J.B. (1991). Hyperacusis and tinnitus. In *Proceedings of the fourth international tinnitus seminar* (pp. 245-248). Amsterdam: Kugler Publications.

Hazell, J.W.P., Sheldrake, J.B., and Graham, R.L. (2002). Decreased sound tolerance: Predisposing factors, triggers, and outcomes after. In R. Patuzzi (Ed.), *Proceedings of the seventh international tinnitus seminar* (pp. 255-261). Perth, Australia: University of Western Australia.

Hogan, C.A., and Turner, C.W. (1998). High-frequency audibility: Benefits for hearing-impaired listeners. *Journal of the Acoustical Society of America, 104*(1), 432-441.

Lewis, J.E., Stephens, S.D., and McKenna, L. (1994). Tinnitus and suicide. *Clinical Otolaryngology, 19,* 50-54.

McCabe, B.F. (1979). Autoimmune sensorineural hearing loss. *Annals of Otology, Rhinology, and Laryngology, 88*(5 Pt. 1), 585-589.

Merchant, S.N., McKenna, M.J., Nadol, J.B., Jr., Kristiansen, A.G., Tropitzsch, A., Lindal, S., and Tranebjaerg, L. (2001). Temporal bone histopathologic and genetic studies in Mohr-Tranegjaerg Syndrome (DFN-1). *Otology and Neurotology, 22,* 506-511.

Nadol, J.B., Jr. (2001). Primary cochlear neuronal degeneration. In Y.S. Sininger, and A. Starr (Eds.), *Auditory Neuropathy: A new perspective on hearing disorders* (pp. 99-140). New York: Thompson Learning.

Nance, W.E. (2003). The genetics of deafness. *Mental Retardation and Development Disabilities Research Reviews, 9*(2), 109-119.

National Research Council. (1982). *Tinnitus: Facts, theories, and treatments.* Washington, DC: National Academy Press.

Occupational Safety and Health Administration. (2002). *Hearing conservation* (revised). Washington, DC: U.S. Department of Labor.

Peterson, A., Shallop, J., Driscoll, C., Breneman, A., Babb, J., Stoeckel, R., and Fabry, L. (2003). Outcomes of coclear implantation in children with auditory neuropathy. *Journal of the American Academy of Audiology, 14*(4), 188-201.

Rapin, I., and Gravel, J. (2003). "Auditory neuropathy": Physiologic and pathologic evidence calls for more diagnostic specificity. *International Journal of Pediatric Otorhinolaryngology, 67*(7), 707-728.

Shallop, J.K., Peterson, A., Facer, G.W., Fabry, L.B., and Driscoll, C.L. (2001). Cochlear implants in five cases of auditory neuropathy: Postoperative findings and progress. *Laryngoscope, 111*(4, pt. 1), 555-562.

Sininger, Y.S., and Oba, S. (2001). Patients with auditory neuropathy: Who are they and what can they hear? In Y.S. Sininger, and A. Starr (Eds.), *Auditory neuropathy: A new perspective on hearing disorders* (pp. 15-35). San Diego, CA: Singular.

Snow, J.B., Jr. (2004). *Tinnitus: Theory and management.* Hamilton, ON, Canada: B.C. Decker.

Spoendlin, H. (1974). Optic and cochleovestibular degenerations in hereditary ataxias II. Temporal bone pathology in two cases of Friedreich's ataxia with vestibulo-cochlear disorders. *Brain, 97,* 41-48.

Starr, A., Michalewski, H., Zeng, F.G., Fujikawa-Brooks, S., Linthicum, F., Kim, C.S., Winnier, D., and Keats, B. (2003). Pathology and physiology of auditory neuropathy with a novel mutation in the MPZ gene (Tyrl45>Ser). *Brain, 126,* 1-15.

Starr, A., Picton, T.W., and Kim, R. (2001). Pathophysiology of auditory neuropathy. In Y.S. Sininger, and A. Starr (Eds.), *Auditory neuropathy: A new perspective on hearing disorders* (pp. 67-82). San Diego, CA: Singular.

Starr, A., Picton, T.W., Sininger, Y., Hood, L.J., and Berlin, C.I. (1996). Auditory neuropathy. *Brain, 119*(Pt 3), 741-753.

Starr, A., Sininger, Y.S., Winter, M., Derebery, J., Oba, S., and Michalewski, H. (1998). Transient deafness due to temperature-sensitive auditory neuropathy. *Ear and Hearing, 19,* 169-179.

Stouffer, J.L., and Tyler, R.S. (1990). Characterization of tinnitus by tinnitus patients. *Journal of Speech and Hearing Disorders, 55*(3), 439-453.

Sullivan, M.D., Katon, W., Dobie, R., Sakai, C., Russo, J., and Harrop-Griffiths, J. (1988). Disabling tinnitus. Association with affective disorder. *General Hospital Psychiatry, 10*(4), 285-291.

Tyler, R.S. (2000). *Tinnitus handbook.* San Diego, CA: Singular Thomson Learning.

Tyler, R.S., and Baker, L.J. (1983). Difficulties experienced by tinnitus sufferers. *Journal of Speech and Hearing Disorders, 48*(2), 150-154.

Vernon, J.A., and Meikle, M.B. (2000). Tinnitus masking. In R.S. Tyler (Ed.), *Tinnitus handbook* (pp. 313-356). San Diego, CA: Singular Thomson Learning.

Yost, W.A. (2000). *Fundamentals of hearing: An introduction* (4th ed.). New York: Academic Press.

Zoger, S., Svedlund, J., and Holgers, K.M. (2002). Psychiatric profile of tinnitus patients with high risk of severe and chronic tinnitus. In *Proceedings of the seventh international tinnitus seminar.* Perth, Australia: University of Western Australia.

CHAPTER 3

Aleksandrovsky, I.V., McCullough, J.K., and Wilson, R.H. (1998). Development of suprathreshold word recognition test for Russian-speaking patients. *Journal of the American Academy of Audiology, 9*(6), 417-425.

American National Standards Institute. (1969). ANSI S3.5-1969. *Method for the calculation of the articulation index.* New York: American National Standards Institute.

American National Standards Institute. (1996). ANSI S3.6-1996. *Specification for audiometers.* New York: American National Standards Institute.

American National Standards Institute. (1997). ANSI S3.21-1978 (R1997). *Method for manual pure-tone threshold audiometry.* New York: American National Standards Institute.

American National Standards Institute. (2002a). ANSI S3.39-1987 (R2002). *Specifications for instruments to measure aural acoustic impedance and admittance* (Aural Acoustic Immittance). New York: American National Standards Institute.

American National Standards Institute. (2002b). ANSI S3.5-1997 (R2002). *Method for the calculation of the Speech Intelligibility Index.* New York: American National Standards Institute.

American Speech-Language-Hearing Association. (1978). Guidelines for manual pure-tone threshold audiometry. *ASHA, 20,* 297-301.

American Speech-Language-Hearing Association. (1988). Guidelines for determining the threshold level of speech. *ASHA, 30,* 85-89.

American Speech-Language-Hearing Association. (1990). Guidelines for screening for hearing impairment and middle ear disorders. *ASHA, 32*(Suppl 2), 17-24.

Beattie, R.C., Forrester, P.W., and Ruby, B.K. (1977). Reliability of the Tillman-Olsen procedure for determination of spondee threshold using recorded and live voice presentations. *Journal of the American Audiological Society, 2*(4), 159-162.

Bentler, R.A. (2000). List equivalency and test-retest reliability of the Speech in Noise test. *American Journal of Audiology, 9*(2), 84-100.

Bess, F.H., and Humes, L.E. (2003). *Audiology: The fundamentals* (3rd ed.). Baltimore, MD: Lippincott Williams and Wilkins.

Bilger, R.C., Nuetzel, J.M., Rabinowitz, W.M., and Rzeczkowski, C. (1984). Standardization of a test of speech perception in noise. *Journal of Speech and Hearing Research, 27*(1), 32-48.

Boothroyd, A., Hanin, L., and Hnath, T. (1985). *CUNY laser videodisk of everyday sentences.* New York: Speech and Hearing Sciences Research Center, City University of New York.

Boothroyd, A., Hnath-Chisolm, T., Hanin, L., and Kishon-Rabin, L. (1988). Voice fundamental frequency as an auditory supplement to the speechreading of sentences. *Ear and Hearing, 9*(6), 306-312.

Brownell, W.E., Bader, C.R., Bertrand, D., and de Ribaupierre, Y. (1985). Evoked mechanical responses of isolated cochlear outer hair cells. *Science, 227*(4683), 194-196.

Cakiroglu, S., and Danhauer, J.L. (1992). Effects of listeners' and talkers' linguistic backgrounds on W-22 test performance. *Journal of the American Academy of Audiology, 3*(3), 186-192.

Carhart, R. (1971). Observations on relations between thresholds for pure tones and for speech. *Journal of Speech and Hearing Disorders, 36*(4), 476-483.

Carhart, R., and Jerger, J. (1959). Preferred method for clinical determination of pure-tone thresholds. *Journal of Speech and Hearing Disorders, 24,* 330-345.

Clarke, J.B. (1981). The uses and abuses of hearing loss classification. *ASHA, 23,* 493-500.

Clemis, J.D., Ballad, W.J., and Killion, M.C. (1986). Clinical use of an insert earphone. *Annals of Otology, Rhinology, and Laryngology, 95*(5 Pt. 1), 520-524.

Cokely, J.A., and Yager, C.R. (1993). Scoring Spanish word-recognition measures. *Ear and Hearing, 14*(6), 395-400.

Coles, R.R.A., and Mason, S.M. (1984). The results of cortical electrical response audiometry in medico-legal investigations. *British Journal of Audiology, 18,* 71-78.

Comstock, C.L., and Martin, F.N. (1984). A children's Spanish word discrimination test for non-Spanish-speaking clinicians. *Ear and Hearing, 5*(3), 166-170.

Cox, R.M., Alexander, G.C., and Gilmore, C. (1987). Development of the Connected Speech Test (CST). *Ear and Hearing, 8*(5 Suppl), 119S-126S.

Cox, R.M., Alexander, G.C., Gilmore, C., and Pusakulich, K.M. (1988). Use of the Connected Speech Test (CST) with hearing-impaired listeners. *Ear and Hearing, 9*(4), 198-207.

Cox, R.M., Gray, G.A., and Alexander, G.C. (2001). Evaluation of a Revised Speech in Noise (RSIN) test. *Journal of the American Academy of Audiology, 12*(8), 423-432.

Danhauer, J.L., Crawford, S., and Edgerton, B.J. (1984). English, Spanish, and bilingual speakers' performance on a nonsense syllable test (NST) of speech sound discrimination. *Journal of Speech and Hearing Disorders, 49*(2), 164-168.

Dimitrijevic, A., John, M.S., Van Roon, P., Purcell, D.W., Adamonis, J., Ostroff, J., Nedzelski, J. M., and Picton, T. (2002). Estimating the audiogram using multiple auditory steady-state responses. *Journal of the American Academy of Audiology, 13,* 205-224.

Dirks, D., Bell, T., Rossman, R., and Kincaid, G. (1986). Articulation index predictions of contextually dependent words. *Journal of the Acoustical Society of America, 80,* 82-92.

Dirks, D.D., Morgan, D.E., and Dubno, J.R. (1982). A procedure for quantifying the effects of noise on speech recognition. *Journal of Speech and Hearing Disorders, 47*(2), 114-123.

Dirks, D.D., Takayanagi, S., Moshfegh, A., Noffsinger, P.D., and Fausti, S.A. (2001). Examination of the neighborhood activation theory in normal and hearing-impaired listeners. *Ear and Hearing, 22*(1), 1-13.

Dubno, J.R., and Dirks, D.D. (1982). Evaluation of hearing-impaired listeners using a Nonsense-Syllable Test. I. Test reliability. *Journal of Speech and Hearing Research, 25*(1), 135-141.

Dubno, J.R., Dirks, D.D., and Langhofer, L.R. (1982). Evaluation of hearing-impaired listeners using a Nonsense-Syllable Test. II. Syllable recognition and consonant confusion patterns. *Journal of Speech and Hearing Research, 25*(1), 141-148.

Erber, N.P. (1975). Auditory-visual perception of speech. *Journal of Speech and Hearing Disorders, 40*(4), 481-492.

Erber, N.P. (1979). Auditory-visual perception of speech with reduced optical clarity. *Journal of Speech and Hearing Research, 22*(2), 212-223.

Etymotic Research. (1993). *The SIN test (compact disk)*. Elk Grove Village, IL: Etymotic Research.

Etymotic Research. (2001). *QuickSIN speech-in-noise test, version 1.3 manual*. Elk Grove Village, IL: Etymotic Research.

Fletcher, H. (1950). A method of calculating hearing loss for speech from an audiogram. *Journal of the Acoustical Society of America, 22*, 1-5.

Gat, I.B., and Keith, R.W. (1978). An effect of linguistic experience. Auditory word discrimination by native and non-native speakers of English. *Audiology, 17*(4), 339-345.

Goodman, A. (1965). Reference zero levels for pure-tone audiometer. *ASHA, 7*, 262-263.

Hardick, E.J., Oyer, H.J., and Irion, P.E. (1970). Lipreading performance as related to measurements of vision. *Journal of Speech and Hearing Research, 13*(1), 92-100.

Hargus, S.E., and Gordon-Salant, S. (1995). Accuracy of speech intelligibility index predictions for noise-masked young listeners with normal hearing and for elderly listeners with hearing impairment. *Journal of Speech and Hearing Research, 38*(1), 234-243.

Hirsh, I., Davis, H., Silverman, S.R., Reynolds, E.G., Eldert, E., and Benson, R.W. (1952). Development of materials for speech audiometry. *Journal of Speech and Hearing Disorders, 17*, 321-337.

Hodgson, W.R., and Skinner, P.H. (1981). *Hearing aid assessment and use in audiologic habilitation*. Baltimore, MD: Williams and Wilkins.

Hone, S.W., Norman, G., Keogh, I., and Kelly, V. (2003). The use of cortical evoked response audiometry in the assessment of noise-induced hearing loss. *Otolaryngology, Head and Neck Surgery, 128*, 257-262.

Hyde, M., Alberti, P., Matsumoto, N., and Yao-Li, L. (1986). Auditory evoked potentials in audiometric assessment of compensation and medicolegal patients. *Annals of Otology, Rhinology, and Laryngology, 95*, 514-519.

Jerger, J., and Herer, G. (1961). An unexpected dividend in Bekesy audiometry. *Journal of Speech and Hearing Disorders, 26*, 390-391.

Kalikow, D.N., Stevens, K.N., and Elliott, L.L. (1977). Development of a test of speech intelligibility in noise using sentence materials with controlled word predictability. *Journal of the Acoustical Society of America, 61*(5), 1337-1351.

Kemp, D.T. (1986). Otoacoustic emissions, travelling waves and cochlear mechanisms. *Hearing Research, 22*, 95-104.

Kirk, K.I., Pisoni, D.B., and Osberger, M.J. (1995). Lexical effects on spoken word recognition by pediatric cochlear implant users. *Ear and Hearing, 16*, 470-481.

Lasky, R.E., and Yang, E. (1986). Methods for determining auditory evoked brain-stem response thresholds in human newborns. *Electroencephalogaphy and Clinical Neurophysiology, 65*(4), 276-281.

Lloyd, L.L., and Price, J.G. (1971). Sentence familiarity as a factor in visual speech reception (lipreading) of deaf college students. *Journal of Speech and Hearing Research, 14*(2), 291-294.

Luce, P.A., and Pisoni, D.B. (1998). Recognizing spoken words: The neighborhood activation model. *Ear and Hearing, 19*(1), 1-36.

Margolis, R.H., and Hunter, L.L. (1999). Tympanometry: Basic principles and clinical applications. In F.E. Musiek and W.F. Rintelmann (Eds.), *Contemporary perspectives in hearing assessment* (pp. 89-130). Boston: Allyn and Bacon.

Martin, F.N., and Champlin, C.A. (2000). Reconsidering the limits of normal hearing. *Journal of the American Academy of Audiology, 11*(2), 64-66.

Martin, F.N., Champlin, C.A., and Chambers, J.A. (1998). Seventh survey of audiometric practices in the United States. *Journal of the American Academy of Audiology, 9*(2), 95-104.

Mayo, L.H., Florentine, M., and Buus, S. (1997). Age of second-language acquisition and perception of speech in noise. *Journal of Speech-Language-Hearing Research, 40*(3), 686-693.

McCullough, J.A., Wilson, R.H., Birck, J.D., and Anderson, L.G. (1994). A multimedia approach for estimating space recognition of multilingual clients. *American Journal of Audiology, 3*, 19-22.

Mineau, S.M., and Schlauch, R.S. (1997). Threshold measurement for patients with tinnitus: Pulsed or continuous tones. *American Journal of Audiology, 7*, 50-54.

Newby, H.A. (1964). *Audiology* (2nd ed.). New York: Appleton-Century Crofts.

Nilsson, M., Soli, S.D., and Sullivan, J.A. (1994). Development of the Hearing in Noise Test for the measurement of speech reception thresholds in quiet and in noise. *Journal of the Acoustical Society of America, 95*(2), 1085-1099.

Owens, E., and Schubert, E.D. (1977). Development of the California Consonant Test. *Journal of Speech and Hearing Research, 20*(3), 463-474.

Owens, E., Kessler, D.K., Raggio, M.W., and Schubert, E.D. (1985). Analysis and revision of the minimal auditory capabilities (MAC) battery. *Ear and Hearing, 6*(6), 280-290.

Perez-Abalo, M.C., Savio, G., Torres, A., Martin, V., Rodriguez, E., and Galan, L. (2001). Steady state responses to multiple amplitude-modulated tones: an optimized method to test frequency-specific thresholds in hearing-impaired children and normal-hearing subjects. *Ear and Hearing, 22*(3), 200-211.

Picton, T.W., Durieux-Smith, A., Champagne, S.C., Whittingham, J., Moran, L.M., Giguere, C., and Beauregard, Y. (1998). Objective evaluation of aided thresholds using auditory steady-state responses. *Journal of the American Academy of Audiology, 9*(5), 315-331.

Plomp, R. (1986). A signal-to-noise ratio model for the speech-reception threshold of the hearing impaired. *Journal of Speech and Hearing Research, 29*, 146-154.

Plomp, R., and Duquesnoy, A.J. (1980). Room acoustics for the aged. *Journal of the Acoustical Society of America, 68*, 1616-1621.

Prieve, B.A., and Fitzgerald, T.S. (2002). Otoacoustic emissions. In J. Katz (Ed.), *Handbook of clinical audiology* (pp. 440-466). Philadelphia: Lippincott, Williams and Wilkins.

Ramkissoon, I., Proctor, A., Lansing, C.R., and Bilger, R.C. (2002). Digit speech recognition thresholds (SRT) for non-native speakers of English. *American Journal of Audiology, 11*(1), 23-8.

Resnick, S.B., Dubno, J.R., Hoffnung, S., and Levitt, H. (1975). Phoneme errors on a nonsense syllable test. *Journal of the Acoustical Society of America, 58*(Suppl 1), 114.

Rickards, F.W., Tan, L.E., Cohen, L.T., Wilson, O.J., Drew, J.H., and Clark, G.M. (1994). Auditory steady-state evoked potential in newborns. *British Journal of Audiology, 28*(6), 327-337.

Rintelmann, W.F., and Harford, E.R. (1963). The detection and assessment of pseudohypoacusis among school-aged children. *Journal of Speech and Hearing Disorders, 10*, 733-744.

Ross, M. (1964). The variable intensity pulse count method (VIPCM) for the detection and measurement of the pure-tone thresholds of children with functional hearing losses. *Journal of Speech and Hearing Disorders, 29*, 477-482.

Ruhm, H.B., and Cooper, W.A. (1964). Delayed feedback audiometry. *Journal of Speech and Hearing Disorders, 29*, 448-455.

Russell, I.J., and Sellick, P.M. (1978). Intracellular studies of hair cells in the mammalian cochlea. *Journal of Physiology, 284*, 261-290.

Schlauch, R.S., Arnce, K.D., Olson, L.M., Sanchez, S., and Doyle, T.N. (1996). Identification of pseudohypacusis using speech recognition thresholds. *Ear and Hearing, 17*(3), 229-236.

Schrott, A., Puel, J.L., and Rebillard, G. (1991). Cochlear origin of 2f1-f2 distortion products assessed by using 2 types of mutant mice. *Hearing Research, 52*(1), 245-254.

Schum, D.J., Matthews, L.J., and Lee, F.S. (1991). Actual and predicted word-recognition performance of elderly hearing-impaired listeners. *Journal of Speech and Hearing Research, 34*, 36-42.

Silman, S., and Gelfand, S.A. (1981). The relationship between magnitude of hearing loss and acoustic reflex threshold levels. *Journal of Speech and Hearing Disorders, 46*(3), 312-316.

Silverman, S.R., and Hirsh, I.J. (1955). Problems related to the use of speech in clinical audiometry. *Annals of Otology, Rhinology, and Laryngology, 64*(4), 1234-1244.

Sims, D.G., and Hirsh, I. (1982). Hearing and speechreading evaluation for the deaf adult. In D.G. Sims, G.G. Walter, and R.L. Whitehead (Eds.), *Deafness and communication assessment and training* (pp. 177-185). Baltimore, MD: Williams and Wilkins.

Sininger, Y.S., and Abdala, C. (1998). Otoacoustic emissions for the study of auditory function in infants and children. In C.I. Berlin (Ed.), *Otoacoustic emissions: Basic science and clinical applications* (pp.182). San Diego, CA: Singular.

Sininger, Y.S., Abdala, C., and Cone-Wesson, B. (1997). Auditory threshold sensitivity of the human neonate as measured by the auditory brainstem response. *Hearing Research, 104*(1-2), 27-38.

Sininger, Y.S., and Oba, S. (2001). Patients with auditory neuropathy: Who are they and what can they hear? In Y.S. Sininger and A. Starr (Eds.), *Auditory neuropathy: A new perspective on hearing disorders* (pp. 15-35). San Diego, CA: Singular.

Snyder, J.M. (2001). Audiological evaluation of exaggerated hearing loss. In R. Dobie (Ed.), *Medico-legal evaluation of hearing loss* (pp. 49-88). San Diego, CA: Singular.

Social Security Administration. (2003). *Disability evaluation under Social Security.* (Blue Book) SSA Pub. No. 64-039. Available: http://www.ssa.gov/disability/professionals/bluebook/2003-version.pdf. [Accessed August 2004.]

Speaks, S., and Jerger, J. (1965). Method for measurement of speech identification. *Journal of Speech and Hearing Research, 8*, 185-194.

Spitzer, J.B. (1980). The development of a picture speech reception threshold test in Spanish for use with urban U.S. residents of Hispanic background. *Journal of Communication Disorders, 13*(2), 147-151.

Stapells, D.R., Gravel, J.S., and Martin, B.A. (1995). Thresholds for auditory brain stem responses to tones in notched noise from infants and young children with normal hearing or sensorineural hearing loss. *Ear and Hearing, 16*(4), 361-371.

Stuart, A., Yang, E.Y., and Green, W.B. (1994). Neonatal auditory brainstem response thresholds to air-and bone-conducted clicks: 0 to 96 hours postpartum. *Journal of the American Academy of Audiology, 5*(3), 163-172.

Studebaker, G.A. (1985). A "rationalized" arcsine transform. *Journal of Speech and Hearing Research, 28*, 455-462.

Studebaker, G.A., Sherbecoe, R.L., and Gilmore, C. (1993). Frequency-importance and transfer functions for the Auditec of St. Louis recordings of the NU-6 word test. *Journal of Speech and Hearing Research, 36*, 799-807.

Suter, A.H. (1985). Speech recognition in noise by individuals with mild hearing impairments. *Journal of the Acoustical Society of America, 78*(3), 887-900.

Thornton, A.R., and Raffin, M.J. (1978). Speech-discrimination scores modeled as a binomial variable. *Journal of Speech and Hearing Research, 21*(3), 507-18.

Tillman, T.W., and Carhart, R. (1966). An expanded test for speech discrimination utilizing CNC monosyllabic words. Northwestern University Auditory Test No. 6. [SAM-TR-66-55.] (pp. 1-12).

Tillman, T.W., and Olsen, W.O. (1973). Speech audiometry. In J. Jerger (Ed.), *Modern developments in audiology* (pp. 37-74). New York: Academic Press.

Tsui, B., Wong, L.L.N., and Wong, E.C.M. (2002). Accuracy of cortical evoked response audiometry in the identification of non-organic hearing loss. *International Journal of Audiology, 41*, 330-333.

Tye-Murray, N. (1998). *Foundations of aural rehabilitation*. San Diego, CA: Singular.

Tyler, R., Preece, J., and Tye-Murray, N. (1986). *The Iowa phoneme and sentence tests*. Iowa City: The University of Iowa Hospitals and Clinics.

Tyler, R.S., Gantz, B.J., McCabe, B.F., Lowder, M.W., Otto, S.R., and Preece, J.P. (1985). Audiological results with two single channel cochlear implants. *Annals of Otology, Rhinology, and Laryngology, 94*(2 Pt 1), 133-139.

Wall, L.G., Davis, L.A., and Myers, D.K. (1984). Four spondee threshold procedures: A comparison. *Ear and Hearing, 5*(3), 171-174.

Weislander, P., and Hodgson, W.R. (1989). Evaluation of four Spanish word-recognition-ability lists. *Ear and Hearing, 10*, 387-392.

Wilson, R.H., Morgan, D.E., and Dirks, D.D. (1973). A proposed SRT procedure and its statistical precedent. *Journal of Speech and Hearing Disorders, 38*(2), 184-191.

Wilson, R.H., Zizz, C.A., Shanks, J.E., and Causey, G.D. (1990). Normative data in quiet, broadband noise, and competing message for Northwestern University Auditory Test No. 6 by a female speaker. *Journal of Speech and Hearing Disorders, 55*(4), 771-778.

Yang, E.Y., and Stuart, A. (1990). A method of auditory brainstem rsponse testing of infants using bone-conducted clicks. *Journal of Speech-Language Pathology and Audiology, 14*, 69-76.

Yang, E.Y., Rupert, A.L., and Moushegian, G. (1987). A developmental study of bone conduction auditory brain stem response in infants. *Ear and Hearing, 8*(4), 244-251.

CHAPTER 4

American National Standards Institute. (1993). ANSI/AAMI ESI: 1993. *Safe current limits for electromedical apparatus* (3rd. ed.). New York: American National Standards Institute.

American National Standards Institute. (1996). ANSI S3.6-1996. *Specification for audiometers.* New York: American National Standards Institute.

American National Standards Institute. (2002a). ANSI S3.13-1987 (R2002). *Mechanical coupler for measurement of bone vibrators.* New York: American National Standards Institute.

American National Standards Institute. (2002b). ANSI S3.39-1987 (R2002). *Specifications for instruments to measure aural acoustic impedance and admittance* (Aural Acoustic Immittance). New York: American National Standards Institute.

American National Standards Institute. (2002c). ANSI S3.42-1992 (R2002). *Testing hearing aids with a broadband noise signal.* New York: American National Standards Institute.

American National Standards Institute. (2002d). ANSI S3.46-1997 (R2002). *Methods of measurement of real-ear performance characteristics of hearing aids.* New York: American National Standards Institute.

American National Standards Institute. (2002e). ANSI S3.5-1997 (R2002). *Method for the calculation of the Speech Intelligibility Index.* New York: American National Standards Institute.

American National Standards Institute. (2003a). ANSI S3.1-1999 (R2003). *Maximum permissible ambient noise levels for audiometric test rooms.* New York: American National Standards Institute.

American National Standards Institute. (2003b). ANSI S3.22-2003. *Specification of hearing aid characteristics.* New York: American National Standards Institute.

American Speech-Language-Hearing Association. (1988). Guidelines for determining the threshold level of speech. *ASHA, 30*, 85-89.

American Speech-Language-Hearing Association. (1991a). Guidelines for the audiological assessment of children from birth through 36 months of age. *ASHA, 33*(5 Suppl), 37-43.

American Speech-Language-Hearing Association. (1991b). Sound field measurement tutorial. Working group on sound field calibration of the committee on audiologic evaluation *ASHA, 33*(3), 25-38.

American Speech-Language-Hearing Association. (1993). Preferred practice patterns for the professions of speech-language pathology and audiology. *ASHA Supplement, 11*(Suppl to 35, No. 3), 1-102.

American Speech-Language-Hearing Association (2002). *Communication facts: Incidence and prevalence of communication disorders and hearing loss in children—2002 edition*. Rockville, MD: ASHA.

Blanchfield, B.B., Feldman, J.J., Dunbar, J.L., and Gardner, E.N. (2001). The severely to profoundly hearing-impaired population in the United States: Prevalence estimates and demographics. *Journal of the American Academy of Audiology, 12*(4), 183-189.

Brown, R.E.C. (1948). Experimental studies on the reliability of audiometry. *Journal of Laryngology and Otology, 62*, 467-524.

Campbell, K. (1998). *Essential audiology for physicians*. San Diego, CA: Singular.

Carhart, R., and Jerger, J. (1959). Preferred method for clinical determination of pure-tone thresholds. *Journal of Speech and Hearing Disorders, 24*, 330-345.

Cohen, M.R., and McCullough, T.D. (1996). Infection control protocols for audiologists. *American Journal of Audiology, 5*, 20-22.

Corthals, P., Vinck, B., De Vel, E., and Van Cauwenberge, P. (1997). Audiovisual speech reception in noise and self-perceived hearing disability in sensorineural hearing loss. *Audiology, 36*(1), 46-56.

Etymotic Research. (2001). *QuickSIN speech-in-noise test, version 1.3 manual*. Elk Grove Village, IL: Etymotic Research.

Fishman, K., Shannon, R.V., and Slattery, W. (1997). Speech recognition as a function of the number of electrodes used in the SPEAK cochlear implant strategy. *Journal of Speech Language and Hearing Research, 40*, 1201-1215.

Fletcher, H. (1950). A method of calculating hearing loss for speech from an audiogram. *Journal of the Acoustical Society of America, 22*, 1-5.

Flynn, M.C., Dowell, R.C., and Clark, G.M. (1998). Aided speech recognition abilities of adults with a severe or severe-to-profound hearing loss. *Journal of Speech Language and Hearing Research, 41*(2), 285-299.

Hardick, E.J., Melnick, W., Hawes, N.A., et al. (1980). *Compensation for hearing loss for employees under jurisdiction of the U.S. Department of Labor: Benefit formula and assessment procedures*. Columbus, OH: Ohio State University.

Houtenville, A.J. (2002). Employment and economic consequences of visual impairment. In Committee on Disability Determination for Individuals with Visual Impairments, P. Lennie and S.B. Van Hemel (Eds.), *Visual impairments: Determining eligibility for Social Security benefits* (pp. 275-321). Washington, DC: National Academy Press.

International Organization for Standardization. (1986). *Danger signals for workplaces-auditory danger signals*. (ISO 7731-1986 (E)). Geneva: International Standards Organization.

King, P.F., Coles, R.R.A., Lutman, M.E., and Robinson, D.W. (1992). *Assessment of hearing disability: Guidelines for medicolegal practice*. London, England: Whurr.

Larson, V.D., Williams, D.W., Henderson, W.G., Luethke, L.E., Beck, L.B., Noffsinger, D., Wilson, R.H., Dobie, R.A., Haskell, G.B., Bratt, G.W., Shanks, J.E., Stelmachowicz, P., Studebaker, G.A., Boysen, A.E., Donahue, A., Canalis, R., Fausti, S.A., and Rappaport, B.Z. (2000). Efficacy of 3 commonly used hearing aid circuits: A crossover trial. *Journal of the American Medical Association, 284*(14), 1806-1813.

Nilsson, M., Soli, S.D., and Sullivan, J.A. (1994). Development of the Hearing in Noise Test for the measurement of speech reception thresholds in quiet and in noise. *Journal of the Acoustical Society of America, 95*(2), 1085-1099.

Pahor, A.L. (1981). The ENT problems following Birmingham bombings. *Journal of Laryngology and Otology, 95*, 1085-1099.

Pearsons, K., Bennett, R., and Fidell, S. (1977). *Speech levels in various noise environments.* (Report No. EPA-60011-77-025). Washington, DC: U.S. Environmental Protection Agency.

Robinson, D.W. (1960). Variability in the realization of the audiometric zero. *Annals of Occupational Hygiene, 2,* 107-126.

Segal, S., Harell, M., Shahar, A., and Englender, M. (1988). Acute acoustic trauma: Dynamics of hearing loss following cessation of exposure. *American Journal of Otology, 9*(4), 293-298.

Skinner, M.W., Holden, L.K., Whitford, L.A., Plant, K.L., Psarros, C., and Holden, T.A. (2002). Speech recognition with the Nuecleus 24 SPEAK, ACE, and CIS speech coding strategies in newly implanted adults. *Ear and Hearing, 23*(3), 207-223.

Stoppenbach, D.T., Craig, J.M., Wiley, T.L., and Wilson, R.H. (1999). Word recognition performance for Northwestern University Auditory Test No. 6 word lists in quiet and in competing message. *Journal of the American Academy of Audiology, 10*(8), 429-435.

Suter, A.H. (1985). Speech recognition in noise by individuals with mild hearing impairments. *Journal of the Acoustical Society of America, 78*(3), 887-900.

Swets, J.A. (1988). Measuring the accuracy of diagnostic systems. *Science, 240*(4857), 1285-1293.

Thornton, A.R., and Raffin, M.J. (1978). Speech-discrimination scores modeled as a binomial variable. *Journal of Speech and Hearing Research, 21*(3), 507-518.

Tillman, T.W., and Carhart, R., (1966). *An expanded test for speech discrimination utilizing CNC monosyllabic words.* Northwestern University Auditory Test No. 6 (pp. 1-12). Brooks Air Force Base, TX: USAF School of Aerospace Medicine Technical Report-66-55.

Tyler, R.S., Fryauf-Bertchy, H., Gantz, B.J., Kelsay, D.M., and Woodworth, G.G. (1997). Speech perception in prelingually implanted children after four years. *Advances in Otorhinolaryngology, 52*, 187-192.

U.S. Census Bureau. (2003). *Language use and English-speaking ability: 2000, Census 2000 brief.* Washington, DC: U.S. Census Bureau.

Webster, J.C. (1964). Important frequencies in noise-masked speech. *Archives of Otolaryngology—Head & Neck Surgery, 80,* 494-502.

Wilson, R., and Strouse, A. (1999). Auditory measures with speech skills. In F.E. Musiek, and W.F. Rintelmann (Eds.), *Contemporary perspectives in hearing assessment* (pp. 21-66). Boston: Allyn and Bacon.

Wilson, R.H., Zizz, C.A., Shanks, J.E., and Causey, G.D. (1990). Normative data in quiet, broadband noise, and competing message for Northwestern University Auditory Test No. 6 by a female speaker. *Journal of Speech and Hearing Disorders, 55*(4), 771-778.

CHAPTER 5

Advanced Bionics. (2004). *Advanced Bionics Clarion CI: Candidates for cochlear implants.* Available: http://www.hearinglossweb.com/res/ci/ab/htm. [Accessed March 2004.]

American Academy of Pediatrics. (2004). Recommendations for the administration of catch-up doses of pneumococcal conjugate vaccine. Available: http://www.aap.org/member/pcv0503.htm. [Accessed May 2004.]

American National Standards Institute. (2002). ANSI S3.5-1997. *Method for the calculation of the Speech Intelligibility Index.* New York: American National Standards Institute.

American Speech-Language-Hearing Association (2004). Technical Report: Cochlear implants. *ASHA Supplement 24.*

Battmer, R.D., Gupta, S.P., Alllum-Mecklenburg, D.J., and Lenarz, T. (1995). Factors influencing cochlear implant perceptual performance in 132 adults. *Annals of Otology, Rhinology, and Laryngology, 166*, 185-187.

Bentler, R.A., and Kramer, S.E. (2000). Guidelines for choosing a self-report outcome measure. *Ear and Hearing, 21*(4, Suppl), 37S-49S.

Bowe, F.G. (2002). Deaf and hard of hearing Americans' instant messaging and e-mail use: A national survey. *American Annals of the Deaf, 147*(4), 6-10.

Brown, C.J., Abbas, P.J., and Gantz, B.J. (1990). Electrically evoked whole-nerve action potentials: Data from human cochlear implant users. *Journal of the Acoustical Society of America, 88*, 1385-1391.

Busby, P.A., Roberts, S.A., Tong, Y.C., and Clark, G.M. (1991). Results of speech perception and speech production training for three prelingually deaf patients using a multiple-electrode cochlear implant. *British Journal of Audiology, 25*, 291-302.

Byrne, D., and Dillon, H. (1986). The National Acoustics Laboratories new procedure for selecting the gain and frequency response of a hearing aid. *Ear and Hearing, 7*, 257-265.

Byrne, D., Dillon, H., Ching, T., Katsch, R., and Keidser, G. (2001). NAL-NL1 procedure for fitting non-linear hearing aids: Characteristics and comparisons with other procedures. *Journal of the American Academy of Audiology, 12*(1), 37-51.

Centers for Disease Control and Prevention (CDC). (2003). *Use of vaccines for the prevention of meningitis in persons with cochlear implants: Fact sheet.* Available: http://www.cdc.gov/nip/issues/cochlear/cochlear-gen.htm. [Accessed May 2004.]

Cheng, A., Rubin, H., Powe, N., Mellon, N., Francis, H., and Niparko, J. (2000). Cost-utility analysis of the cochlear implant in children. *Journal of the American Medical Association, 284*, 850-856.

Chung, S.M., and Stephens, S.D.G. (1986). Factors influencing binaural hearing aid use. *British Journal of Audiology, 20*, 129-140.

Clark, G.M., Black, R., Dewhurst, D.J., Forster, I.C., Patrick, J.F. and Tong, Y.C. (1977). A multiple-electrode hearing prosthesis for cochlea implantation in deaf patients. *Medical Progress through Technology, 5*(3), 127-140.

Cochlear Corporation. (2004). *FDA releases next generation cochlear implant system: Candidacy requirements.* Available: http://www.cochlearamericas.com/About/341.asp. [Accessed March 2004.]

Cohen, N.L., Waltzman S.B., and Fisher, S.G. (1993). A prospective, randomized study of cochlear implants. *New England Journal of Medicine, 328*, 233-237.

Compton, C.L. (2000). Assistive technology for the enhancement of receptive communication. In J.G. Alpiner and P.A. McCarthy (Eds.), *Rehabilitative audiology: Children and adults* (3rd ed., pp. 501-555). Philadelphia: Lippincott, Williams and Wilkins.

Cornelisse, L.E., Seewald, R.C., and Jamieson, D.G. (1995). The input/output formula: A theoretical approach to the fitting of personal amplification devices. *Journal of the Acoustical Society of America, 97*(3), 1854-1864.

Dawson, P.W., Blamey, P.J., Rowland, L.C., Dettman, S.J., Clark, G.M., Busby, P.A., Dowell, R.C., and Rickards, F.W. (1992). Cochlear implants in children, adolescents, and prelingually deafened adults: Speech perception. *Journal of Speech and Hearing Research, 35*, 401-417.

Fishman., K., Shannon, R.V., and Slattery, W. (1998). Speech recognition as a function of the number of electrodes used in the SPEAK cochlear implant strategy. *Journal of Speech and Hearing Research, 40*, 1201-1215.

Flynn, M.C., Dowell, R.C., and Clark, G.M. (1998). Aided speech recognition abilities of adults with a severe or severe-to-profound hearing loss. *Journal of Speech Language and Hearing Research, 41,* 285-299.

Food and Drug Administration. (2001). Letter to Mr. Thomas A. Doyle, Med-El Corporation, announcing completion of review of MED-EL COMBI 40+ Cochlear Implant System. Available: http://www.FDA.gov.

Food and Drug Administration. (2003). *FDA public health web notification: Risk of bacterial meningitis in children with cochlear implants.* Available: http://www.fda.gov/cdrh/safety/cochlear.html. [Accessed May 2004.]

Francis, H., Chee, N., Yeagle, J., Cheng, A., and Niparko, J. (2002). Impact of cochlear implants on the functional health status of older adults. *Laryngoscope, 112,* 1482-1488.

Fu, Q.J., Shannon, R.V., and Wang, X. (1998). Effects of noise and spectral resolution on vowel and consonant recognition: Acoustic and electric hearing. *Journal of the Acoustical Society of America, 104,* 3586-3596.

Gantz, B.J., and Turner, C.W. (2003). Combining electrical and acoustical hearing. *Laryngoscope, 103,* 1726-1730.

Gantz, B.J., McCabe, B.F., and Tyler, R.S. (1988a). Use of multichannel cochlear implants in obstructed and obliterated cochleas. *Otolaryngology—Head and Neck Surgery, 98*(1), 72-81.

Gantz, B.J., Tyler, R.S., Knutson, J.F., Woodworth, G., Abbas, P., McCabe, B.F., Hinrichs, J., Tye-Murray, N., Lansing, C., Kuk, F., and Brown, C. (1988b). Evaluation of five different cochlear implant designs: Audiologic assessment and predictors of performance. *Laryngoscope, 98*(10), 1100-1106.

Gantz, B.J., Tyler, R.S., Rubinstein, J.T., Wolaver, A., Lowder, M., Abbas, P., Brown, C.J., Hughes, M., and Preece, J.P. (2002). Binaural cochlear implants placed during the same operation. *Otology and Neurotology, 23,* 169-180.

Gantz, B.J., Woodworth, G.G., Abbas, P.J., Knutson, J.F., and Tyler, R.S. (1993). Multivariate predictors of audiological success with multichannel cochlear implants. *Annals of Otology, Rhinology, and Laryngology, 102,* 909-916.

Geir, L., Barker, M., Fisher, L., and Opie, J. (1999). The effect of long-term deafness on speech recognition in postlingually deafened adult Clarion cochlear implant users. *Annals of Otology, Rhinology, and Laryngology, 108*(Suppl 177), 80-83.

Gfeller, K., Turner, C.W., Woodworth, G., Mehr, M., Fearn, R., Knutson, J.F., Witt, S., and Stordahl, J. (2002). Recognition of familiar melodies by adult cochlear implant recipients and normal hearing adults. *Cochlear Implants International, 3*(1), 31-55.

Haskell, G.B., Noffsinger, D., Larson, V.D., Williams, D.W., Dobie, R.A., and Rogers, J.L. (2002). Subjective measures of hearing aid benefit in the NIDCD/VA clinical trial. *Ear and Hearing, 23*(4), 301-307.

Hollow, R.D., Dowell, R.C., Cowan, R.S.C., Skok, M.C., Pyman, B.C., and Clark, G.M. (1995). Continuing improvements in speech processing for adult cochlear implant patients. *Annals of Otology, Rhinology, and Laryngology, 166*(Suppl.), 292-294.

House, W. (1976). Cochlear implants. *Annals of Otology Rhinology and Laryngology, 85*(Suppl 27), 1.

House, W.F., and Hitselberger, W.E. (2001). Twenty-year report of the first auditory brain stem nucleus implant. *Annals of Otology, Rhinology, and Laryngology, 110,* 103.

Humes, L.E., Wilson, D.L., Barlow, N.N., and Garner, C. (2002). Changes in hearing aid benefit following 1 or 2 years of hearing-aid use by older adults. *Journal of Speech, Language, and Hearing Research, 45,* 772-782.

Jackler, R.K., Luxford, W.M., and House, W.F. (1987). Sound detection with the cochlear implant in five ears of four children with congenital malformations of the cochlea. *Laryngoscope, 97*(Suppl 40),15-17.

Jerger, J., Chmiel, R., Florin, E., Pirozzolo, F., and Wilson, N. (1996). Comparison of conventional amplification and an assistive listening device in elderly persons. *Ear and Hearing, 17*(6), 490-504.

Kobler, S., Rosenhall, U., and Hansson, H. (2001). Bilateral hearing aids-effects and consequences from a user perspective. *Scandinavian Audiology, 30*, 223-235.

Kochkin, S. (2001). The VA and direct mail sales spark growth in hearing aid market. *Hearing Review, 8*(12), 16-24, 63-65.

Kochkin, S. (2002). Factors impacting consumer choice of dispenser and hearing aid: Use of ALDs and computers. *Hearing Review, 9*(12), 14-23.

Kuk, F.K., Potts, L., Valente, M., Lee, L., and Picirrillo, J. (2003). Evidence of acclimatization in persons with severe-to-profound hearing loss. *Journal of the American Academy of Audiology, 14*(2), 84-99.

Larson, V.D., Williams, D.W., Henderson, W.G., Luethke, L.E., Beck, L.B., Noffsinger, D., Wilson, R.H., Dobie, R.A., Haskell, G.B., Bratt, G.W., Shanks, J.E., Stelmachowicz, P., Studebaker, G.A., Boysen, A.E., Donahue, A., Canalis, R., Fausti, S.A., and Rappaport, B.Z. (2000). Efficacy of 3 commonly used hearing aid circuits: A crossover trial. *Journal of the American Medical Association, 284*(14), 1806-1813.

Leake, P.A., Hradek, G.T., and Snyder, R.L. (1999). Chronic electrical stimulation by a cochlear implant promotes survival of spiral ganglion neurons in neonatally deafened cats. *Journal of Comparative Neurology, 412*(4), 543-562.

Loizou, P.C., Stickney, G., Mishra, L., and Assman, P. (2003). Comparison of speech processing strategies used in the Clarion implant processor. *Ear and Hearing, 24*(1), 12-19.

Loovis, C.F., Schall, D.G., and Teter, D.L. (1997). The role of assistive devices in the rehabilitation of hearing impairment. *Otolaryngologic Clinics of North America, 30*(5), 803-847.

Michelson R. (1971). Electrical stimulation of the human cochlea: A preliminary report. *Archives of Otolaryngology—Head and Neck Surgery, 9*, 317.

Miyamoto, R.T., Robbins, A.J., Myres, W.A., and Pope, M.L. (1986). Cochlear implantation in the Mondini inner ear malformation. *American Journal of Otolaryngology, 4*, 258-261.

Moore, B. (2000). Use of a loudness model for hearing aid fitting IV. Fitting hearing aids with multi-channel compression so as to restore "normal" loudness for speech at different levels. *British Journal of Audiology, 34*(3), 165-177.

Mueller, H.G., Hawkins, D.B., and Northern, J.L. (1992). *Probe microphone measurements: Hearing aid selection and assessment.* San Diego, CA: Singular.

Noble, W. (1998). *Self-assessment of hearing and related functions.* London, England: Whurr.

Otto, S.R., Brackmann, D.E., Hitselberger, W.E., Shannon, R.V., and Kuchta, J. (2002). Multi-channel auditory brainstem implant: Update on performance in 61 patients. *Journal of Neurosurgery, 96*(6), 1063-1071.

Rubinstein, J.T., and Miller, C.A. (1999). How do cochlear prostheses work? *Current Opinion in Neurobiology, 9*, 399-404.

Rubinstein, J.T., Parkinson, W.S., Tyler, R.S., and Gantz, B.J. (1999). Residual speech recognition and cochlear implant performance: Effects of implantation criteria. *American Journal of Otology, 20*(4), 445-452.

Shanks, J.E., Wilson, R.H., Larson, V., and Williams, D. (2002). Speech recognition performance of patients with sensorineural hearing loss under aided and unaided conditions using linear and compression hearing aids. *Ear and Hearing, 23*(4), 280-290.

Shipp, D., Nedzelski, J., Chen, J., and Hanusaik, L. (1997). Prognostic indicators of speech recognition performance in postlingually deafened adult cochlear implant users. In I. Honjo and H. Takahashi (Eds.), *Cochlear implant and related sciences update, Advances in otorhinolaryngology* (pp. 74-77). Basel, Switzerland: Karger.

Simmons, B.F (1965). Auditory nerve: Electrical stimulation in man. *Science, 148*, 104-106.

Simmons, B.F. (1966). Electrical stimulation in the auditory nerve in man, *Archives of Oto-laryngology-Head and Neck Surgery, 84,* 2-54.

Skinner, M.W., Holden, L.K., Whitford, L.A., Plant, K.L., Psarros, C., and Holden, T.A. (2002). Speech recognition with the Nucleus 24 SPEAK, ACE, and CIS speech coding strategies in newly implanted adults. *Ear and Hearing, 23*(3), 207-223.

Souza, P.E., Yueh, B., Sarubbi, M., and Loovis, C.F. (2000). Fitting hearing aids with the Articulation Index: Impact on hearing aid effectiveness. *Journal of Rehabilitation Research and Development, 37*(4), 473-481.

Tyler, R.S., Fryauf-Bertchy, H., Gantz, B.J., Kelsay, D.M., and Woodworth, G.G. (1997). Speech perception in prelingually implanted children after four years. *Advances in Otorhinolaryngology, 52,* 187-192.

van Hoesel, R.J.M., and Tyler, R.S. (2003). Speech perception, localization, and lateralization with bilateral cochlear implants. *Journal of the Acoustical Society of America, 113*(3), 1617-1630.

Walden, B.E., Surr, R.K., Cord, M.T., Edwards, B., and Olsen, L. (2000). Comparison of benefits provided by different hearing aid technologies. *Journal of the American Academy of Audiology, 11*(10), 540-560.

Wheeler-Scruggs, K. (2002). Assessing the employment and independence of people who are deaf and low functioning. *American Annals of the Deaf, 147*(4), 11-17.

Wilson, B.S., Lawson, D.T., Finley, C.C., and Wolford, R.D. (1991). Coding strategies for multichannel cochlear prostheses. *American Journal of Otology, 12,* 56-61.

Wilson, B.S., Lawson, D.T., Finley, C.C., and Wolford, R.D. (1993). Importance of patient and processor variables in determining outcomes with cochlear implants. *Journal of Speech and Hearing Research, 36,* 373-379.

Yueh, B., Souza, P., McDowell, J., Collins, M., Loovis, C., Hedrick, S., Ramsey, S., and Deyo, R. (2001). Randomized trial of amplification strategies. *Archives of Otolaryngology-Head and Neck Surgery, 127*(10), 1197-1204.

Zwolan, T.A. (2000). Selection criteria and evaluation. In S. Waltzman and N. Cohen (Eds.), *Cochlear implants* (pp. 63-73). New York: Theime.

Zwolan, T.A., Kileny, P.R., and Telian, S.A. (1996). Self-report of cochlear implant use and satisfaction by prelingually deafened adults. *Ear and Hearing, 17,* 198-210.

CHAPTER 6

American Medical Association. (2001). *Guides to the evaluation of permanent impairment* (5th ed.). Chicago, IL: American Medical Association.

Andrews, J.F., Leigh, I.W., and Weiner, M. (2004). *Deaf people: Evolving perspectives in psychology, sociology, and education.* Boston: Allyn and Bacon.

Bain, L., Scott, S., and Steinberg, A. (2004). Socialization experiences and coping strategies of adults raised using spoken language. *Journal of Deaf Studies and Deaf Education, 9,* 120-128.

Baldwin, W. (2000). Information no one else knows: The value of self-report. In A.A. Stone, J.S. Turkkan, C.A. Bachrach, J.B. Jobe, H.S. Kurtzman, and V.S. Cain (Eds.), *The science of self-report* (pp. 3-7). Mahwah, NJ: Erlbaum.

Barnartt, S., Seelman, K., and Gracer, B. (1990). Policy issues in communication accessibility. *Journal of Disability Studies Policy, 1*(2), 47-63.

Bentler, R.A., and Kramer, S.E. (2000). Guidelines for choosing a self-report outcome measure. *Ear and Hearing, 21*(Suppl), 37S-49S.

Bess, F.H. (2000). The role of generic health-related quality of life measures in establishing audiological rehabilitation outcomes. *Ear and Hearing, 21*(4 Suppl), 74S-79S.

Bess, F. H., Lichtenstein, M. J., Logan, S. A., Burger, M. C., and Nelson, E. (1989). Hearing impairment as a determinant of function in the elderly. *Journal of the American Geriatrics Society, 37*(2), 123-128.

Blamey, P. (2003). Development of spoken language by deaf children. In M. Marschark, and P. Spencer (Eds.), *Oxford handbook of deaf studies, language, and education* (pp. 232-246). New York: Oxford.

Blanchfield, B.B., Feldman, J.J., Dunbar, J.L., and Gardner, E.N. (2001). The severely to profoundly hearing-impaired population in the United States: Prevalence estimates and demographics. *Journal of the American Academy of Audiology, 12*(4), 183-189.

Bowling, A. (1995). What things are important in people's lives? A survey of the public's judgements to inform scales of health related quality of life. *Social Science and Medicine, 41*(10), 1447-1462.

Bregner, M., Bobbitt, R.A., Carter, W.B., and Gilson, B.S. (1981). The sickness impact profile: Development and final revision of a health status measure. *The Journal of Medical Care, 19*, 787-805.

Buchanan, R. (1999). *Illusions of equality: Deaf Americans in school and factory 1850-1950.* Washington, DC: Gallaudet University Press.

Christiansen, J.B., and Leigh, I.W. (2002). *Cochlear implants in children: Ethics and choices.* Washington, DC: Gallaudet University Press.

Clarcq, J., and Walter, G. (1997-1998). Supplemental Security Income payments made to young adults who are deaf and hard of hearing. *Journal of the American Deafness and Rehabilitation Association, 31*, 1-9.

Cox, R.M. (1999a). Measuring hearing aid outcomes: Part 1. *Journal of the American Academy of Audiology, 10.*

Cox, R.M. (1999b). Measuring hearing aid outcomes: Part 2. *Journal of the American Academy of Audiology, 10.*

Dalton, D.S., Cruickshanks, K.J., Klein, B.E.K., Klein, R., Wiley, T.L., and Nondahl, D.M. (2003). The impact of hearing loss on quality of life in older adults. *The Gerontologist, 43*, 661-668.

Demorest, M.E., and DeHaven, G.P. (1993). Psychometric adequacy of self-assessment scales. *Seminars in Hearing, 14*, 314-325.

Demorest, M.E., and Erdman, S.A. (1989). Factor structure of the communication profile for the hearing impaired. *Journal of Speech and Hearing Disorders, 54*, 541-549.

Demorest, M.E., and Walden, B.E. (1984). Psychometric principles in the selection, interpretation, and evaluation of communication self-assessment inventories. *Journal of Speech and Hearing Disorders, 49*(3), 226-240.

Dillon, H., Birtles, G., and Lovegrove, R. (1999). Measuring the outcomes of a national rehabilitation program: Normative data for the Client Oriented Scale of Improvement (COSI) and the Hearing Aid User's Questionnaire (HAUQ). *Journal of the American Academy of Audiology, 10*, 67-79.

Dobie, R.A. (1996). Compensation for hearing loss. *Audiology, 35*(1), 1-7.

Dobie, R.A., and Sakai, C.S. (2001). Estimation of hearing loss severity from the audiogram. In D. Henderson, D. Prasher, R. Kopke, R. Salvi, and R. Hamernik (Eds.), *Noise induced hearing loss basic mechanisms, prevention and control* (pp. 351-363). London, England: Noise Research Network Publications.

Dorman, M. (1998). An overview of cochlear implants. In B. Tucker (Ed.), *Cochlear implants: A handbook* (pp. 5-28). Jefferson, NC: McFarland and Company.

Dowler, D.L., and Walls, R.T. (1996). Accommodating specific job functions for people with hearing impairments. *Journal of Rehabilitation, 62*, 35-43.

Ebrahim, S. (1995). Clinical and public health perspectives and applications of health-related quality of life measurement. *Social Science and Medicine, 41*(10), 1383-1394.

Erdman, S.A., and Demorest, M.E. (1998). Adjustment to hearing impairment II: Audiological and demographic correlates. *Journal of Speech, Language, and Hearing Research, 41*(1), 123-136.

The EuroQol Group. (1990). EuroQol—A new facility for the measurement of health-related quality of life. *Health Policy, 16*(3), 199-208.

Flanagan, J.C. (1978). A research approach to improving our quality of life. *American Psychologist, 33,* 138-147.

Gatehouse, S. (1999). Glasgow hearing aid benefit profile: Derivation and validation of a client-centered outcome measure for hearing aid services. *Journal of the American Academy Audiology, 10,* 80-103.

Glass, L.E., and Elliott, H.H. (1993). Workplace success for persons with adult-onset hearing impairment. *Volta Review, 95,* 403-415.

Hallberg, L.R., and Barrenas, M.L. (1995). Coping with noise-induced hearing loss: Experiences from the perspective of middle-aged male victims. *British Journal of Audiology, 29*(4), 219-230.

Hetu, R. (1994). Mismatches between auditory demands and capacities in the industrial work environment. *Audiology, 33,* 1-14.

Hetu, R., Getty, L., and Waridel, S. (1994). Attitudes towards co-workers affected by occupational hearing loss II: Focus group interviews. *British Journal of Audiology, 28,* 313-325.

Hetu, R., Riverin, L., Getty, L., Lalande, N.M., and St-Cyr, C. (1990). The reluctance to acknowledge hearing difficulties among hearing-impaired workers. *British Journal of Audiology, 24*(4), 265-276.

Hetu, R., Riverin, L., Lalande, N., Getty, L., and St-Cyr, C. (1988). Qualitative analysis of the handicap associated with occupational hearing loss. *British Journal of Audiology, 22*(4), 251-264.

High, W.S., Fairbanks, G., and Glorig, A. (1964). Scale for self-assessment of hearing handicap. *Journal of Speech and Hearing Disorders, 29,* 215-230.

Humes, L.E. (1999). Dimensions of hearing aid outcome. *Journal of the American Academy of Audiology, 10*(1), 26-39.

Hyde, M.L. (2000). Reasonable psychometric standards for self-report outcome measures in audiological rehabilitation. *Ear and Hearing, 21*(4 Suppl), 24S-36S.

Knutson, J.F., Murray, K.T., Husarek, S., Westerhouse, K., Woodworth, G., Gantz, B.J., and Tyler, R.S. (1998). Psychological change over 54 months of cochlear implant use. *Ear and Hearing, 19*(3), 191-201.

Kochkin, S. (2001). The VA and direct mail sales spar growth in hearing aid market. *Hearing Review, 8*(12), 16-24, 63-65.

Lane, H.L., Hoffmeister, R., and Bahan, B.J. (1996). *A journey into the deaf-world.* San Diego, CA: DawnSignPress.

Laroche, C., Garcia, L.J., and Barrette, J. (2000). Perceptions by persons with hearing impairment, audiologists, and employers of the obstacles to work integration. *Journal of the Academy of Rehabilitative Audiology, 23,* 63-90.

Laroche, C., Soli, S., Giguere, C., Lagace, J., Vaillancourd, V., and Fortin, M. (2003). An approach to the development of hearing standards for hearing-critical jobs. *Noise and Health, 6*(21), 17-37.

Linn, M.W., and Linn, B.S. (1984). Self-evaluation of life function (self) scale: A short, comprehensive self-report of health for elderly adults. *Journal of Gerontology, 39*(5), 603-612.

Meadow-Orlans, K.P. (1985). Social and psychological effects of hearing loss in adulthood: A literature review. In H. Orlans (Ed.), *Adjustment to adult hearing loss* (pp. 35-57). San Diego, CA: College-Hill Press.

Middlebrooks, J.C., and Green, D.M. (1991). Sound localization by human listeners. *Annual Review of Psychology, 42*, 135-159.

Mital, A. (1994). Issues and concerns in accommodating the elderly in the workplace. *Journal of Occupational Rehabilitation, 4*, 253-268.

National Association of the Deaf. (2000). *Legal rights: The guide for deaf and hard of hearing people* (5th ed.). Washington, DC: Gallaudet University Press.

National Research Council and the Institute of Medicine. (2004). *Health and safety needs of older workers.* Committee on the Health and Safety Needs of Older Workers. D.H. Wegman and J.P. McGee (Eds.). Washington, DC: The National Academies Press.

Nelson, E.C., Wasson, J.H., Johnson, D., and Hays, R. (1996). Dartmouth COOP functional health assessment charts: Brief measures for clinical practice. In B. Spiker (Ed.), *Quality of life and pharmacoeconomics in clinical trials* (2nd ed.). Philadelphia: Lippincott-Raven.

Nilsson, M., Soli, S.D., and Sullivan, J.A. (1994). Development of the Hearing in Noise Test for the measurement of speech reception thresholds in quiet and in noise. *Journal of the Acoustical Society of America, 95*(2), 1085-1099.

Noble, W. (1998). *Self-assessment of hearing and related functions.* London, England: Whurr.

Noble, W.G., and Atherley, G.R.C. (1970). The hearing measure scale: A questionnaire for the assessment of auditory disability. *Journal of Auditory Research, 10*, 229-250.

Padden, C. (1980). The deaf community and the culture of deaf people. In C. Baker and R. Battison (Eds.), *Sign language and the deaf community* (pp. 89-103). Silver Spring, MD: National Association of the Deaf.

Padden, C., and Humphries, T. (1988). *Deaf in America: Voices from a culture.* Cambridge, MA: Harvard University Press.

Palmore, E., and Luikart, C. (1972). Health and social factors related to life satisfaction. *Journal of Health and Social Behavior, 13*(1), 68-80.

Phillippe, T., and Auvenshine, D. (1985). Career development among deaf persons. *Journal of Rehabilitation of the Deaf, 19*, 9-17.

Pollard, R. (1994). Public mental health service and diagnostic trends regarding individuals who are deaf or hard of hearing. *Journal of Rehabilitation Psychology, 39*, 147-160.

Rogerson, R.J. (1995). Environmental and health-related quality of life: Conceptual and methodological similarities. *Social Science and Medicine, 41*(10), 1373-1382.

Rosen, J.K. (1979). Psychological and social aspects of the evaluation of acquired hearing impairment. *Audiology, 18*(3), 238-252.

Ross, M. (1994). *Communication access for persons with hearing loss.* Baltimore, MD: York Press.

Schein, S., Bottum, E.B., Lawler, J.T., Madory, R., and Wantuch, E. (2001). Psychological challenges encountered by hearing impaired adults and their families. *Rehabilitation Psychology, 46*, 322-323.

Scherich, D., and Mowry, R.L. (1997). Accommodations in the workplace for people who are hard of hearing: Perceptions of employees. *Journal of the American Deafness and Rehabilitation Association, 31*, 31-43.

Schroedel, J.G., and Geyer, P.D. (2000). Long-term career attainments of deaf and hard of hearing college graduates: Results from a 15-year follow-up survey. *American Annals of the Deaf, 145*(4), 303-314.

Shontz, F.C. (1971). Physical disability and personality. In W.S. Neff (Ed.), *Rehabilitation psychology* (pp. 33-73). Washington, DC: American Psychological Association.

Stika, F.C. (1997). Living with hearing loss-focus group results; Part II: Career development and vocational experiences. *Hearing Loss, 18*(6), 29-32.

Thomas, A. (1984). *Acquired hearing loss: Psychological and psychosocial implications.* London: Academic Press.

Thomas, A.J. (1988). Rehabilitation of adults with acquired hearing loss: The psychological dimension. *British Journal of Audiology, 22*(2), 81-83.

Ware, J.E.Jr, and Sherbourne, C.D. (1992). The MOS 36-item short-form health survey (SF-36). I. Conceptual framework and item selection. *Medical Care, 30*(6), 473-483.

Welsh, W.A. (1993). Factors influencing career mobility of deaf adults. *Volta Review, 95,* 329-339.

World Health Organization. (1980). *International classification of impairments, disabilities and handicaps: A manual of classification relating to the consequences of disease.* Geneva: World Health Organization.

World Health Organization. (1993). Study protocol for the World Health Organization project to develop a Quality of Life assessment instrument (WHOQOL). *Quality of Life Research, 2*(2), 153-159.

CHAPTER 7

Abberton, E., and Fourcin, A.J. (1975). Visual feedback and the acquisition of intonation. In E.H. Lenneberg and E. Lennenberg (Eds.), *Foundations of language development* (pp. 157-165). New York: Academic Press.

Acoustical Society of America. (2000). *Classroom acoustics: A resource for creating learning environments with desirable listening conditions.* Melville, NY: Acoustical Society of America.

Adelman, C., Levi, H., Linder, N., and Sohmer, H. (1990). Neonatal auditory brain-stem response threshold and latency: 1 hour to 5 months. *Electroencephalography and Clinical Neurophysiology, 77*(1), 77-80.

Allen, M.C., Nikolopoulos, T.P., and O'Donoghue, G.M. (1998). Speech intelligibility in children after cochlear implantation. *American Journal of Otology, 19,* 742-746.

American Academy of Audiology. (2003). *Pediatric amplification protocol.* Available: http://www.audiology.org/professional/positions/pedamp.pdf. [Accessed June 2004.]

American Academy of Pediatrics. (1999). *Pediatricians make new recommendations on hearing screening.* Chicago, IL: American Academy of Pediatrics.

American Academy of Pediatrics. (2000). Year 2000 position statement: Principles and guidelines for early hearing detection. *Pediatrics, 106*(4), 798-817.

American Academy of Pediatrics Task Force on Newborn and Infant Hearing. (1999). Newborn and infant hearing loss: Detection and intervention (RE9846). *Pediatrics, 103,* 527-530.

American National Standards Institute. (1969). ANSI S3.5-1969. *Method for the calculation of the articulation index.* New York: American National Standards Institute.

American Speech-Language Hearing Association. (2004). *Cochlear implants.* (Supplement 24). New York: American Speech-Language Hearing Association.

Anderson, K. (1989). *Screening instrument for targeting educational risk (SIFTER).* Austin, TX: Pro-Ed.

Anderson, K., and Matkin, N. (1996). *Screening Instrument for targeting educational risk in preschool children (age 3-kindergarten) (Preschool S.I.F.T.E.R.).* Tampa, FL: Educational Audiology Association.

Angelocci, A.A., Kopp, G.A., and Holbrook, A. (1964). The vowel formats of deaf and normal-hearing eleven to fourteen-year-old boys. *Journal of Speech and Hearing Disorders, 29*(2), 156-170.

Bangs, T.E. (1968). *Language and learning disorders of the pre-academic child.* Englewood Cliffs, NJ: Prentice-Hall.

Bat-Chava, Y., and Deignan, E. (2001). Peer relationships of children with cochlear implants. *Journal of Deaf Studies and Deaf Education, 6*(2), 186-199.

Bench, J., and Bamford, J. (1979). *Speech-hearing tests and the spoken language of hearing-impaired children.* London, England: Academic Press.

Bench, J., Bamford, J., Wilson, I., and Clift, L. (1979). A comparison of the VKV sentence lists for children with other speech audiometry tests. *Australian Journal of Audiology, 1*, 61-66.

Bess, F.H., Tharpe, A.M., and Gibler, A.M. (1986). Auditory performance of children with unilateral sensorineural hearing loss. *Ear and Hearing, 7*(1), 20-26.

Bess, F.H., Dodd-Murphy, J., and Parker, R.A. (1998). Children with minimal sensorineural hearing loss: Prevalence, educational performance, and functional status. *Ear and Hearing, 19*(5), 339-354.

Binnie, C.A., Daniloff, R.G., and Buckingham, H.W., Jr. (1982). Phonetic disintegration in a five-year-old following sudden hearing loss. *Journal of Speech and Hearing Disorders, 47*(2), 181-189.

Boothroyd, A., and Boothroyd-Turner, D. (2002). Postimplantation audition and educational attainment in children with prelingually acquired profound deafness. *Annals of Otology, Rhinology, and Laryngology, 189*, 79-84.

Boothroyd, A., and Iglehart, F. (1998). Experiments with classroom FM amplification. *Ear and Hearing, 19*(3), 202-217.

Boyd, R.C., Knutson, J.F., and Dahlstrom, A.J. (2000). Social interaction of pediatric cochlear implant recipients with age-matched peers. *Annals of Otology, Rhinology, and Laryngology, 185*, 105-109.

Brackett, D., and Zara, C.V. (1998). Communication outcomes related to early implantation. *American Journal of Otology, 19*, 453-459.

Brannon, J., and Murray, T. (1966). The spoken syntax of normal, hard of hearing, and deaf children. *Journal of Speech and Hearing Research, 9*, 604-610.

Briscoe, J., Bishop, D.V., and Norbury, C.F. (2001). Phonological processing, language, and literacy: A comparison of children with mild-to-moderate sensorineural hearing loss and those with specific language impairment. *Journal of Child Psychology and Psychiatry, 42*(3), 329-340.

Bunch, G., and Clarke, B. (1978). The deaf child's learning of English morphology. *Audiology and Hearing Education, 4*, 12-24.

Calvert, D.R. (1962). Speech sound duration and the surd-sonant error. *Volta Review, 64*, 401-402.

Carhart, R. (1965). Considerations in the measurement of speech discrimination. *Aeromedical Review, 3*, 1-22.

Carney, A.E., and Moeller, M.P. (1998). Treatment efficacy: Hearing loss in children. *Journal of Speech, Language, and Hearing Research, 41*(1), S61-S84.

Christiansen, J.B., and Leigh, I.W. (2002). *Cochlear implants in children: Ethics and choices.* Washington, DC: Gallaudet University Press.

Cohen, N.L., Waltzman, S.B., Roland, T.Jr., Staller, S.J., and Hoffman, R.A. (1999). Early results using the Nucleus CI24M in children. *American Journal of Otology, 20*, 198-204.

Cooper, R. (1967). The ability of deaf and hearing children to apply morphological rules. *Journal of Speech and Hearing, 10*, 77-86.

Cornelisse, L.E., Seewald, R.C., and Jamison, D.G. (1995). The input/output formula: A theoretical approach to the fitting of personal amplification devices. *Journal of the Acoustical Society of America, 97*(3), 1854-1864.

Cowan, R.S.C., DelDot, J., Barker, E.J., Sarant, J.Z., Pegg, P., Dettman, S., Galvin, K.L., Rance, G., Hollow, R., Dowell, R.C., Pyman, B., Gibson, W. P.R., and Clark, G.M. (1997). Speech perception results for children with implants with different levels of preoperative residual hearing. *American Journal of Otology, 18*, 125-126.

Cox, R.M., and Alexander, G.C. (1995). The Abbreviated Profile of Hearing Aid Benefit. *Ear and Hearing, 16*, 176-186.

Crandell, C.C. (1993). Speech recognition in noise by children with minimal degrees of sensorneural hearing loss. *Ear and Hearing, 14*(3), 210-216.

Davis, H. (1965). The young deaf child: Identification and management. *Acta Otolaryngologica,* (Suppl 206), 1-258.

Davis, J. (1974). Performance of young hearing-impaired children on a test of basic concepts. *Journal of Speech and Hearing Research, 17,* 342-352.

Davis, J.M., Elfenbein, J., Schum, R., and Bentler, R.A. (1986). Effects of mild and moderate hearing impairments on language, educational, and psychosocial behavior of children. *Journal of Speech and Hearing Disorders, 51*(1), 53-62.

Dawson, P.W., Nott, P.E., Clark, G.M., and Cowan, R.S. (1998). A modification of play audiometry to assess speech discrimination ability in severe-profoundly deaf 2- to 4-year-old children. *Ear and Hearing, 19*(5), 371-384.

de Quiros, J.B. (1980). Influence of hearing disorders on language development. *Folia Phoniatrica (Basel), 32*(2), 103-118.

Dillon, H., Birtles, G., and Lovegrove, R. (1999). Measuring the outcomes of a national rehabilitation program: Normative data for the Client Oriented Scale of Improvement (COSI) and the Hearing Aid User's Questionnaire (HAUQ). *Journal of the American Academy of Audiology, 10,* 67-79.

Dunn, L., and Dunn, L. (1997). *Peabody picture vocabulary test-III.* Circle Pines, MN: American Guidance Service.

Eisenberg, L.S., and Dirks, D.D. (1995). Reliability and sensitivity of paired comparisons and category rating in children. *Journal of Speech and Hearing Research, 38*(5), 1157-1167.

Elfenbein, J.L., Hardin-Jones, M.A., and Davis, J.M. (1994). Oral communication skills of children who are hard of hearing. *Journal of Speech and Hearing Research, 37*(1), 216-226.

Elliott, L.L., and Katz, D. (1980). *Development of a new children's test of speech discrimination.* (Technical manual). St. Louis, MO: Auditec.

English, K., and Church, G. (1999). Unilateral hearing loss in children: An update for the 1990's. *Language Speech and Hearing Services in School, 30,* 26-31.

Fryauf-Bertschy, H., Tyler, R.S., Kelsay, D.M., and Gantz, B.J. (1992). Performance over time of congenitally deaf and postlingually deafened children using a mulitchannel cochlear implant. *Journal of Speech and Hearing Research, 35,* 913-920.

Fryauf-Bertschy, H., Tyler, R.S., Kelsay, D.M.R., Gantz, B.J., and Woodworth, G.G. (1997). Cochlear implant use by prelingually deafened children: The influences of age at implant use and length of device use. *Journal of Speech and Hearing Research, 40,* 183-199.

Gallaudet Research Institute. (2002). *Regional and national summary report of data from the 2000-2001 annual survey of deaf and hard of hearing children and youth.* Washington, DC: GRI, Gallaudet University.

Gantz, B.J., Tyler, R.S., Woodworth, G.G., Tye-Murray, N., and Fryauf-Bertschy, H. (1994). Results of multichannel cochlear implants in congenital and acquired prelingual deafness in children: Five-year follow up. *American Journal of Otology, 15*(2), 1-7.

Geers, A.E. (2003). Predictors of reading skill development in children with early cochlear implantation. *Ear and Hearing, 24,* 59S-68S.

Geers, A.E., and Brenner, C. (2003). Background and educational characteristics of prelingually deaf children implanted by five years of age. *Ear and Hearing, 24*(1 Suppl), 2S-14S.

Geers, A.E., and Moog, J. (1994). Description of the CID study. *Volta Review, 96,* 1-14.

Geers, A.E., Brenner, C., and Davidson, L. (2003a). Factors associated with development of speech perception skills in children implanted by age five. *Ear and Hearing, 24*(1 Suppl), 24S-35S.

Geers, A.E., Nicholas, J.G., and Sedey, A.L. (2003b). Language skills of children with early cochlear implantation. *Ear and Hearing, 24*(1 Suppl), 46S-58S.

Gilbertson, M., and Kamhi, A.G. (1995). Novel word learning in children with hearing impairment. *Journal of Speech and Hearing Research, 38*(3), 630-642.

Gravel, J.S., and Hood, L.J. (1999). Pediatric audiology assessment. In F.E. Musiek and W.F. Rintelmann (Eds.), *Contemporary perspectives in hearing assessment* (pp. 305-326). Needham Heights, MA: Allyn and Bacon.

Gravel, J.S., Fausel, N., Liskow, C., and Chobot, J. (1999). Children's speech recognition in noise using omni-directional and dual-microphone hearing aid technology. *Ear and Hearing, 20* (1), 1-11.

Harrison, M., and Roush, J. (1996). Age of suspicion, identification, and intervention for infants and young children with hearing loss: A national study. *Ear and Hearing, 17*(1), 55-62.

Haskins, H. (1949). *A phonetically balanced test of speech discrimination for children.* Evanston, IL: Northwestern University.

Hawkins, D.B. (1984). Comparisons of speech recognition in noise by mildly-to-moderately hearing-impaired children using hearing aids and FM systems. *Journal of Speech and Hearing Disorders, 49*(4), 409-418.

Hodges, A.V., Ash, M.D., Balkany, T.J., Scholffman, J.J., and Butts, S.L. (1999). Speech perception results in children with cochlear implants: Contributing factors. *Otolaryngology-Head and Neck Surgery, 121*, 31-34.

Holden-Pitt, L., and Diaz, J.A. (1998). Thirty years of the annual survey of deaf and hard of hearing children and youth: A glance over the decades. *American Annals of the Deaf, 143*(72-76).

Hood, R.B., and Dixon, R.F. (1969). Physical characteristics of speech rhythm of deaf and normal-hearing speakers. *Journal of Communication Disorders, 2*, 20-28.

Hudgins, C.V., and Numbers, F.C. (1942). An investigation of the intelligibility of the speech of the deaf. *Genetic Psychology Monographs, 25*, 289-392.

Hyde, M., Zevenbergen, R., and Power, D. (2003). Deaf and hard of hearing students' performance on arithmetic word problems. *American Annals of the Deaf, 148*(1), 56-64.

Illg, A., Lesinski-Schiedat, A., von der Haar-Heise, S., Battmer, R.D., Glodring, J.E., and Lenarz, T. (1999). Speech perception results for children implanted with the Clarion cochlear implant at the Medical University of Hannover. *Annals of Otology, Rhinology and Laryngology, 108*, 93-98.

Itoh, M., Horii, Y., Daniloff, R.C., and Binnie, C.A. (1982). Selected aerodynamic characteristics of deaf individuals during various speech and nonspeech tasks. *Folia Phoniatrica, 34*(4), 191-209.

Jensema, C.J., Karchmer, M.A., and Trybus, R.J. (1978). *The rated speech intelligibility of hearing-impaired children: Basic relationships and a detailed analysis.* (Ser. R, No. 6) Office of Demographic Studies. Washington, DC: Gallaudet College.

Jerger, S. (1983). Speech audiometry. In J. Jerger (Ed.), *Recent advances series in speech, hearing, and language. Pediatric audiology* (pp. 71-93). San Diego: College Hill Press.

Jerger, S., and Jerger, J. (1984). *The Pediatric Speech Intelligibility Test (PSI).* St. Louis, MO: Auditec.

Jerger, S., Jerger, J., and Abrams, S. (1983). Speech audiometry in the young child. *Ear and Hearing, 4*(1), 56-66.

Jerger, S., Lai, L., and Marchman, V.A. (2002). Picture naming by children with hearing loss: I. Effect of semantically related auditory distracters. *Journal of the American Academy of Audiology, 13*(9), 463-477.

Jerger, S., Lewis, S., Hawkins, J., and Jerger, J. (1980). Pediatric Speech Intelligibility Test. I. Generation of test materials. *International Journal of Pediatric Otorhinolaryngology, 2*(3), 217-230.

John, J.E.J., and Howarth, J.N. (1965). The effect of time distortions on the intelligibility of deaf children's speech. *Language and Speech, 8*(2), 127-134.

Johnson, C.E. (2000). Children's phoneme identification in reverberation and noise. *Journal of Speech, Language, and Hearing Research, 43*(1), 144-157.

Karchmer, M.A., and Mitchell, R.E. (2003). Demographic and achievement characteristics of deaf and hard-of-hearing students. In M. Marschark (Ed.), *Oxford handbook of deaf studies, language, and education* (pp 21-37). London, England: Oxford University Press.

Kenworthy, O.T., Klee, T., and Tharpe, A.M. (1990). Speech recognition ability of children with unilateral sensorineural hearing loss as a function of amplification, speech stimuli and listening condition. *Ear and Hearing, 11*(4), 264-270.

Kirk, K.I. (1999). Lexical Neighborhood Test: Test-retest reliability and interlist equivalency. *Journal of the American Academy of Audiology, 10*, 113-123.

Kirk, K.I. (2000). Challenges in the clinical investigation of cochlear implant outcomes. In J.K. Niparko, K.I. Kirk, N.K. Mellon, A.M. Robbins, D.L. Tucci, and B.S. Wilson (Eds.), *Cochlear implants: Principles and practices* (pp. 225-259). Philadelphia: Lippincott Williams and Wilkins.

Kirk, K.I., Eisenberg, L.S., Martinez, A.S., and Hay-McCutcheon, M. (1999). Lexical Neighborhood Test: Test-retest reliability and interlist equivalency. *Journal of the American Academy of Audiology, 10*, 113-123.

Kirk, K.I., Pisoni, D.B., and Osberger, M.J. (1995). Lexical effects on spoken word recognition by pediatric cochlear implant users. *Ear and Hearing, 16*, 470-481.

Kirk, K.I., Sehgal, S.T., and Hay-McCutcheon, M. (2000). Comparison of children's familiarity with tokens on the PBK, LNT, and MLNT. *Annals of Otology, Rhinology, and Laryngology, 109*(12), 63-64.

Klee, T.M., and Davis-Dansky, E. (1986). A comparison of unilaterally hearing-impaired children and normal-hearing children on a battery of standardized language tests. *Ear and Hearing, 7*(1), 27-37.

Klein, A.J. (1984). Frequency and age-dependent auditory evoked potential thresholds in infants. *Hearing Research, 16*(3), 291-297.

Kluwin, T.N., and Stewart, D.A. (2000). Cochlear implants for younger children: A preliminary description of the parental decision process and outcomes. *American Annals of the Deaf, 145*(1), 26-32.

Knecht, H.A., Nelson, P.B., Whitelaw, G.M., and Feth, L.L. (2002). Background noise levels and reverberation times in unoccupied classrooms: Predictions and measurements. *American Journal of Audiology, 11*(2), 65-71.

Kopun, J., and Stelmachowicz, P.G. (1998). The perceived communication difficulties of children with hearing loss. *American Journal of Audiology, 7*, 30-38.

Kosky, C., and Boothroyd, A.J. (2003). Validation of an on-line implementation of the imitative test of speech pattern contrast perception (IMSPAC). *Journal of the American Academy of Audiology, 14*(2), 72-83.

Kuk, F.K., Kollofski, C., Brown, S., Melum, A., and Rosenthal, A. (1999). Use of a digital hearing aid with directional microphones in school-aged children. *Journal of the American Academy of Audiology, 10*(10), 535-548.

Lachs, L., Pisoni, D.B., and Kirk, K.I. (2001). Use of audiovisual information in speech perception by prelingually deaf children with cochlear implants: A first report. *Ear and Hearing, 22*(3), 236-251.

Lee, D.J., Gomez-Marin, O., and Lee, H.M. (1998). Prevalence of unilateral hearing loss in children: The National Health and Nutrition Examination Survey II and the Hispanic Health and Nutrition Examination Survey. *Ear and Hearing, 19*(4), 329-332.

Lenarz, T., Illg, A., Lesinki-Schiedat, A., Bertram, B., von der Haar-Heise, S., and Battmer, R.D. (1999). Cochlear implantation in children under the age of two: The MHH experience with the Clarion cochlear implant. *Annals of Otology, Rhinology and Laryngology, 108*, 44-49.

Levitt, H., and Stromberg, H. (1983). Segmental characteristics of the speech of hearing-impaired children: Factors affecting intelligibility. In I. Hochberg, H. Levitt, and M.J. Osberger (Eds.), *Speech of the hearing impaired: Research, training, and personnel preparation* (pp. 53-73). Baltimore, MD: University Park Press.

Ling, D. (1979). Principles underlying the development of speech communication skills among hearing-impaired children. *Volta Review, 81*, 211-223.

Litovsky, R.Y. (1997). Developmental changes in the precedence effect: Estimates of minimum audible angle. *Journal of the Acoustical Society of America, 102*(3), 1739-1745.

Luce, P.A., and Pisoni, D.B. (1998). Recognizing spoken words: The neighborhood activation model. *Ear and Hearing, 19*(1), 1-36.

Markides, A. (1970). The speech of deaf and partially-hearing children with special reference to factors affecting intelligibility. *British Journal of Disorders of Communication, 5*(2), 126-140.

Mauk, G., and Mauk, P. (1992). Somewhere out there: Preschool children with hearing impairment and learning disabilities. *Topics in Early Childhood Education, 12*, 174-195.

Mayne, A., Yoshinaga-Itano, C., and Sedey, A. (1998). Receptive vocabulary development of infants and toddlers who are deaf or hard of hearing. *Volta Review, 100*, 29-52.

McCracken, W. (1994). Deaf children with complex needs: A piece of the puzzle. *Journal of the British Association of Teachers of the Deaf, 18*, 54-60.

McFarland, D.J., and Cacace, A.T. (1995). Modality specificity as a criterion for diagnosing central auditory processing disorder. *American Journal of Audiology, 4*, 36-48.

McGarr, N.S., and Osberger, N.J. (1978). Pitch deviancy and intelligibility of deaf speech. *Journal of Communication Disorders, 11*(2-3), 237-247.

McIntosh, R.A., Sulzen, L., Reeder, K., and Kidd, D.H. (1994). Making science accessible to deaf students. The need for science literacy and conceptual teaching. *American Annals of the Deaf, 139*(5), 480-484.

Mendel, L.L., and Danhauer, J.L. (1997). *Audiologic evaluation and management and speech perception assessment*. San Diego, CA: Singular.

Menyuk, P. (1972). *The development of speech*. Indianapolis, IN: Bobbs-Merrill.

Meyer, T.A., Svirsky, M.A., Kirk, K.I., and Miyamoto, R.T. (1998). Improvements in speech perception by children with profound, prelingual hearing loss: Effects of device, communication mode and chronological age. *Ear and Hearing, 41*, 846-858.

Miyamoto, R.T., Osberger, M.J., Myers, W.A., Robbins, A.J., Kessler, K., Renshaw, J., and Pope, M.L. (1989). Comparison of sensory aids in deaf children. *Annals of Otology, Rhinology, and Laryngology, 98*(Suppl 8 Pt. 2), 2-7.

Miyamoto, R.T., Osberger, M.J., Robbins, A.M., Myers, W.A., and Kessler, K. (1993). Prelingually deafened children's performance with the Nucleus multichannel cochlear implant. *American Journal of Otolaryngology, 14*, 437-445.

Miyamoto, R.T., Osberger, M.J., Robbins, A.M., Myers, W.A., Kessler, K., and Pope, M.L. (1991). Comparison of speech perception abilities in deaf children with hearing aids or cochlear implants. *Otolaryngology-Head and Neck Surgery, 104*, 42-46.

Moeller, M.P. (1988). Combining formal and informal strategies for language assessment of hearing-impaired children. *Journal of the Academy of Rehabilitative Audiology, 21*, S73-S99.

Moeller, M.P. (2000). Early intervention and language development in children who are deaf and hard of hearing. *Pediatrics, 106*(3), 43.

Moeller, M.P., Coufal, K., and Hixson, P. (1990). The efficacy of speech-language pathology intervention: Hearing-impaired children. *Seminars in Speech and Language, 11*, 227-240.

Moeller, M.P., Donaghy, K.F., Beauchaine, K.L., Lewis, D.E., and Stelmachowicz, P.G. (1996). Longitudinal study of FM system use in nonacademic settings: Effects on language development. *Ear and Hearing, 17*(1), 28-41.

Moeller, M.P., Osberger, M.J., and Eccarius, M. (1986). Language and learning skills of hearing-impaired students. Receptive language skills. *ASHA Monographs,* (23), 41-53.

Monsen, R.B. (1974). Durational aspects of vowel production in the speech of deaf children. *Journal of Speech and Hearing Research, 17*(3), 386-398.

Monsen, R.B. (1976). The production of English stop consonants in the speech of deaf children. *Journal of Phonetics, 4,* 29-41.

Monsen, R.B. (1978). Toward measuring how well hearing-impaired children speak. *Journal of Speech and Hearing Research, 21*(2), 197-219.

Monsen, R.B. (1979). Acoustic qualities of phonation in young hearing-impaired children. *Journal of Speech and Hearing Research, 22*(2), 270-88.

Monsen, R.B. (1983a). General effects of deafness on phonation and articulation. In I. Hochberg, H. Levitt, and M. Osberger, (Eds.), *Speech of the hearing impaired. Research, training, and personnel preparation* (pp. 23-24). Baltimore, MD: University Park Press.

Monsen, R.B. (1983b). Voice quality and speech intelligibility among deaf children. *American Annals of the Deaf, 128*(1), 12-19.

Monsen, R.B., and Engebretson, A.M. (1977). Study of variations in the male and female glottal wave. *Journal of the Acoustical Society of America, 62*(4), 981-993.

Monsen, R.B., Engebretson, A.M., and Vemula, N.R. (1978). Indirect assessment of the contribution of subglottal air pressure and vocal-fold tension to changes of fundamental frequency in English. *Journal of the Acoustical Society of America, 64*(1), 65-80.

Monsen, R.B., Engebretson, A.M., and Vemula, N.R. (1979). Some effects of deafness on the generation of voice. *Journal of the Acoustical Society of America, 66*(6), 1680-1690.

Moodie, K., Seewald, R., and Sinclair, S. (1994). Procedure for predicting real-ear hearing aid performance in young children. *American Journal of Audiology, 3*(1), 23-31.

Moog, J.S., and Geers, A.E. (1990). *Early speech perception test for profoundly hearing-impaired children.* St. Louis, MO: Central Institute for the Deaf.

Moog, J.S., and Geers, A.E. (1999). Speech and language acquisition in young deaf children after cochlear implantation. *Otolaryngologic Clinics of North America, 32*(6), 1127-1141.

National Institutes of Health Consensus Statement. (1993). *Early identification of hearing impairment in infants and young children.* Vol. 11(1). Washington, DC: National Institutes of Health.

Nelson, P., Soli, S., and Seltz, A. (2002). *Classroom acoustics II: Acoustical barriers to learning.* Melville, NY: Acoustical Society of America.

Nickerson, R.B. (1975). Characteristics of the speech of deaf persons. *Volta Review, 77,* 342-362.

Nikolopoulos, T.P., O'Donoghue, G.M., and Archbold, S. (1998). Age at implantation: Its importance in pediatric cochlear implantation. *Laryngoscope, 109,* 595-599.

Nilsson, M.J., Soli, S.D., and Gelnett, D.J. (1996). *Development of the Hearing in Noise Test for Children (HINT-C).* Los Angeles: House Ear Institute.

Nober, E.H., and Nober, L.W. (1977). Effects of hearing loss on speech and language in the postbabbling stage. In B.F. Jaffe (Ed.), *Hearing loss in children* (pp. 630-639). Baltimore, MD: University Park Press.

O'Donoghue, G.M., Nikolopoulos, T.P., Archbold, S.M., and Tait, M. (1999). Speech perception in children after cochlear implantation. *American Journal of Otology, 19,* 762-767.

Osberger, M.J., Barker, M., Zimmerman-Phillips, S., and Geier, L. (1999). Clinical trials of the Clarion cochlear implant in children. *Annals of Otology, Rhinology, and Laryngology, 108,* 88.

Osberger, M.J., and Fisher, L.M. (1998). *Preoperative predictors of postoperative implant performance in children*. Presented at the 7th Symposium on Cochlear Implants in Children (June 4-7). Iowa City, Iowa.

Osberger, M.J., and Levitt, H. (1979). The effect of timing errors on the intelligibility of deaf children's speech. *Journal of the Acoustical Society of America, 66*(5), 1316-1324.

Osberger, M.J., Todd, S.L., Berry, S.W., Robbins, A.M., and Miyamoto, R.T. (1991). Effect of age at onset of deafness on children's speech perception abilities with a cochlear implant. *Annals of Otology, Rhinology, and Laryngology, 100*, 883-888.

Paul, P.V. (2003). Processes and components of reading. In M. Marschark (Ed.), *Oxford handbook of deaf studies, language, and education* (pp. 97-109). New York: Oxford University Press.

Pediatric Working Group. (1996). Amplification for infants and children with hearing loss. *American Journal of Audiology, 5*, 53-68.

Perez-Abalo, M.C., Savio, G., Torres, A., Martin, V., Rodriguez, E., and Galan, L. (2001). Steady state responses to multiple amplitude-modulated tones: An optimized method to test frequency-specific thresholds in hearing-impaired children and normal-hearing subjects. *Ear and Hearing, 22*(3), 200-211.

Pettersson, E. (1987). Speech discrimination tests with hearing aids in tele-coil listening mode. A comparative study in school children. *Scandinavian Audiology, 16*(1), 13-19.

Pittman, A.L., Lewis, D.E., Hoover, B.M., and Stemachowicz, P.G. (1999). Recognition performance for four combinations of FM system and hearing aid microphone signals in adverse listening conditions. *Ear and Hearing, 20*(4), 279-289.

Power, D.J., and Quigley, S.P. (1973). Deaf children's acquisition of the passive voice. *Journal of Speech and Hearing Research, 16*(1), 5-11.

Prizant, B.M., Audet, L.R., Burke, G.M., Hummel, L.J., Maher, S.R., and Theadore, G. (1990). Communication disorders and emotional/behavioral disorders in children and adolescents. *Journal of Speech and Hearing Disorders, 55*(2), 179-192.

Quigley, S.P., and Paul, P.V. (1984). *Language and deafness*. San Diego, CA: College-Hill Press.

Rhodes, M.C., Margolis, R.H., Hirsch, J.E., and Napp, A.P. (1999). Hearing screening in the newborn intensive care nursery: Comparison of methods. *Otolaryngology-Head and Neck Surgery, 120*(6), 799-808.

Rickards, F.W., Tan, L.E., Cohen, L.T., Wilson, O.J., Drew, J.H., and Clark, G.M. (1994). Auditory steady-state evoked potential in newborns. *British Journal of Audiology, 28*(6), 327-337.

Robbins, A.M., Renshaw, J., and Gerry, S. (1991). Evaluating meaningful auditory integration in profoundly hearing impaired children. *American Journal of Otology, 12*(Suppl), 144-150.

Robbins, A.M., Osberger, M.J., Miyamoto, R.T., and Kessler, K. (1995a). Language development in young children with cochlear implants. *Advances in Oto-Rhino-Laryngology 50*, 160-166.

Robbins, A.M., Renshaw, J.J., and Osberger, M.J. (1995b). *Common Phrases Test*. Indianapolis, IN: Indiana University School of Medicine.

Ross, M., and Lerman, J. (1970). A Picture Identification Test for Hearing-Impaired Children. *Journal of Speech and Hearing Research, 13*(1), 44-53.

Schmitt, N. (2000). *Vocabulary in language teaching*. Cambridge: Cambridge University Press.

Scollie, S.D., Seewald, R.C., Moodie, K.S., and Dekok, K. (2000). Preferred listening levels of children who use hearing aids: Comparison to prescriptive targets. *Journal of the American Academy of Audiology, 11*(4), 230-238.

Seyfried, D., and Kricos, P. (1996). Language and speech of the deaf and hard of hearing. In R. Schow and M. Nerbonne (Eds.), *Introduction to audiologic rehabilitation* (3rd ed.). Boston: Allyn Bacon.

Sikora, D.M., and Plapinger, D.S. (1994). Using standardized psychometric tests to identify learning disabilities in students with sensorineural hearing impairments. *Journal of Learning Disabilities, 27*(6), 352-359.

Silverman, S.R. (1983). Speech training then and now: A critical review. In I. Hochberg, H. Levitt, and M.J. Osberger (Eds.), *Speech of the hearing impaired: Research, training, and personnel preparation* (pp. 1-20). Baltimore, MD: University Park Press.

Sininger, Y.S. (2002). Auditory neuropathy in infants and children: Implications for early hearing detection and intervention programs. *Audiology Today,* (Special Issue–October), 16-23.

Sininger, Y.S., Abdala, C., and Cone-Wesson, B. (1997). Auditory threshold sensitivity of the human neonate as measured by the auditory brainstem response. *Hearing Research, 104*(1-2), 27-38.

Sininger, Y.S., Doyle, K.J., and Moore, J.K. (1999). The case for early identification of hearing loss in children. Auditory system development, experimental auditory deprivation, and development of speech perception and hearing. *Pediatric Clinics of North America, 46*(1), 1-14.

Smaldino, J., and Anderson, K. (1997). *Development of the listening inventory for education.* Presented at the second biannual hearing aid research and development conference. Bethesda, MD.

Smith, C.R. (1975). Residual hearing and speech production in deaf children. *Journal of Speech and Hearing Research, 18,* 795-811.

Soli, S.D., and Sullivan, J.A. (1997). Factors affecting children's speech communication in classrooms. *Journal of the Acoustical Society of America, 101,* S3070.

Spencer, L.J., Barker, B.A., and Tomblin, J.B. (2003). Exploring the language and literacy outcomes of pediatric cochlear implant users. *Ear and Hearing, 24*(3), 236-247.

Staller, S.J., Beiter, A.L., Brimacombe, J., Meckelenburg, D.J., and Arndt, P.L. (1991). Pediatric performance with the Nucleus 22-channel cochlear implant system. *American Journal of Otology, 12*(Suppl), 126-136.

Stapells, D.R. (2002). The tone-evoked ABR. *The Hearing Journal, 55*(11), 14-22.

Stapells, D.R., Picton, T.W., Durieux-Smith, A., Edwards, C.G., and Moran, L.M. (1990). Thresholds for short-latency auditory-evoked potentials to tones in notched noise in normal-hearing and hearing-impaired subjects. *Audiology, 29*(5), 262-274.

Stark, R.E. (1983). Phonatory development in young normally hearing and hearing-impaired children. In I. Hochberg, H. Levitt, and M.J. Osberger (Eds.), *Speech of the hearing-impaired: Research, training, and personal perception* (pp. 251-266). Baltimore, MD: University Park Press.

Starr, A., Amlie, R.N., Martin, W.H., and Sanders, S. (1977). Development of auditory function in newborn infants revealed by auditory brainstem potentials. *Pediatrics, 60*(6), 831-839.

Stelmachowicz, P.G. (1999). Hearing aid outcome measures for children. *Journal of the American Academy of Audiology, 10,* 14-25.

Stelmachowicz, P.G., Lewis, D., Kalberer, A., and Cruetz, T. (1994). *Situational hearing aid response profile (SHARP). Version 2.0 users manual.* Omaha, NE: Boys Town National Research Hospital.

Stelmachowicz, P.G., Pittman, A.L., Hoover, B.M., and Lewis, D.E. (2002). Aided perception of /s/ and /z/ by hearing-impaired children. *Ear and Hearing, 23*(4), 316-324.

Stern, A. (2001) *Deafness and reading* Available: http://www.literacytrust.org.uk/Pubs/stern.htm. [Accessed June 2004].

Stredler-Brown, A., and Johnson, C.D. (2001) *Functional auditory performance indicators: An integrated approach to auditory development.* Available: http://www.cde.state.co.us/cdesped/download/pdf/FAPI_3-1-04g.pdf. [Accessed August 2004.]

Subtelny, J. (1983). Patterns of performance in speech perception and production. In I. Hochberg, H. Levitt and M. Osberger (Eds.), *Speech of the hearing impaired. Research, training, and personnel preparation* (pp. 215-230). Baltimore, MD: University Park Press.

Svirsky, M.A. (2000). Speech intelligibility of pediatric cochlear implant users and hearing aid users. In S.B. Waltzman and N.L. Cohen (Eds.), *Cochlear implants* (pp. 312-314). New York: Thieme.

Svirsky, M.A., and Meyer, T.A. (1999). Comparison of speech perception in pediatric Clarion cochlear implant and hearing aid users. *Annals of Otology, Rhinology, and Laryngology, 108*, 104-109.

Svirsky, M.A., Robbins, A.M., Kirk, K.I., Pisoni, D.B., and Miyamoto, R.T. (2000). Language development in profoundly deaf children with cochlear implants. *Psychological Science, 11*, 153-158.

Templin, M.C. (1957). *Certain language skills in children, their development and interrelationships*. Minneapolis: University of Minnesota Press.

Templin, M.C. (1966). *A study of cognitive development and performance in children with normal and defective hearing*. Minneapolis: University of Minnesota, Minneapolis Institute of Child Development.

Tharpe, A.M., Fino-Szumski, M.S., and Bess, F.H. (2001). Survey of hearing aid fitting practices for children with multiple impairments. *American Journal of Audiology, 10*(1), 32-40.

Tobey, E., Geers, A., and Brenner, C. (1994). Speech production results: Speech feature acquisition. *Volta Review, 96*, 109-130.

Tobey, E.A., Geers, A.E., Brenner, C., Altuna, D., and Gabbert, G. (2003). Factors associated with development of speech production skills in children implanted by age five. *Ear and Hearing, 24*(1 Suppl), 36S-45S.

Tomblin, J.B., Spencer, L., Flock, S., Tyler, R., and Gantz, B. (1999). A comparison of language achievement in children with cochlear implants and children using hearing aids. *Journal of Speech, Language, and Hearing Research, 42*, 496-511.

Tomblin, J.B., Spencer, L.J., and Gantz, B.J. (2000). Language and reading acquisition in children with and without cochlear implants. *Advances in Otorhinolaryngology, 57*, 300-304.

Traxler, C.B. (2000). The Stanford Achievement Test, 9th edition: National norming and performance standards for deaf and hard-of-hearing students. *Journal of Deaf Studies and Deaf Education, 5*(4), 337-348.

Tyler, R.S. (1993). Cochlear implants and the deaf culture. *American Journal of Audiology, 2*(1), 26-32.

Tyler, R.S., Fryauf-Bertchy, H., Gantz, B.J., Kelsay, D.M., and Woodworth, G.G. (1997). Speech perception in prelingually implanted children after four years. *Advances in Otorhinolaryngology, 52*, 187-192.

Tyler, R.S., Rubinstein, J.T., Teagle, H., Kelsay, D., and Gantz, B.J. (2000). Prelingually deaf children can perform as well as postlingually deaf adults using cochlear implants. *Cochlear Implants International, 1*(1), 39-44.

Waltzman, S., and Cohen, N.L. (1998). Cochlear implantation in children younger than 2 years old. *American Journal of Otology, 19*, 158-162.

Waltzman, S., Cohen, N.L., Gomolin, R., Green, J., Shapiro, W., Brackett, D., and Zara, C. (1997). Perception and production results in children implanted between two and five years of age. In I. Honjo and H. Takahashi (Eds.), *Cochlear implant and related sciences update: Advances in otorhinolaryngology* (vol. 52, pp. 125-128). Basel, Switzerland: Karger.

Waltzman, S., Cohen, N.L., and Shapiro, W. (1995). Effects of cochlear implantation on the young deaf child. In A.S. Uziel and M. Mondain (Eds.), *Cochlear implants in children: Advances in otorhinoloaryngology* (vol. 50, pp. 125-128). Basel, Switzerland: Karger.

Whitehead, R.L. (1983). Some respiratory and aerodynamic patterns in the speech of the hearing-impaired. In I. Hochberg, H. Levitt, and M.J. Osberger (Eds.), *Speech of the hearing impaired: Research, training, and personnel preparation* (pp. 97-116). Baltimore, MD: University Park Press.

Widen, J.E., and O'Grady, G. (2002). Using visual reinforcement audiometry in the assessment of hearing in infants. *The Hearing Journal 55*, 28-36.

Wirz, S.L., Subtelny, J.D., and Whitehead, R.L. (1981). Perceptual and spectrographic study of tense voice in normal hearing and deaf subjects. *Folia Phoniatrica (Basel), 33*(1), 23-36.

Wolgemuth, K., Kamhi, A., and Lee, R. (1998). Metaphor performance in children with hearing impairment. *Language, Speech, and Hearing Services in Schools, 29*, 216-231.

Yoshinaga-Itano, C. (1994). Language assessment of infants and toddlers with significant hearing loss. *Seminars in Hearing, 15*, 128-147.

Yoshinaga-Itano, C., and Apuzzo, M.L. (1998a). Identification of hearing loss after age 18 months is not early enough. *American Annals of the Deaf, 143*(5), 380-387.

Yoshinaga-Itano, C., and Apuzzo, M.L. (1998b). The development of deaf and hard of hearing children identified early through the high-risk registry. *American Annals of the Deaf, 143*(5), 416-424.

Yoshinaga-Itano, C., Sedey, A.L., Coulter, D.K., and Mehl, A.L. (1998). Language of early- and later-identified children with hearing loss. *Pediatrics, 102*(5), 1161-1171.

Young, N.M., Carrasco, V.N., Grohne, K.M., and Brown, C. (1999). Speech perception of young children using Nucleus 22-channel or Clarion cochlear implants. *Annals of Otology, Rhinology, and Laryngology, 108*, 99-103.

Zimmerman, G.N., and Rettaliata, P. (1981). Articulatory patterns of an adventitiously deaf speaker: Implications for the role of auditory information in speech production. *Journal of Speech and Hearing Research, 24*, 169-178.

Zimmerman-Phillips, S., Robbins, A.M., and Osberger, M.J. (2000). Assessing cochlear implant benefit in very young children. *Annals of Otology, Rhinology, and Laryngology Supplement, 185*, 42-43.

Zwolan, T.A., Zimmerman-Phillips, S., Ashbaugh, C.J., Hieber, S.J., Kileny, P.R., and Teliam, S.A. (1997). Cochlear implantation of children with minimal open-set speech recognition. *Ear and Hearing, 18*, 240-251.

Appendix A

Definitions and Technical Terms

This appendix consists of two glossaries. The first is a list of Social Security terms relevant to disability. The source is http://www.socialsecurity.gov/glossary.htm. The glossary is provided so that the reader can understand exactly how the Social Security Administration defines and uses each term.

The second glossary is a list of technical terms related to the science of hearing. The sources include glossaries from web sites maintained by the National Institute on Deafness and Other Communication Disorders, FreeHearingTest.com, and the Hope for Hearing Foundation. Some definitions have been adapted by the committee to specifically address terms as they are used in this report.

SOCIAL SECURITY TERMS

Term	Explanation
Appeal (Appeal Rights)	Whenever Social Security makes a decision that affects your eligibility for Social Security or Supplemental Security Income (SSI) benefits, we send you a letter explaining our decision. If you disagree with our decision, you have the right to appeal it (ask us to review your case). If our decision was wrong, we'll change it.

Application for Benefits To receive Social Security or Black Lung benefits, Supplemental Security Income payments, or Medicare, you must complete and sign an application. You can apply for retirement benefits and spouse's benefits online at http://www.socialsecurity.gov/applytoretire, in person, or by telephone at 1-800-772-1213. Our TTY number is 1-800-325-0778. Many other services now are available through the Internet at http://www.socialsecurity.gov/

For more information see *How To* on our home page or go to http://www.ssa.gov/howto.htm.

Base Years A worker's (wage earner) base years for computing Social Security benefits are the years after 1950 up to the year of entitlement to retirement or disability insurance benefits. For a survivor's claim, the base years include the year of the worker's death.

Benefits Social Security provides five major categories of benefits:

- Retirement,
- Disability,
- Family (dependents),
- Survivors, and
- Medicare.

The retirement, family (dependents), survivor, and disability programs provide monthly cash benefits and Medicare provides medical coverage.

Child We use the term "child" to include your biological child or any other child who can inherit your personal property under state law or who meets certain specific requirements under the Social Security Act; such as:

- A legally adopted child,
- An equitably adopted child,

- A stepchild, or
- A grandchild.

See *Benefits* for additional information.

Credits (Social Security Credits)

Previously called *"Quarters of Coverage."* As you work and pay taxes, you earn credits that count toward your eligibility for future Social Security benefits. You can earn a maximum of four credits each year. Most people need 40 credits to qualify for benefits. Younger people need fewer credits to qualify for disability or survivors' benefits. For more information see *How You Earn Credits* (05-10072).

Decision Notice (Award Letter or Denial Letter)

When you file for Social Security, we decide if you will receive benefits. We send you an official letter explaining our decision and, if benefits are payable, we tell you the amount you will get each month.

Disability Benefits

You can get disability benefits if you:

- Are under full retirement age,
- Have enough Social Security credits, and
- Have a severe medical impairment (physical or mental) that's expected to prevent you from doing "substantial" work for a year or more, or have a condition that is expected to result in death.

Earnings Record (Lifetime Record of Earnings)

A chronological history of the amount you earn each year during your working life time. The credits you earned remain on your Social Security record even when you change jobs or have no earnings.

Evidence (Proofs)

"Proofs." The documents you must submit to support a factor of entitlement or payment amount. The people in your Social Security office can explain what evidence is required to establish entitlement and help you to get it. For more information see our *How To* page.

**Family Benefits
(Dependent Benefits)**

When you're eligible for retirement or disability benefits, the following people may receive benefits on your record:

• Spouse if he or she is at least 62 years old (or any age but caring for an entitled child under age 16),
• Children if they are unmarried and under age 18, under age 19 and a full-time elementary or secondary student,
• Children age 18 or older but disabled,
• Divorced ex-spouse.

**Health Insurance
(Medicare)**

The federal health insurance program is for:

• People 65 years of age or older,
• Certain younger people with disabilities, and
• People with permanent kidney failure with dialysis or a transplant, sometimes called ESRD (End-Stage Renal Disease).
For more information see *Medicare* or the *Official U.S. Government Site for Medicare Information.*

Insured Status

If you earned enough Social Security credits to meet the eligibility requirement for retirement or disability benefits or enable your dependents to establish eligibility for benefits due to your retirement, disability, or death, you have insured status. For more information see *How You Earn Credits* (05-10072).

Medicaid

A joint federal and state program that helps with medical costs for people with low incomes and limited resources. Medicaid programs vary from state to state, but most health care costs are covered if you qualify for both Medicare and Medicaid. For more information see the *Official U.S. Government Site for Medicare and Medicaid Information.*

Medical Listings (Listing of Impairments)

The Listing of Impairments describes, for each major body system, impairments that are considered severe enough to prevent a person from doing any gainful activity (or in the case of children under age 18 applying for SSI, cause marked and severe functional limitations). Most of the listed impairments are permanent or expected to result in death, or a specific statement of duration is made. For all others, the evidence must show that the impairment has lasted or is expected to last for a continuous period of at least 12 months. The criteria in the Listing of Impairments are applicable to evaluation of claims for disability benefits or payments under both the Social Security Disability Insurance and SSI programs.

Medicare

A nationwide, federally administered health insurance program that covers the cost of hospitalization, medical care, and some related services for most people over age 65, people receiving Social Security Disability Insurance benefits for 2 years, and people with end-stage renal disease. Medicare consists of two separate but coordinated programs—Part A (Hospital Insurance) and Part B (Supplementary Medical Insurance). See *Health Insurance*. For more information see *Medicare* and the *Official U.S. Government Site for Medicare Information*.

OASDI (Old Age Survivors and Disability Insurance)

The Social Security programs that provide monthly cash benefits to you and your dependents when you retire, to your surviving dependents, and to disabled worker beneficiaries and their dependents.

For more information see *Evidence* or *Evidence Required to Establish Right to Benefits*.

QC (Quarter of Coverage)

Social Security "credits." As you work and pay taxes, you earn credits that count toward eligibility for future Social Security benefits. You can earn a maximum of four credits each year. Most people need 40 credits to qualify for benefits. Younger people need fewer credits to qualify for disability or for their spouse or children to qualify for survivors' benefits. During their working lifetime most workers earn more credits than needed to be eligible for Social Security. These extra credits do not increase eventual Social Security benefits. However, the income earned may increase the benefit amount. For more information see *How You Earn Credits* (05-10072) and *Credits, Social Security*.

Social Security

Social Security is based on a simple concept: While you work, you pay taxes into the Social Security system, and when you retire or become disabled, you, your spouse, and your dependent children receive monthly benefits that are based on your reported earnings. Also, your survivors can collect benefits if you die. For more information see *A Snapshot* (05-10006).

Spouse

You are the spouse of the worker if, when he or she applied for benefits:

• You and the worker were validly married or
• You would have the status of a husband or a wife for that person's personal property if they had no will or
• You went through a marriage ceremony in good faith, which would have been valid except for a legal impediment.

Supplemental Security Income (SSI)

A federal supplemental income program funded by general tax revenues (*not* Social Security taxes). It helps aged, blind, and disabled people who have little or no income by providing monthly cash payments to meet basic needs for food, clothing, and shelter.

Wage Earner

A person who earns Social Security credits while working for wages or self-employment income. Sometimes referred to as the "Number Holder" or "Worker."

Widow

You are the widow/widower of the insured person if, at the time the insured person died:

- You and the insured person were validly married or
- You would have the status of a husband or a wife for that person's personal property if they had no will or
- You went through a marriage ceremony in good faith that would have been valid except for a legal impediment.

The minimum age for

- Disabled widows benefits is age 50.
- Retirement for widows is age 60.

GLOSSARY OF TECHNICAL TERMS RELATED TO HEARING

Term	Explanation
Acoustic Immittance	A series of tests, including tympanometry and acoustic reflex measures, that assess the transfer of acoustic energy through the middle ear system. These measures provide information about the integrity of the middle ear system and the structures comprising the acoustic reflex pathway.
Acoustic Nerve	The eighth cranial nerve, the nerve concerned with hearing and balance; also called the **Vestibulocochlear Nerve**.
Acoustic Neurinoma or Neuroma	Tumor, usually benign, which may develop on the hearing and balance nerves and can cause gradual hearing loss, tinnitus, and/or dizziness (sometimes called vestibular schwannoma). Also see **Neurofibromatosis Type 2**.
Acoustic Trauma	The term for damage to hearing due to a single exposure to extremely loud noise. (cf.See **Noise-Induced Hearing Loss**).
Acquired Deafness	Loss of hearing that occurs or develops some time during the lifespan but is not present at birth.
Air Conduction	The term for the transmission of sound through the outer ear, the bones of the middle ear, and into the inner ear.
Air-Bone Gap	The difference between the pure-tone thresholds assessed by air conduction (reflects the sensitivity of the entire peripheral auditory system) and bone conduction (reflects the sensitivity of the sensorineural system only).
Alerting Device	See **Visual Alarm Signal.**

Alport Syndrome   Hereditary condition characterized by kidney disease, sensorineural hearing loss, and sometimes eye defects.

American Sign Language (ASL)   Manual language with its own syntax and grammar, used in the United States primarily by people who are deaf.

Americans with Disabilities Act   The Americans with Disabilities Act (ADA), passed in 1990, which defines certain rights and requires certain accommodations for people with disabilities. The ADA definitions of a person with a disability are "(1) An individual with a physical or mental impairment that substantially limits one or more major life activities; (2) An individual with a record of a substantially limiting impairment; (3) An individual who is perceived to have such an impairment."

Amplified Phone   Phone equipped with volume control in the handset. Public coin-operated phones have a volume control button on the wall unit.

Amplitude (Sound)   The magnitude of a sound wave, associated with the loudness of a perceived sound.

Assistive Listening Device (ALD)   A variety of electronic devices to assist hard-of-hearing people, with or without a hearing aid. Includes group and personal FM amplification systems, inductive loop amplification systems, infrared amplification systems, telephone amplifiers, etc.

Audio Loop (Induction Loop)   System that uses electromagnetic waves for transmission of sound. The sound from an amplifier is fed into a wire loop surrounding the seating area (or worn on the listener's neck), which broadcasts to a telecoil that serves as a receiver. Hearing aids without a T-switch to activate a telecoil can use a special induction receiver to pick up the sound.

Audiogram   The diagrammatic representation of hearing
                                as the result of an audiological examination.
                                An audiogram shows pure-tone thresholds
                                by air and bone conduction for each ear. It is
                                usually part of a report including results of
                                other tests, such as immitance testing and
                                speech recognition testing.

Audiologist   A health care professional who is trained to
                                evaluate hearing loss and related disorders,
                                including balance (vestibular) disorders and
                                tinnitus, and to rehabilitate individuals with
                                hearing loss and related disorders. An audi-
                                ologist uses a variety of tests and procedures
                                to assess hearing and balance function and to
                                fit and dispense hearing aids and other
                                assistive devices for hearing.

Audiometry   The measurement of hearing function.

Auditory Brainstem   A test for hearing in infants, young children,
Response (ABR) Test   and others who cannot cooperate for behav-
                                ioral testing, and for ear and brainstem
                                function in all patients. ABR involves attach-
                                ing electrodes to the head to record electrical
                                activity from the hearing nerve and other
                                parts of the brain.

Auditory Evoked   Electrical potential (voltage) changes usually
Potentials   measured on the scalp that occur when
                                sound stimuli activate the sensory cells of the
                                auditory system and then the hearing centers
                                of the brain. Some of these potentials can be
                                used to diagnose hearing loss.

Auditory Nerve   Former name for the eighth cranial nerve,
                                now called the **Vestibulocochlear Nerve**,
                                that connects the inner ear to the brainstem
                                and is responsible for hearing and balance.

Auditory Neuropathy   A condition involving hearing loss, often
                                unstable, thought to be associated with
                                damage to the eighth cranial nerve.

Auditory Perception   Ability to identify, interpret, and attach
                              meaning to sound.

Auditory Prosthesis   Device that aids or enhances the ability to
                              hear.

Auditory Steady-   The auditory steady-state response (ASSR),
State Response   previously known as the steady-state evoked
                              potential (SSEP), is a way of objectively
                              assessing frequency-specific responses.
                              ASSR uses pure-tone (carrier) stimuli that are
                              amplitude modulated with another tone at
                              an appropriate modulation frequency. When
                              the neural activity shows a preference for the
                              modulation frequency over other frequencies
                              in the analysis, it is assumed that the audi-
                              tory system is responding to the carrier
                              frequency.

Aural Rehabilitation   Techniques used with people who have
                              hearing loss to improve their ability to re-
                              ceive spoken communication.

Auricle   Outer flap of the ear. Also called the **Pinna**.

Autoimmune Deafness   Condition in which an individual's immune
                              system produces abnormal antibodies or
                              cellular responses that attack the body's
                              healthy tissues and cause hearing loss.

Azimuth   Direction from the listener in the horizontal
                              plane; expressed as angular degrees on a
                              circle whereby 0° is directly in front of the
                              listener, and 180° is directly behind him or
                              her.

Basilar Membrane   Thin sheet of tissue in the scala media that
                              vibrates in response to movements in the
                              liquid that fills the cochlea.

Bone Conduction   The term for the transmission of sound
                              perceived through bones of the skull and
                              lower jaw.

Bony Labyrinth   The cavity in the skull that encloses the
                              Membranous Labyrinth.

Brainstem Implant   Auditory prosthesis that bypasses the co-
                              chlea and auditory nerve. This type of im-
                              plant helps individuals who cannot benefit
                              from a cochlear implant because the auditory
                              nerves are not working.

Brainstem Testing   Test that measures hearing sensitivity with-
                              out requiring responses from very young
                              patients or persons who are unable to coop-
                              erate with behavioral tests. See **Auditory
                              Brainstem Response.**

Captioning   Text display of spoken words, presented on a
                              television or a movie screen, that allows a
                              deaf or hard-of-hearing viewer to follow the
                              dialogue and the action of a program simul-
                              taneously.

Central Auditory   Inability to differentiate, recognize, or under-
Processing Disorder   stand sounds due to abnormal brain function
                              despite normal inner ear and eighth nerve
                              function.

Cerumen   See **Ear Wax.**

Cholesteatoma   Accumulation of dead skin cells in the
                              middle ear, caused by repeated middle ear
                              infections or negative pressure in the middle
                              ear. May be congenital.

Closed Captions (CC)   Text display of spoken dialogue and sounds
                              on TV and videos, visible only to those using
                              a caption decoder or TV built-in decoder chip.

Closed-Set Speech   Speech recognition test in which the possible
Recognition   stimulus items (words, syllables, etc.) are
                              limited to a set of items known to the lis-
                              tener, e.g., when a list of several possible
                              words is given and the listener indicates
                              which he or she heard.

Cochlea	Snail-shaped structure in the inner ear that contains the organ of hearing.
Cochlear Implant	A surgically implanted electronic device that bypasses damaged structures in the inner ear and directly stimulates the auditory nerve, allowing some deaf individuals to learn to hear and interpret sounds and speech.
Conductive Hearing Loss	Hearing loss caused by a problem of the outer or middle ear, resulting in the inability of sound to be conducted to the inner ear.
Congenital Hearing Loss	Hearing loss that is present from birth and may or may not be hereditary.
Cued Speech	Method of communication that combines the mouth movements of speech with visual cues (hand shapes distinguish consonants, hand locations near the mouth distinguish vowels) to help deaf or hard-of-hearing individuals differentiate words that look similar on the lips (e.g., bunch vs. punch) or are hidden from view (e.g., gag).
Cycles Per Second	Measurement of frequency, or a sound's pitch. See **Hertz**.
Cytomegalovirus (Congenital)	One group of herpes viruses that infects humans and can cause a variety of clinical symptoms, including deafness or hearing impairment; infection with the virus may be either before or after birth, but only prenatal infection causes hearing loss.
Deaf	A term (with a capital D) used by some people who have little or no useful residual hearing to identify themselves as members of Deaf Culture. Most Deaf people use sign language to communicate.
deaf	A term (with a lower-case d) used in this report to describe people who have little or

no useful residual hearing (i.e., severe or profound hearing loss), whether or not they identify themselves as Deaf.

Decibel (dB)   Unit used to express the intensity of a sound wave in logarithmic ratios to the base of 10. A 20-dB change is equivalent to a 100-fold change in acoustic intensity (energy flow per unit time per unit area) or a 10-fold change in sound pressure level.

Ear Canal   The short tube that conducts sound from the outer ear to the eardrum.

Ear Infection   Tissue-invasive growth of microorganisms, usually bacteria, viruses, or fungi, in the ear.

Ear Wax   Yellow secretion (**Cerumen**) from glands in the outer ear that keeps the skin of the ear dry and protected from infection.

Eardrum   The **Tympanic Membrane,** separating outer ear from middle ear. Vibrations of the air (sound) are transmitted by the eardrum to the bones of the middle ear.

Effusion   Fluid in the middle ear behind an intact tympanic membrane, usually seen in association with infection of the middle ear (**Otitis Media**).

Endolymph   Extracellular fluid inside the membranous labyrinth, including the balance organs (three semicircular canals, utricle, and saccule) and the cochlear duct or scala media of the cochlea. Endolymph is relatively high in potassium and low in sodium.

Eustachian Tube   Tube running from the nasal cavity to the middle ear, which opens during yawning and swallowing to allow air to flow to the middle ear. Helps keep middle ear pressure equal to ambient air pressure.

Exaggeration

A term used by the medical community to describe a patient's claim of impairment or distress that is out of proportion to the medical findings that can be objectively documented. The term is preferred to "malingering" or other words that imply intent to deceive on the part of the patient.

Floor Effect

A floor effect occurs in a study when the tests used are so difficult that both experimental and control (for example, normally hearing and hard-of-hearing) groups score very poorly on them, obscuring any difference between the groups that might be attributed to the effect of independent variables.

Frequency

The number of vibrations per second (usually expressed in Hertz) of a sound.

Hair Cells

Sensory cells of the inner ear, which are topped with hair-like structures, the stereocilia, and which aid in the transduction of the mechanical energy of sound waves into nerve impulses.

Haptic Sense

Sense of physical contact or touch.

Hard-of-Hearing

Describes people with any degree of hearing loss ranging from mild to profound. They can understand some speech sounds, with or without a hearing aid. Most people who identify themselves as hard-of-hearing use oral speech, although a small number learn sign language. Generally, they are committed to participating in society by using their residual hearing plus hearing aids, speech-reading, and assistive technology to aid communication.

Hearing

Sensory function in which sound waves in the air are converted to bioelectric signals, which are sent as nerve impulses to the brain, where they are interpreted.

Hearing Aid

Electronic device that brings amplified sound to the ear. A hearing aid usually consists of a microphone, an amplifier, and a receiver.

Hearing Disorder

Disruption in the normal hearing process that may occur in the outer, middle, or inner ear, whereby sound waves are not converted to electrical signals and nerve impulses are not transmitted to the brain to be interpreted.

Hearing Impaired

Generic term sometimes used to describe all persons with hearing loss. The term "people with hearing loss" is preferred.

Hereditary (or Genetic) Hearing Loss

Hearing loss passed down through generations of a family.

Hertz (Hz)

The unit used to express the frequency of a sound in cycles per second. One cycle per second equals 1 Hz.

Immitance Audiometry

Measurement of the function of the middle ear, used to diagnose conductive hearing loss.

Incus

One of three bones of the middle ear that help transmit sound waves from the outer ear to the cochlea.

Inner Ear

Part of the ear that contains both the organ of hearing (the cochlea, containing the organ of Corti) and the organ of balance (the labyrinth, containing the cristae and the maculae).

Interpreter, Sign Language

An interpreter who translates from voice to sign or from sign to voice (or both) in situations in which some people use spoken language and others sign.

Kilohertz (kHz)

Unit of frequency equal to 1000 Hz, or 1000 cycles per second.

Labyrinth

See **Bony Labyrinth** and **Membranous Labyrinth.**

Lesion	Any damage to an anatomical structure.
Lexical	Pertaining to words and their characteristics.
Malleus	One of three bones of the middle ear that help transmit sound waves from the outer ear to the cochlea.
Mastoid	The bone behind the ear canal, usually hollowed out by multiple air cells that communicate with the middle ear; part of the larger temporal bone.
Membranous Labyrinth	An interconnecting system of fluid-filled tubes inside the **Bony Labyrinth** that encloses the inner ear's organs of hearing and balance.
Ménière's Disease	Inner ear disorder that can affect both hearing and balance. It can cause episodes of vertigo, hearing loss, **Tinnitus**, and the sensation of fullness in the ear.
Meningitis	Inflammation of the meninges, the membranes that envelop the brain and the spinal cord; may cause hearing loss or deafness.
Middle Ear	The part of the ear that includes the eardrum and three tiny bones of the middle ear, ending at the oval and round windows that lead to the inner ear, and connected to the nasal cavity by the Eustachian tube.
Neural Prostheses	Devices, such as the cochlear implant, that substitute for an injured or diseased part of the nervous system.
Neurofibromatosis Type 1 (NF-1, von Recklinghausen's)	Group of inherited disorders in which noncancerous tumors grow on several nerves that may include the hearing nerve. The symptoms of NF-1 include coffee-colored spots on the skin, enlargement and deformation of bones, and neurofibromas.

Neurofibromatosis Type 2 (NF-2)
Group of inherited disorders in which non-cancerous tumors grow on several nerves that usually include the hearing nerve. The symptoms of NF-2 include tumors on the hearing nerve that can affect hearing and balance. NF-2 may occur in the teenage years with hearing loss. Also see **Acoustic Neurinoma**.

Noise-Induced Hearing Loss
Hearing loss caused by exposure to loud sounds, usually over an extended period of time, that damage the sensitive structures of the inner ear. See **Acoustic Trauma**.

Nonsyndromic Hereditary Hearing Impairment
Hearing loss or deafness that is inherited and is not associated with other inherited clinical characteristics.

Open-Set Speech Recognition
Understanding speech when the set of possible stimulus items (words, syllables, etc.) is not known or limited.

Organ of Corti
The organ, located in the cochlea, which contains the hair cells that transduce sound waves into neural impulses that travel through the auditory nerve to the brain.

Ossicles
Collective name for the three bones of the middle ear.

Otitis Media
The term describing an inflammation or infection of the middle ear.

Otoacoustic Emissions (OAEs)
Low-intensity sounds produced by the inner ear that can be quickly measured with a sensitive microphone placed in the ear canal. Otoacoustic emissions testing can be used as one of a battery of physiological tests to diagnose hearing disorders.

Otolaryngologist
Physician or surgeon who specializes in diseases of the ears, nose, throat, and head and neck.

Otologist Physician or surgeon who specializes in diseases of the ear.

Otosclerosis A disease affecting the middle ear in which the stapes is fixed to the oval window so that it cannot move easily, leading to a conductive hearing loss that can be corrected by surgery or a hearing aid. Sometimes the inner ear is also affected, with a resultant mixed hearing loss (conductive plus sensorineural).

Ototoxic Drugs Drugs such as aminoglycoside antibiotics and others that can damage the hearing and balance organs located in the inner ear in some individuals.

Outer Ear The external portion of the ear that collects sound waves and directs them into the ear. Consists of the pinna (auricle) and the ear canal and is separated from the middle ear by the ear drum.

Oval Window Opening in the bony wall of the cochlea to which is attached the footplate of the stapes bone; stapes vibration transmits sound into the cochlea.

Perception (Hearing) See **Auditory Perception**.

Perilymph Extracellular fluid between the bony and membranous labyrinths, filling the outer tubes (scala tympani and scala vestibuli) of the cochlea; also surrounds the semicircular canals, utricle, and saccule. Perilymph is relatively high in sodium and low in potassium.

Phoneme The smallest unit of speech sound that serves to distinguish one utterance from another in a language.

Pinna   The outer, visible part of the ear, also called
                                  the **Auricle**.

Postlingually Deafened   Term for an individual who becomes deaf
                                  after having acquired language (defined as
                                  after age 2 years in this report).

Prelingually Deafened   Term for an individual who is born deaf or
                                  who loses his or her hearing early in child-
                                  hood, before acquiring language (defined as
                                  before age 2 years in this report).

Presbycusis   The term describing hearing loss produced
                                  by degenerative changes of aging. Because
                                  there are so many causes of hearing loss, this
                                  label is tenable only when no other specific
                                  cause for older adult hearing loss can be
                                  found on careful otological evaluation.

Relay Service   Sometimes called dual-party telephone relay
                                  service. Enables text telephone users to
                                  communicate with a voice telephone user by
                                  use of a communications assistant who
                                  voices what the TTY user types to the voice
                                  phone user and types what the voice phone
                                  user says to the TTY user. The ADA man-
                                  dated a nationwide relay service by 1993.
                                  Also see **Text Telephone.**

Retrocochlear   Term describing a structure or lesion beyond
                                  the cochlea in the auditory pathway from ear
                                  to brain.

Root-Mean-Square   The root mean square (or RMS) is a statistical
or RMS   measure of the magnitude of a varying
                                  quantity. It can be calculated for a series of
                                  discrete values or for a continuously varying
                                  function. The name comes from the fact that
                                  it is the *square root* of the *mean* of the *squares*
                                  of the values.

Round Window   One of two membranes separating the
                                  middle ear and the inner ear.

Semantic
Pertaining to the meaning of words or other units of speech.

Sensorineural Hearing Loss
Hearing loss caused by damage to the sensory cells or nerve fibers (or both) of the inner ear.

Sign Language
Method of communication for people who are deaf or hard of hearing in which hand movements, gestures, and facial expressions convey grammatical structure and meaning. Also see **American Sign Language.**

Signal-to-Noise Ratio
A term that refers to the relative decibel levels of a signal and a noise. A signal-to-noise ratio of +10 dB means that the level of the signal is 10 dB higher than that of the noise, and a signal-to-noise ratio of −10 dB means that the level of the signal is 10 dB lower that that of the noise.

Sound Wave
Alternating low- and high-pressure areas moving through the air, which are interpreted as sound when collected in the ear.

Spectrum (Sound Spectrum)
The array of frequencies into which a complex sound can be analyzed. A sound spectrogram shows the relative intensities of the various frequencies as a function of time.

Speech Processor
Part of a cochlear implant that converts speech sounds into electrical impulses to stimulate the auditory nerve, allowing an individual to understand sound and speech.

Spondee
A two-syllable word with equal emphasis on both syllables; usually each syllable is a word in its own right (e.g., baseball, cowboy, railroad).

Stapes
One of three bones of the middle ear that help transmit sound waves from the outer ear to the cochlea.

Sudden Hearing Loss/Sudden Deafness	Loss of hearing that occurs quickly due to such causes as exposure to very intense noise, a viral infection, a rupture of one of the membranes connecting the middle ear to the inner ear, or the use of some drugs.
Syndromic Hearing Impairment	Hearing loss or deafness that, along with other characteristics, is inherited or passed down through generations of a family.
Syntactic	Pertaining to the grammatical features of speech, that is, how words and other semantic units are combined and arranged to communicate meaning.
Tactile Devices	Mechanical instruments that make use of touch to help individuals who have certain disabilities, such as deaf-blindness, to communicate.
Tectorial Membrane	Thin strip of membrane in the organ of Corti. It is in contact with sensory hairs, which are moved by sound vibrations, producing nerve impulses.
Text Telephone	Formerly TDD or TTY; a text telephone is a telecommunications device used by those who cannot understand speech on the phone. A typewriter-like unit shows the conversation on a screen so that it can be read. A text telephone must "talk" with another text telephone or a computer. Also see **Relay Service.**
Tinnitus	Sensation of a ringing, roaring, or buzzing sound in the ears or head that exists when no external sound stimulus is present. It is often associated with many forms of hearing impairment and noise exposure.
Tonotopic	Constructed so that specific frequencies are associated with corresponding neural places; the cochlea has a tonotopic organization.

Transducer	Any device that changes an input of one form of energy into an output of another, such as a microphone that changes the mechanical energy of sound waves into electrical energy.
T-Switch	A setting on a hearing aid that can be used with a hearing-aid-compatible telephone, assistive listening device, and audio loop system. When the hearing aid is switched to "T" it activates the induction telecoil (the technical name for the "T" switch), causing the hearing aid to pick up the magnetic field generated by the hearing-aid-compatible telephone, assistive device, or audio loop system being used.
TTY	See **Text Telephone.**
Tympanic Membrane or Tympanum	Membrane separating the outer ear from the middle ear; the ear drum.
Usher Syndrome	Hereditary disease that affects hearing and vision and sometimes balance.
Vestibular System	System in the body that is responsible for maintaining balance, posture, and the body's orientation in space. This system also regulates locomotion and other movements and keeps objects in visual focus as the head moves.
Vestibule	The part of the bony labyrinth that houses the utricle and saccule.
Vestibulocochlear Nerve	The eighth cranial nerve, formerly called the auditory nerve, that connects the inner ear to the brainstem and is responsible for hearing and balance.
Vibrotactile Aids	Mechanical instruments that help individuals who are deaf to detect and interpret sound through the sense of touch.

Visual Alarm Signal   A visual signal (flashing light) alerting a
                             person about a sound, such as a doorbell, fire
                             alarm, ringing telephone. Some systems
                             monitor a single event; others can monitor
                             several events and indicate which event has
                             occurred.

Waardenburg Syndrome   Hereditary disorder that is characterized by
                             hearing impairment, a white shock of hair
                             and/or distinctive blue color to one or both
                             eyes, and wide-set inner corners of the eyes.
                             Balance problems are also associated with
                             some types of Waardenburg syndrome.

Wavelength   Distance between the peaks of successive
                             sound waves.

White Noise   A complex sound made up of sounds of all
                             frequencies, used to mask other sounds.

Appendix B

American National Standards
on Acoustics

The content of each of ten standards of the American National Standards Institute (ANSI) pertaining to bioacoustics (S3) and referenced in this report is briefly described here. The standards can be obtained from the Acoustical Society of America (ASA), Standards Secretariat, 35 Pinelawn Rd., Suite 114E, Melville, NY 11747, or https://asastore.aip.org/ (under S3 Bioacoustics).

ANSI S3.1-1999 (R2003) *American National Standard Maximum Permissible Ambient Noise Levels for Audiometric Test Rooms.* This Standard specifies maximum permissible ambient noise levels (MPANLs) allowed in an audiometric test room that produce negligible masking (less than or equal to 2 dB) of test signals presented at reference equivalent threshold levels specified in American National Standard S3.6-1996 American National Standard Specification of Audiometers. The MPANLs are specified from 125 to 8000 Hz in octave and one-third octave band intervals for two audiometric testing conditions (ears covered and ears not covered) and for three test frequency ranges (125 to 8000 Hz, 250 to 8000 Hz, and 500 to 8000 Hz). The Standard is intended for use by all persons testing hearing and for distributors, installers, designers, and manufacturers of audiometric testrooms. This standard is a revision of ANSI S3.1-1991 American National Standard Maximum Permissible Ambient Noise Levels for Audiometric Test Rooms

ANSI S3.4-1980 (R2003) *American National Standard Procedure for the*

Computation of Loudness of Noise. This standard specifies a procedure for calculating the loudness of certain classes of noise. In applications of the procedure, it is assumed that the spectrum of the sound has been measured in terms of sound pressure levels in 1/3-octave or 1/1-octave bands in either a diffuse or free field. The procedure is derived from three empirical relations: (1) A set of equal-loudness contours for bands of noise in a diffuse sound field. (2) A rule relating the total loudness of a sound to the loudness indexes of the frequency bands composing it. (3) A loudness function relating loudness in sones to loudness level in phons. This relation is such that loudness is a simple power function of sound pressure at 1000 Hz. On the basis of these empirical relations, the total loudness of a sound may be calculated with the aid of a table or a chart, together with a linear equation. (An appendix provides a computer program in the FORTRAN language for calculations based on 1/3-octave band sound pressure levels.) Loudness as herein computed, depends upon the acoustic properties of a sound that impinges upon a normal-hearing listener. Loudness is also a prime determinant of a person's affective response to sound. The affective response may be expressed in terms such as noisiness, annoyance, and unacceptability. An appendix describes the extent to which the procedure of this standard applies to subjective judgments of noise made in the laboratory when listeners are instructed to judge aspects of the sound other than loudness.

ANSI S3.5-1997 (R2002) *American National Standard Methods for Calculation of the Speech Intelligibility Index.* This Standard defines a method for computing a physical measure that is highly correlated with the intelligibility of speech as evaluated by speech perception tests given to a group of talkers and listeners. The measure is called the Speech Intelligibility Index, or SII. The SII is calculated from acoustical measurements of speech and noise. This standard is not a substitute for ANSI S3.2-1989 (R1995) American National Standard Method for Measuring the Intelligibility of Speech over Communications Systems.

ANSI S3.6-1996 *American National Standard Specification for Audiometers.* The audiometers covered in this specification are devices designed for use in determining the hearing threshold of an individual in comparison with a chosen standard reference threshold level. This standard provides specifications and tolerances for pure-tone, speech, and masking levels and describes the minimum test capabilities of different types of audiometers. The standard also specifies standardized threshold for detecting pure tones.

ANSI S3.13-1987 (R2002) *American National Standard Mechanical Cou-*

pler for Measurement of Bone Vibrators. This standard specifies requirements for mechanical couplers used for calibrating bone-conduction audiometers and making measurements on bone vibrators and bone-conduction hearing aids. Specific design features are given for the mechanical coupler when driven by a vibrator with a prescribed plane circular tip area and applied with a specific static force. An appendix provides an example of a specific construction of a mechanical coupler.

ANSI S3.21-1978 (R1997) *American National Standard Methods for Manual Pure-Tone Threshold Audiometry.* Pure-tone threshold audiometry is the procedure used in the assessment of an individual's threshold of hearing for pure tones. Pure-tone threshold audiometry includes manual air-conduction measurements at octave intervals from 250 through 8000 Hz and at intermediate frequencies as needed. When abrupt differences of 20 dB or more occur between adjacent octave frequencies, additional frequencies may be included at the discretion of the tester. Bone-conduction measurements may be carried out if indicated by the test requirements at octave intervals from 250 through 4000 Hz. Also, when required, masking is to be used. The purpose of this standard is to present procedures for conducting manual pure-tone threshold audiometry whose use will minimize intertest differences based on test method.

ANSI S3.22-2003 *American National Standard Specification of Hearing Aid Characteristics.* This standard describes air-conduction hearing-aid measurement methods that are particularly suitable for specification and tolerance purposes. Among the test methods described are output sound pressure level (SPL) with a 90-dB input SPL, full-on gain, frequency response, harmonic distortion, equivalent input noise, current drain, induction-coil sensitivity, and static and dynamic characteristics of automatic gain control (AGC) hearing aids. Specific configurations are given for measuring the input SPL to a hearing aid. Allowable tolerances in relation to values specified by the manufacturer are given for certain parameters. Appendices are provided to describe equivalent substitution methods, characteristics of battery simulators, and additional tests to characterize the electroacoustic performance of hearing aids more completely.

ANSI S3.39-1987 (R2002) *American National Standard Specifications for Instruments to Measure Aural Acoustic Impedance and Admittance (Aural Acoustic Immittance).* This standard provides specifications for instruments designed to measure acoustic impedance, acoustic admittance, or both quantities, within the human external ear canal. Terms that apply to these instruments and to related measurements are defined. Four types of instruments are classified. Characteristics, specifications, and recommended calibration procedures then are provided. Material within this standard is intended both for users and for manufacturers of instruments that measure aural acoustic impedance and admittance.

ANSI S3.42-1992 (R2002) *American National Standard Testing Hearing Aids with a Broad-Band Noise Signal.* This standard describes techniques for characterizing the steady-state performance of hearing aids with a broad-band noise signal. The need for such a standard arises from the importance of assessing the performance of hearing aids in environments more nearly representing their real-world use. The noise test signal specified herein has been employed by the National Bureau of Standards for over 20 years in testing hearing aids. Among the tests described are noise saturation SPL, noise gain, frequency response, family of frequency response curves, and output versus input characteristic. Additionally, the appendix recommends use of the coherence function to indicate the validity of frequency response measures and distinguishes between use of random and pseudo-random noise and asynchronous versus synchronous analysis.

ANSI S3.46-1997 (R2002) *American National Standard Methods of Measurement of Real-Ear Performance Characteristics of Hearing Aids.* This standard provides definitions for terms used in the measurement of real-ear performance characteristics of hearing aids, provides procedural and reporting guidelines, and identifies essential characteristics to be reported by the manufacturer of equipment used for this purpose. Acceptable tolerances for the control and measurement of SPLs are indicated. Where possible, sources of error have been identified and suggestions provided for their management.

Appendix C

Public Forum Participation

The committee held a public forum on May 7, 2003, and invited organizations in the scientific, service, and advocacy communities to attend. The organizations invited by the committee to nominate speakers for the forum are listed below. Organizations listed in **bold type** nominated speakers, although not all nominees accepted our invitation.

ORGANIZATIONS INVITED TO NOMINATE SPEAKERS

AARP Public Policy Institute/Federal Affairs Department
Academy of Dispensing Audiologists
Academy of Rehabilitative Audiology
Acoustic Neuroma Association
ADARA (advocacy for deaf and hard-of-hearing individuals)
Alexander Graham Bell Association for the Deaf and Hard of Hearing
Alliant University Foundation
AMBUCS (national service organization for people with disabilities)
American Academy of Audiology
American Academy of Disability Evaluating Physicians
American Academy of Otolaryngology
American Association of the Deaf-Blind
American Auditory Society
American Hearing Research Foundation
American Neurotologic Society
American Otological Society

American Society for Deaf Children
American Speech-Language-Hearing Association
American Tinnitus Association
Association of Administrative Law Judges
Association of Late Deafened Adults
Association on Higher Education and Disability
Auditory-Verbal International, Inc.
Autism Network for Hearing and Visually Impaired Persons
Better Hearing Institute
CAOHC: Council for Accreditation in Occupational Hearing
    Conservation
Captioned Media Program/National Association of the Deaf
Center for Hearing Loss in Children
Cochlear Implant Association, Inc.
Community Legal Services
Conference of Educational Administrators of Schools and Programs for
    the Deaf
Convention of American Instructors of the Deaf
Council for Exceptional Children
Council on Education of the Deaf, Gallaudet University
Deaf Community Advocacy Network
Deafness Research Foundation
Department of Veterans Affairs, VA Medical Center
Disability, Inc./Sign Language USA, Inc.
The EAR Foundation
Educational Equity Concepts, Inc.
Galler & Atkins
Hard of Hearing Advocates
Hear Me Foundation
HEAR NOW
Helen Keller National Center for Deaf-Blind Youths and Adults
Hope for Hearing Foundation
The Hyperacusis Network
International Hearing Society
Intertribal Deaf Council
Laurent Clerc National Deaf Education Center
Mainstream, Inc.
National Asian Deaf Congress
National Association of Disability Examiners
National Association of the Deaf
National Association of State Directors of Special Education, Inc.
National Black Association for Speech-Language and Hearing
National Black Deaf Advocates

National Board for Certification in Hearing Instrument Sciences
National Cued Speech Association
National Family Association for Deaf-Blind
National Hearing Conservation Association
National Information Clearinghouse on Children Who Are Deaf-Blind
NISH: National Industries for the Severely Handicapped
National Organization for Hearing Research Foundation
Neurofibromatosis, Inc.
National Institute on Deafness and Other Communication Disorders,
    National Institutes of Health
National Technical Institute for the Deaf, Rochester Institute of
    Technology
Postsecondary Education Consortium
Registry of Interpreters for the Deaf
Rehabilitation Engineering and Assistive Technology Society of North
    America (RESNA)
Rehabilitation Services Administration, Deafness and Communicative
    Disorders Branch
Self Help for Hard of Hearing People (SHHH)
Society for Ear, Nose and Throat Advance in Children, Inc.
Society of Otorhinolaryngology and Head-Neck Nurses, Inc.
TASH (advocacy organization for people with disabilities)
The Triological Society

FORUM SPEAKERS

Dan Malcore, The Hyperacusis Network, Green Bay, Wisconsin
Susan Gold, M.A., CCC-SLP/A, University of Maryland Medical
    Center, Baltimore
Jane Madell, Ph.D., Beth Israel Medical Center, NYC
Sandra MacLean, M.A., CCC-A, Washington Audiology Services,
    Seattle, Washington
Robert Ruben, M.D., FACS, FAAP, Albert Einstein Medical College,
    New York
Cheryl McGinnis, American Tinnitus Association, Portland, Oregon
Richard Tyler, Ph.D., University of Iowa
Warren Hanna, Hard of Hearing Advocates, Framingham,
    Massachusetts (on videotape)

Appendix D

Biographical Sketches of Committee Members and Staff

Robert A. Dobie *(Chair)* is clinical professor in the Department of Otolaryngology at the University of California at Davis, as well as a partner in Dobie Associates. His current professional activities include clinical practice, teaching, research, and consultation in otology (ear disorders), with special interest in medical-legal issues. He is the author of *Medical-Legal Evaluation of Hearing Loss* (2001) and numerous other publications. He is the recipient of multiple research grants from the National Institutes of Health (NIH) and past president of the Association for Research in Otolaryngology. He is a past member of the boards and executive councils of the National Hearing Conservation Association, the Deafness Research Foundation, and the Council on Accreditation in Occupational Hearing Conservation, as well as a member of the editorial board of several scientific journals. At the National Research Council (NRC), he served on the Committee on Hearing, Bioacoustics, and Biomechanics. He has an M.D. degree from Stanford University (1971).

Robyn Cox is professor at the University of Memphis (formerly Memphis State University), where she has worked since 1977, as well as director of the Hearing Aid Research Laboratory. Her early research was in the development of fitting methods for hearing aids. Since 1986, she has conducted research in amplification, focused on improving methods for fitting hearing aids on older adults and determining the long-term outcomes of the hearing aid fitting and other audiological rehabilitation. Her recent work has involved the study of self-report and subjective outcomes, and she has participated in the development of standardized questionnaires to measure hearing aid fitting outcomes. She served on the NRC's Committee on Hearing, Bioacoustics, and Biomechanics and serves as editorial consultant for national and international journals in the field of hearing health care. She has B.S. (1968) and M.A. (1971) degrees from Ball State University and a Ph.D. in audiology from Indiana University (1974).

Robert R. Davila is a member of the National Council on Disability, an independent federal agency that advises the U.S. president and the Congress on matters related to disability issues. He also holds the Jerry C. Lee endowed chair of studies in technology and the adult learner at National University in La Jolla, California. Davila served as chief executive officer of the National Technical Institute for the Deaf at the Rochester Institute of Technology from 1996 to 2003. He also served as assistant secretary for special education and rehabilitative services in the U.S. Department of Education. Other previous positions include headmaster of the New York School for the Deaf, vice president of Gallaudet University, and president of several national and international organizations related to the education of deaf persons. He has a Ph.D. in educational technology from Syracuse University, an M.A. in special education from Hunter College, and a B.A. in education from Gallaudet University. He has honorary degrees from Stonehill College, Hunter College, Rochester Institute of Technology, and Gallaudet University.

Marilyn E. Demorest is professor of psychology and vice provost for faculty affairs at the University of Maryland, Baltimore County. Her academic and research interests are in psychometrics, quantitative methods, and rehabilitative audiology. She is co-developer of the Communication Profile for the Hearing Impaired, a self-assessment tool that measures psychosocial adjustment in adults with hearing impairment. She is a fellow of the American Psychological Association, the American Psychological Society, and the American Speech-Language-Hearing Association, as well as a past president of the Academy of Rehabilitative Audiology. She has a Ph.D. in experimental psychology from the Johns Hopkins University (1969).

Bruce J. Gantz is the Brian F. McCabe distinguished chair and head of the Department Otolaryngology—Head and Neck Surgery, at the University of Iowa Carver College of Medicine. His research interests include cochlear implant outcomes and device development, as well as clinical trials involving the treatment of ear disease. He is on the editorial boards of several publications relating to otology, head and neck surgery, cochlear implants, and otorhinolaryngology. He has received numerous grants and awards, including grants from the NIH to study cochlear implantation, autoimmune ear disease, sudden deafness, and research training in otolaryngology. He was elected to the National Academies'

Institute of Medicine in 2000. He is a director of the American Board of Otolaryngology, has been president of the American Neurotology Society and the Association for Research in Otolaryngology, and is a member of several other professional organizations and serves on many of their committees. He has M.D. (1974) and M.S. (1980) degrees from the University of Iowa.

Sandra Gordon-Salant is professor in the Department of Hearing and Speech Sciences at the University of Maryland, College Park. She is a member of the Association for Research in Otolaryngology and has obtained continuous funding over the past 20 years from the National Institutes of Health for her research on age-related hearing loss. Other memberships include the Acoustical Society of America, the American Speech-Language-Hearing Association, the American Auditory Society, and the American Academy of Audiology. She has published numerous articles and book chapters pertaining to age-related hearing loss, speech perception, auditory temporal processing, and hearing aids. She is a fellow of the American Speech-Language-Hearing Association and served as editor of the hearing section of the *Journal of Speech, Language, and Hearing Research.* She has a Ph.D. from Northwestern University.

Susan Jerger is Ashbel Smith professor and director of the Children's Speech Processing Laboratory in the School of Behavioral and Brain Sciences at the University of Texas at Dallas, as well as research professor in the Department of Otolaryngology—Head and Neck Surgery, Washington University School of Medicine, St. Louis. She has been funded for 19 years by the National Institute on Deafness and Other Communication Disorders, National Institutes of Health, to study the effect of childhood auditory disorders on the development of spoken word recognition. She is a member of numerous national and international professional societies, and has presented the prestigious Carhart lecture at the American Auditory Society. She was editor-in-chief of *Ear and Hearing*, the official journal of the American Auditory Society, for a decade (1992-2002). She has a Ph.D. from Baylor College of Medicine.

William G. Johnson is professor of economics in the School of Health Management and Policy and the Department of Economics in the W.P. Carey School of Business at Arizona State University. His current research focuses on access to care, occupational illness and injury, the effects of health on work and other activities, health care outcomes, and the development of health information systems for use in research. He directs the university's Center for Health Economics and Policy Research and teaches graduate courses in health and economics. He is a member of the NIH Review Panel for Health Services Research and an associate scientist of the Institute of Work and Health in Toronto. He serves on numerous national and international technical advisory committees for health research, as well as on the editorial board of *The Spine Journal*. He has a Ph.D. in economics from Rutgers University.

Karen Iler Kirk is associate professor of otolaryngology—head and neck surgery and the Psi Iota Xi distinguished investigator in pediatric speech and hearing at the Indiana University School of Medicine. Before joining the Indiana faculty in 1991, she held research and academic positions at the House Ear Institute and the University of Iowa, including membership on House's pioneering cochlear implant research team from 1981 to 1985. She is the director of the DeVault Otologic Research Laboratory. Her research, which has been supported by NIH, the American Hearing Research Foundation, the Deafness Research Foundation, and the American Speech-Language-Hearing Foundation, examines speech perception, spoken word recognition, and language development in pediatric cochlear implant users. She recently cochaired the group that produced a technical report on cochlear implants for the American Speech-Language-Hearing Association. She has a Ph.D. in hearing science from the University of Iowa.

Irene W. Leigh is a professor in the Department of Psychology, Clinical Psychology Doctoral Program, at Gallaudet University. With regard to her specialty, deafness, she has conducted research in the areas of attachment, parenting, identity, depression, and adjustment to cochlear implants. She has an extensive publications record in these areas as well as the mental health and psychotherapy of deaf clients. In addition to being a member of various organizations that serve deaf and hard-of-hearing persons, she is also listed in the National Register of Health Service Providers in Psychology. She serves on the American Psychological Association Board for the Advancement of Psychology in the Public Interest, is chair of the deaf and hard of hearing section of the Alexander Graham Bell Association of the Deaf and Hard of Hearing, and is on the editorial board of the *Journal of Deaf Studies and Deaf Education*, *The Volta Review*, and the *Journal of the American Deafness and Rehabilitation Association*. She also chairs the Council on Graduate Education at Gallaudet University and the Gallaudet University Press editorial board. Recent honors include the Estelle Samuelson award from the League for the Hard of Hearing, the Schaefer professorship at Gallaudet University, and distinguished faculty for 2003. She has a Ph.D. from New York University.

Yvonne S. Sininger is a professor in residence in the Division of Head & Neck Surgery of the David Geffen School of Medicine at the University of California, Los Angeles. Her research focus is human infant hearing and pediatric audiological disorders. Previous NIH-funded projects included a study to define auditory sensitivity in healthy newborns using auditory brainstem response and a study on the efficacy of auditory brainstem response and otoacoustic emissions for newborn hearing screening. She has recently completed a project to characterize the nature of auditory neuropathy and edited a book on the subject. Her current research project evaluates factors that influence the auditory outcomes of infants and children with hearing loss who receive amplification. She is a fellow of the American Speech-Language-Hearing Association and a former member of the board of directors of the American Academy of Audiology. She serves as a representative to the Joint Committee on Infant Hearing and is a board member of the International Evoked Response Study Group. She has B.A. and M.A. degrees from Indiana University and a Ph.D. in speech and hearing science from the University of California, San Francisco.

William A. Yost is professor of psychology, adjunct professor at the Parmly Hearing Institute, and adjunct professor of otolaryngology at Loyola University Chicago. He has published numerous reports, articles, book chapters, and books in areas of hearing science. He is a fellow of the Acoustical Society of America, the American Speech-Language-Hearing Association, the American Psychological Society, and the American Association for the Advancement of Science. He received an honorary degree from the Colorado College in 1997 and several service awards from the Association for Research in Otolaryngology; he was faculty member of the year in 1994 and served as associate vice president for research and dean of the Graduate School at Loyola University Chicago. He served as chair of the NRC Committee on Hearing, Bioacoustics, and Biomechanics. He is currently on boards of the Psychonomic Society (associate editor), the National Academies (a national associate), the American National Standards Institute, the Acoustical Society of America (former vice-president), the Association for Research in Otolaryngology (former secretary-treasurer and president), and NIH (former chair of the communication disorders review group). He has a Ph.D. in experimental psychology from Indiana University.

Susan Van Hemel *(Study Director)* is a senior program officer in the Center for the Study of Behavior and Development of the Division of Behavioral and Social Sciences and Education at the NRC. Her recent projects at the NRC include a study of Social Security disability determination for individuals with visual impairments and a workshop on technology for adaptive aging. She has also done work for a previous employer on vision requirements for commercial drivers and on commercial driver fatigue. For over 20 years she managed and performed studies on a variety of topics related to human performance and training. She is a member of the Human Factors and Ergonomics Society and its technical groups on perception and performance and aging. She has a Ph.D. in experimental psychology from the Johns Hopkins University.

Index

A

HEALTH LEARNING CENTER
Northwestern Memorial Hospital
Galter 3-304
Chicago, IL